Handbook
Biologics and Biosimilars
in Dermatology

Handbook of Biologics and Biosimilars in Dermatology

Editors

Shekhar Neema MD (Dermatology)
Assistant Professor
Department of Dermatology
Command Hospital
Kolkata, West Bengal, India

Manas Chatterjee MD DNB (DVL)
Senior Adviser, Professor and Head
Department of Dermatology
INHS Asvini
Mumbai, Maharashtra, India

Assistant Editors

Dipali Rathod MD
Assistant Professor
Department of Dermatology
HBT Medical College and
Dr RN Cooper Municipality General Hospital
Mumbai, Maharashtra, India

Ankan Gupta MD DNB
Assistant Professor
Department of Dermatology
Christian Medical College
Vellore, Tamil Nadu, India

Foreword

Murlidhar Rajagopalan MD

The Health Sciences Publisher
New Delhi | London | Panama

Jaypee Brothers Medical Publishers (P) Ltd

Headquarters
Jaypee Brothers Medical Publishers (P) Ltd
4838/24, Ansari Road, Daryaganj
New Delhi 110 002, India
Phone: +91-11-43574357
Fax: +91-11-43574314
E-mail: jaypee@jaypeebrothers.com

Overseas Offices

JP Medical Ltd
83 Victoria Street, London
SW1H 0HW (UK)
Phone: +44 20 3170 8910
Fax: +44 (0)20 3008 6180
E-mail: info@jpmedpub.com

Jaypee-Highlights Medical Publishers Inc
City of Knowledge, Bld. 235, 2nd Floor, Clayton
Panama City, Panama
Phone: +1 507-301-0496
Fax: +1 507-301-0499
E-mail: cservice@jphmedical.com

Jaypee Brothers Medical Publishers (P) Ltd
17/1-B, Babar Road, Block-B, Shyamoli
Mohammadpur, Dhaka-1207
Bangladesh
Mobile: +08801912003485
E-mail: jaypeedhaka@gmail.com

Jaypee Brothers Medical Publishers (P) Ltd
Bhotahity, Kathmandu, Nepal
Phone +977-9741283608
E-mail: kathmandu@jaypeebrothers.com

Website: www.jaypeebrothers.com
Website: www.jaypeedigital.com

© 2018, Jaypee Brothers Medical Publishers

Inquiries for bulk sales may be solicited at: jaypee@jaypeebrothers.com

Handbook of Biologics and Biosimilars in Dermatology

First Edition: **2018**
ISBN: 978-93-5270-364-7
Printed at Rajkamal Electric Press, Kundli, Haryana.

Dedicated to

*Our families, who tolerate our periods of absence from
their immediate surrounds with equanimity and understanding*

Shekhar Neema
Manas Chatterjee

*My teacher, Col BAK Prasad, who introduced me to scientific reasoning
You will live in our hearts forever*

Shekhar Neema

Contributors

Col D Banerjee
MD (Med), DM (Gastroenterology)
Senior Adviser
Department of Gastroenterology
Command Hospital
Kolkata, West Bengal, India

Col Santanu Banerjee MD DNB
Senior Adviser
Department of Dermatology
Military Hospital
Secunderabad, Telangana, India

Rakesh Bharti MD
Consultant Dermatologist
Bharti Derma Care and Research Centre
Amritsar, Punjab, India

Riti Bhatia MD
Assistant Professor
Department of Dermatology and
Venereology
All India Institute of Medical Sciences
Rishikesh, Uttarakhand, India

Kingshuk Chatterjee
MD MNAMS MRCPS
Calcutta School of Tropical Medicine
Kolkata, West Bengal, India

Manas Chatterjee MD DNB (DVL)
Senior Adviser
Professor and Head
Department of Dermatology
INHS Asvini
Mumbai, Maharashtra, India

Manju Daroach MD
Senior Resident
Department of Dermatology,
Venereology and Leprology
Postgraduate Institute of Medical
Education and Research
Chandigarh, India

Anupam Das MD
Assistant Professor
Department of Dermatology
KPC Medical College and Hospital
Kolkata, West Bengal, India

Dipankar De MD
Associate Professor
Department of Dermatology
Postgraduate Institute of Medical
Education and Research
Chandigarh, India

Sunil Dogra MD DNB FRCP
Professor
Department of Dermatology,
Venereology and Leprology
Postgraduate Institute of Medical
Education and Research
Chandigarh, India

Krupashankar DS MD DVD FAGE
Senior Consultant and Dermatologist
Dr Krupa Shankar Skin Diagnosis Center
Bengaluru, Karnataka, India

Kiran Godse MD PhD FRCP
Professor
Department of Dermatology
DY Patil Hospital
Navi Mumbai, Maharashtra, India

Ankan Gupta MD DNB
Assistant Professor
Department of Dermatology
Christian Medical College
Vellore, Tamil Nadu, India

Vishal Gupta MD
Senior Research Associate
Department of Dermatology and
Venereology
All India Institute of Medical Sciences
New Delhi, India

Swaroop HS MD
Senior Medical Adviser
Biocon

Rajat Kandhari MD
Dr Kandhari's Skin and Dental Clinic
New Delhi, India

Manish Khandare MD
Assistant Professor
Department of Dermatology
INHS Asvini
Mumbai, Maharashtra, India

Sunil Kothiwala MD
Consultant Dermatologist
Skin Eva Clinic
Jaipur, Rajasthan, India

Aneesh KP MBBS
Postgraduate Resident
Department of Dermatology
Base Hospital Lucknow
Lucknow, Uttar Pradesh, India

Lt Col Abhishek Kumar
MD (Med), DNB (Rheumatology)
Assistant Professor
Department of Rheumatology
Command Hospital
Kolkata, West Bengal, India

Bhushan Madke MD
Associate Professor
Department of Dermatology
Jawaharlal Nehru Medical College and
Acharya Vinoba Bhave Rural Hospital
Wardha, Maharashtra, India

Anupama Molpariya MD
Vardhman Mahavir Medical College
and Safdarjung Hospital
New Delhi, India

Lt Col Brijesh Nair MD
Classified Specialist
Department of Dermatology
INHS Sanjivani
Kochi, Kerala, India

Shekhar Neema MD (Dermatology)
Assistant Professor
Department of Dermatology
Command Hospital
Kolkata, West Bengal, India

Lt Col Vijendran P MD DNB
Associate Professor
Department of Dermatology
Base Hospital Lucknow
Lucknow, Uttar Pradesh, India

SG Parasramani MD DDV FAAD
Dermatologist
Lilavati Hospital
Mumbai, Maharashtra, India

Jisha Pillai MD
Dermatologist
Lilavati Hospital
Mumbai, Maharashtra, India

Swetalina Pradhan MD
Senior Resident
Department of Dermatology
All India Institute of Medical Sciences
Bhubaneshwar, Odisha, India

Murlidhar Rajagopalan MD
Senior Consultant Dermatologist
Apollo Hospital
Chennai, Tamil Nadu, India

Dipali Rathod MD
Assistant Professor
Department of Dermatology
HBT Medical College and Dr RN
Cooper Municipality General Hospital
Mumbai, Maharashtra, India

Tanumay Raychaudhury MD
Tata Medical Center
Kolkata, West Bengal, India

Abir Saraswat MD DNB
Indushree Skin Clinic
Lucknow, Uttar Pradesh, India

Nidhi Sharma MD
Consultant Dermatologist
Civil Hospital
Amritsar, Punjab, India

Col Sehdev Singh MD DNB
Senior Adviser
Department of Dermatology
Command Hospital
Kolkata, West Bengal, India

Vinay Singh MD
Vibrance Skin Laser and
Cosmetic Clinic,
New Delhi, India

Muhammed Razmi T MD DNB
Department of Dermatology
Postgraduate Institute of Medical
Education and Research
Chandigarh, India

Col Biju Vasudevan MD
Senior Adviser
Department of Dermatology
Command Hospital
Lucknow, Uttar Pradesh, India

Brig Rajesh Verma MD DNB
Commandant
Professor
Department of Dermatology
Base Hospital Lucknow
Lucknow, Uttar Pradesh, India

Foreword

The 'handbook for biological drug in India' is meant to be a ready reckoner for dermatologists prescribing biological drugs in India and in that sense has restricted itself to those drugs approved for use for dermatological indications in India, in addition to a mention of those, especially small molecules, that are likely to be available in the not too distant future. Its chapters have been formulated keeping in mind the needs of dermatologists prescribing these drugs for the 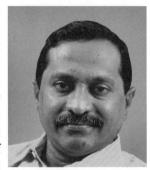 first time as well as those who wish to update themselves on the latest guidelines and procedures for their optimum use. All drugs currently available for dermatological indications in India have been covered along with guidance on the optimum utilization of these drugs for conditions in which they are indicated in terms of choice of agent in view of best practice principles as on date.

Conditions, such as psoriasis are saddled with multiple options in terms of biological therapy and it is frequently difficult to decide which of these drugs would be best fit in a given clinical scenario. Also, some of these drugs have multiple indications and it is only some of these and in certain clinical situations that they are best fit. This brings in the use of biologics in off label indications in dermatology. A clear understanding of the drug and the pathogenesis of the disease is needed for this to happen well, and the results have to be well-documented to get an ethical approval. It is hoped that this book would enable such decision-making to be based on best available evidence as well as the wealth of experience that the authors have summoned to write their respective chapters. As is wont in such cases, opinions would always differ but it is in charting the well-trodden path that ensures the best possible outcome for the patients. That path has to be shown by those who have walked it with success and our distinguished galaxy of authors have done just that.

This book highlights what a clinician needs to know and presents it in as lucid a form as possible for the reader, who would have little time to go through detailed nuances that may not be necessary for the practical prescriber. No essential has been missed and at the same time, superfluities have been avoided to ensure a rapid read of contents required at the time of prescription decision-making. That makes this text most handy and a must have on the table-top of the hands-on clinician for whom this work is primarily meant.

It is ardently hoped and expected that this effort by the authors and editors would bear fruit in terms of the more rational use of these wonderful molecules for the benefit of the patients who should be the final beneficiaries of medical knowledge.

Murlidhar Rajagopalan MD
Senior Consultant Dermatologist
Apollo Hospital
Chennai, Tamil Nadu, India

Preface

The *Handbook of Biologics and Biosimilars in Dermatology* is a work borne out of necessity. The usage of biologics and biosimilars in India as well as other countries in the developing world is steadily increasing. Unlike in the West where expenditure on prescription of biologics is reimbursable, the cost of the same is usually borne by the patient in our situation. More prudence, therefore, becomes imperative in decision-making. A clear understanding which stems out of accurate knowledge of these molecules and their exact mode and mechanism of action becomes necessary.

In addition, this knowledge and understanding must be dovetailed to the comorbidities and financial constraints, which are different in our patient population. This entails a different perspective to biologic and biosimilar usage in our country. This spurred us to attempt to write this handbook which is meant to be a concise guide for dermatology practitioners, who are stepping into the era of biologics, biosimilars and similar targeted therapies.

An attempt has been sincerely made to ensure that concerns that we come across in our day-to-day clinical interactions with our patients are addressed. Things, such as cost-effectiveness have been dealt with to provide perspective to the specialist, as well as provide material to better counsel patients when these medications are prescribed. It was our endeavor to provide up-to-date information to readers. However, the field of biologic is expanding at a rapid pace and it is possible that some newer developments have been missed despite our best efforts. We also disclose that we have no conflict of interest in writing this book and the project has been conceptualized and completed without any grants or support.

It is hoped and expected that this handbook will find its way to the table-tops and not bookshelves of academic and practicing dermatologists alike and be helpful to them in making more informed choices in biologic use.

Jai Hind

Shekhar Neema MD (Dermatology)
Manas Chatterjee MD DNB (DVL)

Acknowledgments

To our institutions where we work and our patients who were willing to be treated by us with whatever we decided to use with complete faith and without question.

We are grateful to Dr Biju Vasudevan for constant support during preparation of the manuscript.

We are grateful to our Assistant Editors, Dr Dipali Rathod and Dr Ankan Gupta. They worked tirelessly the entire year on this project.

We are thankful to Mr Sabysachi Hazra.

Shekhar Neema
Manas Chatterjee

My heartfelt thanks to a most inspirational doctor and a fast friend, Ankan Gupta. This book could not have taken shape without his ideas.

I am grateful to my wife, Dr Sweta Mukherjee for taking her time out for language editing and proofreading some portions of this book.

Shekhar Neema

We especially appreciate the constant support and encouragement of Mr Jitendar P Vij (Group Chairman) and Mr Ankit Vij (Group President), Jaypee Brothers Medical Publishers (P) Ltd, New Delhi, India in publishing this handbook and also their associates particularly Ms Chetna Malhotra Vohra (Associate Director—Content Strategy) and Ms Esha Saini (Development Editor) who have been prompt, efficient and most helpful.

Contents

Chapter 1

History and Development of Biologics

Biju Vasudevan, Ankan Gupta

▊ INTRODUCTION

Biologics are proteins and/or their derivatives that regulate the immune system or support tumor specific defense. They are also known as "biological" or "recombinant therapeutics" and there are multiple definitions to it, being a constant source of controversy amongst the semantic purists. Biologics do not represent one homogeneous drug group, rather includes unrelated molecules like monoclonal antibodies, growth factors, fusion proteins, interferons, and expression vectors generating proteins in situ.[1]

The first documented uses of the term "biologics" was in 1912 when the pharmacological editor of the California State Journal of Medicine, Fred Lackenbach, used it in connection with national health-care legislation and the control of vaccine production in the United States (US).[2] For a long time, there was no equivalent expression in Europe, and terms like Naturstojfe, Wirkstoffe (biologische Arzneimittel) or medicaments biologiques were used; all of them had different meanings and connotations, but sharing a common reference to "natural products". Over the past century, biologics are so ubiquitous that our bodies have increasingly become exposed to them without us realizing the same, e.g. the use of vitamins, vaccines, insulin, etc. In present context, however, the "natural products" of yesteryears cease to be recognized as biologics with new definitions excluding them. The aim of this chapter is not intended to go into the controversial semantics, but to introduce the reader to the history of this therapeutic revolution.

▊ HISTORY OF BIOLOGICS

Under an Act of Congress in 1902, all viruses, sera and toxins used in the United States were required to conform to established standards. It was officially designated as "An Act to Regulate the Sale of Viruses, Serums, Toxins and Analogous Products in the District of Columbia, to Regulate Interstate Traffic in Said Articles, and for Other Purposes".[3] This law marked the beginning of a regime for licensing of drugs that ultimately evolved into the Food and Drug Administration (FDA), which today is responsible for the control of biologics in the US.[4] When the FDA celebrated the 75th anniversary of the Food and Drugs Act of 1920 in 1995, it also celebrated the

"Biologics Control Act" of 1902. Though in the original law of 1st July 1902, there was no mention of "biologics", "biological" or "biological products", which implicitly suggested the continuity in the regulation of biological products. It was with this new legislative framework in place, subsequent years witnessed the emergence of various labels to describe these products.

In 1917, the Biological Department of Eli Lilly (a pharmaceutical bigwig of his times) and Company published a small treatise on "Elements of Biologics" designed to provide the company's representatives with standard knowledge about biological or natural products like antitoxins and vaccines.[5] By 1921, 41 establishments were licensed to sell more than 102 different sera, toxins and analogous products. Of these establishments, 32 were located in the US, one in Canada, one in England, three in France, one in Italy, two in Switzerland and one in Germany, posing a challenge to federal regulators. In 1923, Public Health Reports compiled a list of national agencies and organizations associated with the regulation of "biologics".[6]

The isolation of the first-ever biologic was of the hormone insulin which was achieved by Frederick Banting and Charles Best in Toronto in 1921.[7] The second biologic was erythropoietin, the existence of which was first proposed in 1906 by Paul Carnot based on his transfusion experiments in rabbits.[8] From 1921 to 1934, other biological substances like vitamin D (1927), estrone (1929), androsterone (1931), ascorbic acid (1932) and progesterone (1934) were isolated and synthesized but it was in 1934, when the National Institute of Health (NIH) issued the first licenses to manufacturers for the production of a human blood product, which was a preparation of protein from human placental extract that was designed to immunize against measles.[9,10] In 1937, work on biologics control was granted its own division within the NIH, the Division of Biologics Control. Institutionalizing the control of biologics involved expanding existing regulations on vaccines, sera and antitoxins to include arsenical drugs, blood and blood products. Meanwhile, in Europe, the physician and entrepreneur Gerhard Maclaus (1890–1942) published a famous three-volume textbook of biological remedies (Lehrbuch der biologischen Heilmittel); and in 1939, a research institute for biological remedies was founded at the Paracelsus.[11]

The decades after the Second World War, especially from the 1950s to the 1980s, there were dynamic years for biologics, as the quantity and quality of biologics and the challenges for regulators continued to grow. After the spectacular introduction of penicillin in the 1940s, the biotechnological exploitation of fungal metabolisms invigorated the search for magic bullets. Likewise, the invention of cortisone raised expectations and drove pharmaceutical industries in their search for "natural products" from exotic plants. Another advance in postwar research that significantly influenced the development of biologics was made in 1949 at Boston Children's Hospital, where scientists successfully grew a human virus, the Lansing type 2 poliovirus, in a human tissue cell culture.[12] In the mid-1960s, pionee-ring work resulted in the first experimental live virus vaccine against German measles (rubella).

In July 1972, both the authority to administer the drug provisions of the Federal Food, Drug, and Cosmetic (FD&C) Act for all biological products and the responsibility for implementing the Biologics Act was delegated to the FDA. The Division of Biologics Standards was then transferred from the NIH to the FDA and renamed the Bureau of Biologics (BoB). Insulin was inarguably the first protein that embodied the aspirations of the new biology. A team at the University of California, San Francisco, associated with Herbert Boyer, who in April 1976 founded the small company GeneTech (Genetic Engineering Technology), used the bacterium *Escherichia coli* to produce insulin and claimed success in September 1978. The FDA finally approved the drug in 1982. By 1988, live proteins like insulin, human growth hormone, hepatitis B vaccine, alpha-interferon and tissue plasminogen activator had been approved as drugs by the FDA.

The discovery that revolutionized the antibody therapy came after decoding of the human genome which revealed that there are 30,000 different genes encoding possibly 50,000 different proteins and that disease may result when one of these proteins is defective or present in abnormally high or low concentration. This ability to identify the cause of disease has presented a number of targets for possible therapies. The first monoclonal antibodies (mAb), Ortho Biotech's muromonab-CD3 (Orthoclone), was approved by the FDA in 1986.[13] The original concept of antibodies as molecules that bind to specific targets emerged through the pioneering work of Paul Ehrlich, Emil von Behring, Shibasaburo Kitasato, and Karl Landsteiner.[14] Further, recombinant deoxyribonucleic acid technology has allowed a new generation of protein-based medicines and in Cambridge, the United Kingdom, scientists developed a relatively simple method for custom-producing antibodies in the laboratory.[15] More recent advances led to the development of part-mouse, part-human mAbs called chimeras [e.g. rituximab (Rituxan) and cetuximab (Erbitux)], as well as humanized antibodies [e.g. trastuzumab (Herceptin) and bevacizumab (Avastin)] that contain a bare minimum of nonhuman amino acid sequences. In 2002, the first completely human therapeutic mAb, Abbott's adalimumab (Humira), received market approval. Today, there are over a dozen mAbs, with collective oncology market sales in 2006 of over US $7.8 billion and sharp growth predicted over the next decade.[16]

In 1988, the FDA had again split biologics from the more general drug review process. Since then, the FDA has been busy distributing and redistributing the responsibility for an ever-growing number of biological products. The FDA Center for Biologics Evaluation and Research (CBER) became responsible for some therapeutic proteins, such as monoclonal antibodies, but control of these was later transferred to the Center for Drug Evaluation and Research (CDER).[17]

DEVELOPMENT OF BIOSIMILARS

The realm of biologics has evolved throughout the 20th century. With the advent of biosimilars, there is a big competition to challenge the parent molecules.[18] Biologics and their biosimilars are large complex molecules and require a different regulatory framework to produce constant quality. Most regulations in the 21st century have addressed this by recognizing an intermediate ground of testing for biosimilars which require more testing than for small-molecule generics, but less testing than for registering completely new therapeutics.[19] In 2003, the European Medicines Agency introduced an approval pathway for biosimilars, termed similar biological medicinal products, that is based on a thorough demonstration of "comparability" of the "similar" product to an existing approved product.[20] Within the United States, the Patient Protection and Affordable Care Act of 2010 is developed for biosimilars for comparison with the FDA-licensed reference biological product.[21]

PRESENT DAY BIOLOGICS

Necessity is the mother of invention and new clinical situations where the conventional treatment options fail and/or are contraindicated, newer drugs are being developed and the already existing ones are being tried as a hope rather an expectation. Results are giving rise to research, eventually handling the clinicians a new set of arsenal. Diseases like psoriasis, where target-specific drugs are now universally being used with a more favorable side-effect profile, thus providing an effective and safe alternative choice for treatment. Alefacept (Amevive) was the first biologic approved by the FDA in 2003 for the treatment of moderate-to-severe chronic plaque psoriasis. However, in November 2011, Astellas Pharma US, manufacturer of alefacept, announced its decision to cease sales of the drug. There are currently five other FDA-approved biologics for psoriasis and psoriatic arthritis—adalimumab (Humira®), etanercept (Enbrel®), golimumab (Simponi®), infliximab (Remicade®) and ustekinumab (Stelara®). If there is one biologic in dermatology which is closest to challenging the conventional immunosuppressants as the first choice drug, it would be the use of rituximab in pemphigus. Treatment of hidradenitis suppurativa, pyoderma gangrenosum, skin cancers, collagen vascular dermatoses, severe cutaneous adverse reactions, alopecia areata, chronic urticarial and atopic dermatitis have been a challenge over the years and this "therapeutic revolution" with biologics and biosimilars is expected to make life easier for patients as well as clinicians.

REFERENCES

1. Boehncke WH, Radeke HH. Introduction: definition and classification of biologics. In: Boehncke WH, Radeke HH (Eds). Biologics in General Medicine. Berlin, Heidelberg: Springer; 2007. pp. 1-2.
2. Korwek EL. What are biologics? A comparative legislative, regulatory and scientific analysis. Food Drug Law J. 2007;62:257-304.
3. Carpenter DP. Reputation and gatekeeping authority: the Federal Food, Drug and Cosmetic Act of 1938 and its aftermath. In: Carpenter DP (Ed.). Reputation and Power: Organizational Image and Pharmaceutical Regulation at the FDA. Princeton, NJ: Princeton University Press; 2010. p. 137.
4. Kondratas RA. Biologics Control Act of 1902. In: Young JH (Ed.). The Early Years of Federal Food and Drug Control. Madison, WI: American Institute of the History of Pharmacy; 1982. pp. 8-27.
5. Heiser VG. The health work of the League of Nations. Proceedings of the American Philosophical Society. 1926;65 (Supplement):1-9.
6. Sneader W. (2001). History of insulin. [online] Encyclopedia of Life Sciences. Available from http://mrw.interscience.wiley.com/emrw/9780470015902/els/article/a0003623/current/abstract?hd=All,w&hd=All,sneader [Accessed March, 2010].
7. Jelkmann W. Erythropoietin after a century of research: younger than ever. Eur J Haematol. 2007;78(3):183-205.
8. Miyake T, Kung CK, Goldwasser E. Purification of human erythropoietin. J Biol Chem. 1977;252(15):5558-64.
9. Meng H. Das ärztliche Volksbuc. Gemeinverständliche Darstellung der Gesundheitspflege und Heilkunde. Stuttgart: Hippokrates; 1924-30.
10. Timmermann C. Rationalizing Folk Medicine in Interwar Germany: Faith, Business, and Science at Dr. Madaus & Co. Social History of Medicine, 2001;14:459-82.
11. Bud R. Penicillin: Triumph and Tragedy. Oxford: Oxford University Press; 2007. Gradmann C. Magic bullets and moving targets: antibiotic resistance and experimental chemotherapy 1900-1940. Dynamis. 2011;31,305-21.
12. Fda. gov. (2017) Science and the Regulation of Biological Products. [online] Available at: https://www.fda.gov/AboutFDA/WhatWeDo/History/Product Regulation/100YearsofBiologicsRegulation/ucm070022.htm#TheSt.Louis TragedyandEnactmentofthe1902BiologicsControlAct [Accessed 24 Dec. 2017].
13. Smith S. Ten years of Orthoclone OKT3 (muromonab CD3): a review. J Transpl Coord. 1996;6(3):109-19.
14. Kaufmann SH. Immunology's foundation: the 100-year anniversary of the Nobel Prize to Paul Ehrlich and Elie Metchnikoff. Nat Immunol. 2008;9(7):705-12.
15. Köhler G, Milstein C. Continuous cultures of fused cells secreting antibody of predefined specificity. Nature. 1975;256(5517):495-7.
16. Gricks C, Cann CI, Merrin A. Antibody Therapies in Oncology. Waltham (MA): Decision Resources, Inc.; 2008.
17. Biopharma. Transfer of Biopharmaceuticals (Biologics) within FDA from CBER to CDER. [online] Available from www.biopharma.com/CBERtoCDER.html [Accessed December 2017].
18. Calo-Fernández B, Martínez-Hurtado JL. Biosimilars: company strategies to capture value from the biologics market. Pharmaceuticals. 2012;5(12):1393-408.

19. The US Biosimilars Act: Challenges Facing Regulatory Approval. Pharm Med. 2012;26(3):145-52.
20. Questions and answers on biosimilar medicines (similar biological medicinal products). European Medicines Agency. 2014.
21. United States Food and Drug Administration. Approval Pathway for Biosimilar and Interchangeable Biological Products. Maryland: USFDA; 2010.

Chapter 2

Classification of Biologics

Sunil Kothiwala

INTRODUCTION

The term "biologics" includes wide range of substances such as serum, vaccine, toxin, antitoxin, blood and blood components, allergenic products, somatic cells, gene therapy, tissues and recombinant therapeutic proteins to prevent, treat or cure the diseases. Generally, biologics refer to protein molecules used therapeutically to target specific points in the inflammatory cascade of various immune-mediated diseases.

CLASSIFICATION

Biologics are divided into following groups:[1]
- Monoclonal antibodies
- Fusion antibody proteins
- Recombinant human cytokines and growth factors
- Intravenous immunoglobulins (IVIG).

Monoclonal Antibodies

Monoclonal antibodies are produced by a single clone of cells. They work by targeting specific cell-surface receptors. In early days of biologics, purely murine monoclonal antibodies were used resulting in rapid removal from blood through immune response due to development of antimurine antibodies. The monoclonal antibodies used now have genes that have different amounts of murine sequences in the variable region and may be categorized into three classes:

1. *Chimeric antibodies:* 30% murine genes fused with human antibodies
2. *Humanized antibodies:* 10% murine genes fused with human antibodies
3. *Human antibodies:* Solely derived from human immunoglobulin genes.

Nomenclature of Monoclonal Antibody
It includes following components:

Stem: All monoclonal antibody names end with the stem—*mab*.

Substem: Monoclonal antibody nomenclature uses different parts of the preceding word depending on structure and function. These are officially called as substems.

Source substem: Prefix mentioned below preceding the "-mab" denotes origin of the antibodies.

Chimeric:	'-xi-'	e.g. Infliximab
Humanized:	'-zu-'	e.g. Efalizumab
Human sequence:	'-u-'	e.g. Adalimumab

Target substem: It precedes the source of the antibodies and denotes the medicine's target.

| Immune: | '-li-' (old), '-l-' (new) | e.g. Infliximab |
| Interleukin: | '-ki' (old), '-k-' (new) | e.g. Ustekinumab |

Prefix: The prefix carries no special meaning. It should be unique for each medicine and contributes to a well-sounding name. Antibodies with the same source and target substems are only distinguished by their prefix.

Additional word: A second word following the name of the antibody indicates that another substance is attached.

- An antibody can be PEGylated (attached to molecules of polyethylene glycol) to slow down its degradation by enzymes and to decrease its immunogenicity; this is shown by the word pegol, e.g. Certolizumab pegol.

The principal monoclonal antibodies with therapeutic relevance in dermatology are summarized in Table 2.1.

Fusion Antibody Proteins

Fusion proteins, also known as chimeric proteins, are proteins which are created by the fusion of two or more gene that originally code for separate protein. For example, the fusion of receptor domain of a human protein with the constant region of human immunoglobulin G (IgG) results in formation of fusion antibody protein.[3] It binds specifically to a ligand or co-receptor. Recombinant fusion proteins have also been produced by combining human proteins with bacterial toxins. The name of fusion protein in which human antibodies are bound to human receptors end with "cept", e.g. etanercept.

The fusion proteins most commonly used in dermatology are summarized in Table 2.2.

Recombinant Human Cytokines and Growth Factors

Cytokines are small nonimmunoglobulin proteins and glycoproteins produced by a broad range of cells in the human body. In response to any immune stimulus, cytokines are released transiently into the tissue microenvironment and act through receptors to modulate balance between humoral and cell-mediated immune system. Recombinant cytokines or cytokine antagonists produced by recombinant deoxyribonucleic acid technology have been used as immunomodulators for malignant and inflammatory dermatoses.[4] The principal recombinant cytokines and growth factors used in dermatology are summarized in Table 2.3.

Table 2.1: The principal monoclonal antibodies in dermatology.[2]

Receptor	Name of biologic	Type of monoclonal antibody	Uses
Anti-tumor necrosis factor (TNF) α (Fig. 2.1)	Infliximab	Human-mouse monoclonal antibody	Psoriasis, atopic dermatitis, hidradenitis suppurativa
	Adalimumab	Human immunoglobulin G (IgG)-1 monoclonal antibody	Psoriasis, hidradenitis suppurativa
	Certolizumab pegol	PEGylated antigen binding fragment of humanized monoclonal antibody	Psoriasis, psoriatic arthritis
	Golimumab	Fully human monoclonal antibody	Psoriasis arthritis (under phase III trial)
Anti-lymphocyte function-associated antigen-1(LFA-1) (CD11a)	Efalizumab	Humanized IgG1 monoclonal antibody	Psoriasis, lichen planus, discoid lupus erythematosus, dermatomyositis
Anti CD20	Rituximab	Humanized monoclonal antibody	Lymphoma, systemic lupus erythematosus, autoimmune bullous diseases
Anti-interleukin (IL)-12 and anti-IL-23	Ustekinumab	Fully human monoclonal antibody	Psoriasis
Anti-IL-17	Secukinumab Brodalumab Ixekizumab	Human IgG1κ monoclonal antibody	Psoriasis (Brodalumab, Ixekizumab are under phase III trial)
Anti CD2	Siplizumab	Humanized IgG1 monoclonal antibody	Psoriasis
Anti CD4	Orthoclone	Humanized antihuman IgG4 monoclonal antibody	Psoriasis
Anti CD6	Itolizumab	Humanized recombinant IgG1 monoclonal antibody	Psoriasis
Anti CD25	Basiliximab	Chimeric mouse-human monoclonal antibody	Plaque psoriasis, Palmoplantar pustular psoriasis
	Daclizumab	Humanized monoclonal antibody	Psoriasis

Contd...

Contd...

Receptor	Name of biologic	Type of monoclonal antibody	Uses
Anti-CD80r	Galiximab	Primatized mono-clonal antibody with a human IgG1 constant region	Psoriasis
Anti-immuno-globulin E	Omalizumab	Recombinant, humanized, mono-clonal antibody	Atopic dermatitis Chronic urticaria

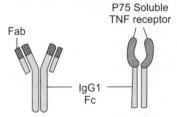
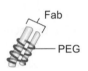

1. Recombinant receptor/Fc fusion protein
 • Etanercept

2. Monoclonal antibody
 • Infliximab (ch.)
 • Adalimumab (h)
 • Golimumab (h)

3. Pegylated fab fragment/Fc-free
 • Certolizumab pegol

Fig. 2.1: TNF blocking agents.

Table 2.2: The principal fusion proteins in dermatology.

Components	Name of biologic	Type of fusion protein	Uses
Two identical TNFα type II (p75) receptor peptides and fragment crystallizable (Fc) portion of the human immunoglobulin G (IgG)-1	Etanercept	Fully human dimeric fusion protein	Psoriasis Hidradenitis suppurativa Scleroderma
First extracellular domain of LFA3 with hinge Ch1 and Ch2 sequences of human IgG1p	Alefacept	Recombinant fusion protein	Psoriasis Graft versus host disease Lichen planus Alopecia areata Atopic dermatitis Hailey–Hailey disease
Extracellular domain of CTLA4 and the Fc region of IgG4	Abatacept	Recombinant fusion protein	Psoriasis
Human interleukin (IL)-2 gene and the enzymatically active ADP-ribosyltransferase domain of the diphtheria toxin	Denileukin diftitox	Recombinant fusion toxin	Cutaneous T-cell lymphoma

Table 2.3: The principal recombinant cytokines and growth factors used in dermatology.

Cytokines/growth factors/enzyme inhibitors	Type of biologic	Uses
Interferons	Interferon α	Verruca vulgaris, cutaneous T cell lymphoma, Kaposi's sarcoma, basal cell carcinoma, melanoma
	Interferon γ	Chronic granulomatous disease
Interleukins	Interleukin 1 receptor antagonist (IL1Ra), Anakinra	Psoriatic arthritis
	Interleukin 2 (IL-2)	Cutaneous T cell lymphoma, metastatic melanoma
	Interleukin 4 (rhIL-4)	Psoriasis
	Interleukin 10 (rhIL-10, Tenovil)	Psoriasis
	Interleukin 11 (rhIL-11, Oprelvekin)	Psoriasis
Granulocyte macrophage colony-stimulating factor (GM-CSF)	Recombinant human GM-CSF	Wound (leg ulcer), melanoma, Sézary syndrome
Platelet-derived growth factor (PDGF)	Recombinant PGDF-BB	Diabetic foot ulcer

Intravenous Immunoglobulins

Intravenous immunoglobulin is a fractioned blood product consisting of IgG antibodies that was first used in antibody deficiency disorders. It is a protein derivative consisting of high concentrations of IgG (>95%) and trace amounts of IgA and IgM made from large pools of human plasma antibodies. IVIG is currently FDA approved in dermatology for graft versus host disease and Kawasaki syndrome. Other uses include connective tissue disorders, autoimmune bullous disorders, toxic epidermal necrolysis and pyoderma gangrenosum.[5]

REFERENCES

1. Stern DK, Tripp JM, Ho VC, et al. The use of systemic immune moderators in dermatology. In: Maclean DI, Maddin WS (Eds). Dermatologic Clinics, Volume 23. Elsevier; 2005. p. 275.

2. Sehgal VN, Pandhi D, Khurana A. Biologics in dermatology: An integrated review. Indian J Dermatol. 2014;59:425-41.
3. Coondoo A. Biologics in dermatologic therapy--an update. Indian J Dermatol. 2009;54:211-20.
4. Trefzer U, Hofmann M, Sterry W, et al. Cytokine and anticytokine therapy in dermatology. Expert Opin Biol Ther. 2003;3:733-43.
5. Smith DI, Swamy PM, Heffernan MP. Off-label uses of biologics in dermatology: Interferon and intravenous immunoglobulin (part 1 of 2). J Am Acad Dermatol. 2007;56(1):e55-79.

Chapter 3

Concept and Development of Biosimilars

Brijesh Nair

▌ INTRODUCTION

Biosimilars are biopharmaceuticals that have been assessed by regulatory agencies to have efficacy and safety similar to their reference products and are expected to be marketed at substantially lower prices. They are not 100% identical, but essentially the same biological substance, though there may be minor differences due to their complex nature and production methods. They have come into the limelight because of patent expiry of originator biological molecules. The new wave of biosimilars will largely consist of monoclonal antibodies, which are mainly used in the oncology and immunology setting. Biologicals have revolutionized the field of medicine and dermatology in particular, with significant impact in the management of psoriasis, psoriatic arthritis (PsA), urticarial and immunobullous disorders. The expected benefits of biosimilars are reductions in costs and consequently better access to biotherapeutics. However, uptake of biosimilars in the market has been slower than expected, which may, at least partly, be attributed to a lack of trust in the efficacy and safety of biosimilars as well as their interchangeability with the originator product by both patients and clinicians, which needs to be addressed meticulously. The difference in philosophy of biosimilar development is the focus on detection of potential differences in efficacy rather than the demonstration of efficacy, per se. "The demonstration of comparability does not necessarily mean that the quality attributes of the pre-change and post-change product are identical, but that they are highly similar and that the existing knowledge is sufficiently predictive to ensure that any differences in quality attributes have no adverse impact upon safety or efficacy of the drug product".

As such, a biosimilar development is therefore not so much "abridged" but rather "tailored" toward a distinct scientific objective—that is, to establish biosimilarity, not to reestablish benefit for the patient. The current concept of development of biosimilar monoclonal antibodies/soluble receptor fusion proteins (mAbs/cepts) follows the principle that extensive state-of-the-art physicochemical, analytical and functional comparison of the molecules is complemented by comparative nonclinical and clinical data that establishes equivalent efficacy and safety in a clinical "model" indication that is most sensitive to detect any minor differences (if these exist) between biosimilar and its reference mAb also at the clinical level.[1,2]

Definition: Biosimilars

The European Medicines Agency (EMA) defines biosimilars as "biological medicinal products that contain a version of the active substance of an already authorized, original biological medicinal product (reference medicinal product). A biosimilar agent is similar to the reference medicinal product in terms of quality characteristics, biological activity, safety and efficacy based on a comprehensive comparability exercise."

The intention of the biosimilar development is to show similarity with the reference product, not to independently demonstrate patient benefit. The scientific principles for establishing biosimilarity are the same as those for demonstrating comparability after a change in the manufacturing process of an already licensed biological originator molecule. According to US legislation, biosimilars must utilize the same mechanism or mechanisms of action for the condition or conditions of use prescribed, recommended, or suggested in the proposed labeling and are prescribed for conditions that have been previously approved for the reference product. Furthermore, the route of administration, the dosage form, and the strength of the biosimilar should be the same as those of the reference product.[3-5]

Why is Biosimilar Development Complex?

Biologicals are derived from living cells or organisms and consist of relatively large and often highly complex molecular entities that may be difficult to fully characterize. Because of inherent variability of the biologic system and the manufacturing process, any resulting biological will display a certain degree of variability (microheterogeneity), even between different batches of the same product. Because of unavoidable differences in the manufacturing processes, a biosimilar and the respective originator product, the reference product, will not be entirely identical. However, the amino acid sequence is expected to be the same, and only small differences in the microheterogeneity pattern of the molecule may be acceptable. A very thorough comparison of the structural and functional characteristics, and the product and process-related impurities of the biosimilar and the reference product is essential. Any differences found will need to be explained and justified with regard to the potential impact on the clinical performance of the biosimilar. Hence, the data requirements for demonstration of biosimilarity will usually be more extensive than for demonstration of comparability of a given biological before and after manufacturing changes by the same manufacturer. Data requirements for the development and licensing of biosimilars are considerably greater than for small chemically synthesized generic molecules. For a generic, physicochemical identification and demonstration of a similar pharmacokinetic profile (bioequivalence) to the originator product are usually sufficient to conclude on therapeutic equivalence. In contrast, a biosimilar needs to be developed based on a more extensive head-to-head comparison with the reference product, to ensure close resemblance in physicochemical and biologic characteristics, safety, and efficacy. The focus of biosimilar development is not to establish patient's benefit per se—this has already been done for the originator product—but to convincingly demonstrate high similarity to the reference product as basis for relying, in part, on its efficacy and safety experience.

Clinicians need to be aware that clinical data are not the only cornerstone of a biosimilar development to be relied on. Extensive characterization and comparison of the physicochemical properties and biologic activity of the biosimilar and the originator product play a fundamental role in this, and close similarity in these aspects is a prerequisite for any reduction in the amount of nonclinical and clinical data requirements. Clinical data provide complementary information. The biosimilar development program is scientifically tailored using up-to-date analytical tools and sensitive test models to best detect even small potential product-related differences between the biosimilar and the reference product.[6-11]

PRECLINICAL ANALYTICAL ASSESSMENT

Preclinical analytical assessments are used to determine similarity to an originator biologic and are critical for regulatory approval of biosimilars. Approximately 40 different analytical methods are utilized to assess 100 different drug attributes. The International Psoriasis Council suggested guidelines for standardization of preclinical assessments of emerging biosimilars through the development of a biosimilar index. Companies in the business of making biosimilars are not in possession of the original cell line utilized for the originator compound, and thus their biologic, derived from a new cell line, is not identical to the original product. Instead of relying on any one key piece of data, the weight of all the analytical assessments is considered when determining whether the biosimilar is "similar" to the originator compound, the choice of the cell line, the culture media, the culture temperature and the purification processes can all be altered, with each change potentially affecting the quality of the end product. The primary amino acid composition of a biosimilar medication is precisely bioengineered, but other features of biologics such as three-dimensional protein folding, glycosylation, charge and presence of impurities are more variable during the manufacturing process. These particular features of a biologically produced product may affect both the antigen binding and immunogenicity of a given drug, and thus may affect both drug efficacy and safety in clinical use. Evaluating posttranslational modifications via mass spectrometry, including testing for glycosylation, acetylation, sulfation, phosphorylation, glycation and charge, is essential in the characterization of biologics and biosimilars. Testing for drug product stability (e.g. shelf life and alterations with temperature) and product devices (e.g. auto-injectors, prefilled syringes) are also needed in order to determine similarity between the biosimilar product and originator biological product.[12-14]

Biosimilar index is an algorithm where each comparison is weighted with regard to its criticality, and where variability for each assay/test (e.g. <10% or 1 SD) is standardized. Using this index, biosimilars would be rated and scored regarding their preclinical analytical similarity to the originator biologic.[15]

▌ SOME TERMINOLOGIES DEFINED

Biomimics: These are versions of mAbs or fusion proteins available in countries where regulation is less strict. Biomimics are also known as 'biocopies', 'intended copies', or 'nonregulated biologics'. Kikuzubam was a rituximab biomimic which demonstrated adverse events different from originator molecule of rituximab, and hence regulatory authorities had to revoke the approval, thus demonstrating the complexity of the biomimic explosion. It also needs to be stated that different adverse effect profile of a biomimic raises questions on its biosimilarity.

Reference product (alternative terms-'originator' or 'innovator' product): The initial biopharmaceutical that has been approved by regulatory agencies for specific indications; preclinical and clinical data regarding the reference product provides the basis for comparison of a biosimilar agent in the approval process.

Biosimilar (alternative terms—'similar biotherapeutic product', 'subsequent entry biologic', 'follow-on biologic' and 'biocomparables'): A mAb or fusion protein that has undergone a complete development process based on comparability to preclinical and clinical data of the reference product, with sufficient bioequivalence to meet regulatory approval.

Interchangeability:[16-19] Interchangeability is the concept that a biosimilar drug and its parent biologic compound are so similar that a patient could be switched from one originator drug to another biosimilar drug and back during chronic therapeutic use, perhaps an indefinite number of times, without any untoward clinical side effects occurring due to this interchange of products. This designation allows a biosimilar agent to be substituted for its reference product by the pharmacist without prescriber input. Unlike small-molecule drugs, a biopharmaceutical that is repeatedly interchanged with a similar biological agent might elicit immunogenicity that could compromise the efficacy and safety of both the medications.

Thus, the prevalent American College of Rheumatology (ACR) and European League Against Rheumatism (EULAR) consensus is that frequent switching between the original protein product and the biosimilar agent should be avoided, as even subtle differences, such as impurities introduced during manufacturing, can trigger an immune response to biosimilar agents.

Switch: Therapeutic transition from a reference product to a biosimilar agent or vice versa, based on prescriber decision. A 'switch' study demonstrating no loss of efficacy or no increase in risk would support the transition from biological to other.

Substitution: Interchange of a biosimilar agent with its reference product by someone other than the prescribing health professional. If a biosimilar agent is determined to be "interchangeable" with its reference product, a pharmacist would be allowed to substitute a prescribed biological therapy for a biosimilar agent without involving the prescribing physician.[20,21]

METHODOLOGY OF PROVING BIOSIMILARITY

For approval, a comprehensive dossier of analytical, preclinical, pharmacokinetic, pharmacodynamics and clinical data that demonstrates comparable efficacy and safety of the biosimilar and its off-patent reference biopharmaceutical is required. EMA has prescribed certain steps which are mandatory for approval of a biosimilar. This process is depicted in Table 3.1.

IMMUNOGENICITY

It is important to understand the complexity of production of both biological reference product and biosimilar, which precludes exact replication. Earlier batches of reference product have also changed due to the process changes and hence the current version of a biological reference product is not identical to the earlier batches of the same product. This underlines the need for rigorous pharmacological equivalence and biocomparability studies (for clinical comparison) in the approval process of a biological/ biosimilar.

Immunogenicity may be influenced by patient-, disease-, or product-related factors. Patient- and disease related factors are already known from the experience gained with the originator product and therefore do not need to be reinvestigated for the biosimilar. The focus of the evaluation is thus on potential product-related factors, such as structural or impurities/contaminants, most of which are readily detected by state-of-the-art analytical methods. Differences in immunogenicity can also be due to extraneous factors like impurities in the manufacturing process of the prefilled syringes. This demonstrates the complexity of biosimilarity confirmation process.

Table 3.1: Steps for approval of biosimilar.

Stages	Steps
Preclinical Stage	
In vitro studies	• Assessing binding to targets • Assess signal transduction and functional activity/viability.
Determine if in vivo studies are needed	Necessary only if factors of concern are identified, e.g. new post-translational modification structures.
In vivo studies	Focus of study depends on the need for additional information.
PHASE 1	
Pharmacokinetic/pharmacodynamics studies	• Single dose crossover or parallel group designs preferred • Pharmacodynamic markers selected on the basis of their clinical relevance • Affinity is a key determinant of the PK and PD profile of mAbs and soluble receptors • Close reproduction of conformational structure for biosimilar mAbs and cepts is needed to ensure comparable biological effect.
PHASE 3	
Safety and efficacy studies	• No clinically significant difference in efficacy to reference product • Compare severity and frequency of adverse events, in particular for immunogenicity/safety

(PK: Pharmacokinetics; PD: Pharmacodynamics; mAbs: Monoclonal antibodies; cepts: Soluble receptor constructs).

In order to gain full insight into the long-term outcomes, particularly the immunogenicity profile of biosimilars, it is recommended that comparative clinical data should be collected for more than 1 year especially for anti-tumor necrosis factor (anti-TNF) therapies. Immunogenicity data beyond 1 year lacks scientific rationale, and would raise the bar for biosimilars above that expected for innovator drugs, with obvious negative consequences for the affordability of these products.[22-26]

PHARMACOVIGILANCE

Pharmacovigilance, embedded in postmarketing surveillance, is of critical importance for biosimilars. As the abbreviated clinical development program of biosimilar agents is less able to identify small safety risks (compared with the development of reference products), appropriate pharmaco-vigilance measures need to be implemented after approval is granted. The means of pharmaco-vigilance are company initiated risk management plans, postmarketing research and surveillance of existing databases (registries) created to monitor patients receiving biologic agents.

The pharmaco-equivalence and bioequivalence of the biosimilar to reference product intuitively suggests similarity in safety profile from product-related and patient-population-related perspectives. However, variability in immunogenicity due to batch to batch variability is a cause for concern. Thus, the safety of biosimilars needs to be actively and comprehensively followed up on an ongoing basis. Adverse event reports, if any, should include, in addition to the International Nonproprietary Name (INN), other indicators, such as brand name, manufacturer's name, lot number, and country of origin of the batch used.[27,28]

Nomenclature

To avoid confusion between biosimilar agents and their reference products during pharmacovigilance, specific nomenclature is necessary to distinguish each biosimilar from its reference drug and from each other. It has been suggested that a Greek letter or a combination of several letters could be appended to the end of the INN of each biopharmaceutical. Alternatively, a "biologic qualifier" (BQ) [a four-digit code proposed by the World Health Organization (WHO)] could be used to distinguish reference products and biosimilars from one another. Overall, the general agreement is that use of the INN alone is insufficient to differentiate biosimilars, and that traceability of each biosimilar needs to be secured. However, even though an internationally standardized system of nomenclature for biosimilars is urgently needed, this system has not yet been established, making postmarketing surveillance, risk evaluation and management strategies for biosimilars more difficult.[29-31]

Extrapolation

Extrapolation is defined as the ability to utilize clinical study data for one disease to gain agency approval for another disease not explicitly studied in clinical trials. Extrapolation is the foundation of the biosimilar regulatory framework and is here defined as granting regulatory approval for indications of the reference medicine that are not specifically studied during the clinical development of the biosimilar medicine. The Food and Drug Administration (US FDA/FDA) issued guidance, stating that data from a clinical trial of a biosimilar agent conducted in one disease could be used to support approval for additional indications for which the reference product has already been licensed. To obtain approval for any additional indication, the licensed biosimilar must follow the traditional regulatory pathway for biopharmaceuticals. FDA mandates two randomized, placebo-controlled clinical trials (conducted in patients with the disease for which the indication is being sought) that demonstrates both efficacy and safety of the biological agent in that disease state. Thus, if a biosimilar agent was not approved initially for all indications for which the reference biopharmaceutical is licensed, the biosimilar manufacturer must conduct clinical trials in each additional individual disease state to support a biological license application for each separate indication. Similarly, if the reference biopharmaceutical is approved for an additional indication after its biosimilar has already been licensed, extrapolation of indications no longer applies: the manufacturer of the licensed biosimilar must conduct new clinical trials in this new indication to get approval. Thus, extrapolation of indication requires convincing scientific justification, which should address the mechanism of action, toxicities, and immunogenicity in each indication of use.[32-38]

For mAb, extrapolation is more complex as their mechanism of action may depend on multiple sites of the molecule. Often, no direct pharmacodynamic marker exists for their activity, which means that clinical studies are designed around (insensitive) clinical end points, which makes it particularly challenging to study these products. How the different structure–activity relationships of antibodies contribute to efficacy and safety in the different indications is often not fully understood.[39,40]

Regulatory Issues

CT-P13 (an infliximab biosimilar) was the first monoclonal antibody biosimilar to be approved, but not all national regulatory agencies granted extrapolation to all infliximab indications. Infliximab biosimilar (Remsima™) had been approved in a total of 47 countries as of May 2014, and marketing applications were pending in an additional 23 countries. Thus, as of May 2015, CT-P13 has been approved for use in approximately 70 countries worldwide. Agencies allowed extrapolation of indications for CT-P13 to six additional diseases for which the reference infliximab is approved but in which CT-P13 was not studied, namely psoriatic arthritis (PsA), psoriasis, adult and juvenile Crohn's disease, and adult and juvenile ulcerative colitis. This decision established a regulatory precedent for the extrapolation of indications for a therapeutic monoclonal antibody based on results of one successful phase III trial in a sensitive population [in rheumatoid arthritis (RA)] and on additional pharmacokinetic, efficacy, safety and immunogenicity data acquired in a phase I trial of patients with a different disease [ankylosing spondylitis (AS)]. Extrapolation of indications for biosimilars is possible, but concerns have been raised regarding the potential efficacy and safety of a biosimilar in diseases for which it has not been studied. It is opined that the outcome of a biosimilarity exercise should be binary: you either are, or you are not biosimilar to a given reference product. Selective approval for extrapolation to indications is at odds with this concept. Allowing products on the market that do not have the same authorized indications will create considerable confusion about the concept of biosimilarity. The success of biosimilars will depend on how they will be able to be interchanged with the reference product and other biosimilars in clinical practice. If multiple biosimilars are allowed in the market with different approved uses, this will create a complex situation that will add hurdles for the successful practitioner uptake of biosimilars.[41-44]

INDIAN SCENARIO FOR BIOSIMILARS

There has been burgeoning interest in biosimilars in Indian dermatology scenario. Biosimilars of infliximab, etanercept, rituximab and adalimumab have been launched. The permissive nature of regulation in India has resulted in proliferation of intended copies without published biocomparability research supporting their use. The possibility of revoking an approval on recognition of inefficacy or adverse events is a definite possibility in the current scenario. Indian guidelines allow a biosimilar product to be authorized if the reference product is licensed and widely marketed for at least 4 years in a country with a well-established regulatory framework, although not marketed in India (e.g.: Humira).[45] The biosimilars currently approved for use in India are depicted in Table 3.2.

ZRC-3197, developed and marketed by Zydus Cadila (India) in India as Exemptia™ to treat RA, juvenile inflammatory arthritis, PsA and AS, is described as a "fingerprint match" of the reference adalimumab (Humira®, Abbvie Inc., USA) "in terms of safety, purity and potency." The primary and secondary structures of ZRC-3197 and reference adalimumab are identical, and no differences were detected in aggregation or in the profile

Table 3.2: Biosimilars currently approved for use in India.

Product	Brand name/manufacturer	Biosimilarity status
Adalimumab	Exemptia (Zydus)	Biosimilarity proven
	Adalirel (Reliance), Adfrar P (Torrent)	Intended copies/biomimics
Etanercept	Etacept (Cipla), Intacept (Intas)	Intended copies/biomimics
Rituximab	Reditux (Dr Reddy's), Rituxirel (Reliance), Mabtas RA (Intas)	Intended copies/biomimics
Infliximab	Infimab (Sun/Epirus/Reliance)	Biocomparability studies with switching carried out in rheumatoid arthritis. Similar study in psoriasis planned
Omalizumab	On patent	No biosimilar

of low-molecular-weight fragments between these two biopharmaceuticals. Based on this, ZRC-3197 was approved for RA, juvenile idiopathic arthritis, AS, PsA, hidradenitis suppurativa, ulcerative colitis and Crohn's disease, but interestingly not for the treatment of psoriasis. The reason for not authorizing the product for psoriasis is not clear.[46-48]

BIOSIMILARS IN PSORIASIS

There is a paucity of biosimilar trials pertaining to psoriasis. In dermatology, direct data on psoriasis patients is missing. Most approvals are based on extrapolation. The question has been raised whether results obtained from such diverse patient populations treated with the same biologic may be compared at all. In general, psoriasis patients have been exposed to previous treatment protocols [e.g. Ultraviolet (UV) therapy]. They also tend to exhibit different patient characteristics that may make them more susceptible to adverse drug reactions than other patient groups (e.g. alcohol abuse, liver toxicity). The fact that, for instance, inflammatory bowel diseases respond to infliximab and adalimumab but not to etanercept, whereas etanercept, on the other hand, is effective in psoriasis and RA also clearly underlines the differences between the mechanistic of various autoimmune diseases. The underpowered biosimilarity studies are ill-equipped to detect safety signals. Although not all ongoing biosimilar trials may have been registered, the present situation in terms of registered trials is unsatisfactory and will leave clinicians with a high degree of uncertainty with respect to their treatment decisions. It is now up to the clinical community to start collecting data on efficacy and particularly safety with independent trials and patient registries.

Biosimilars ideally must be studied in the preferred ('most sensitive') indication to assess comparable safety and efficacy. In case of TNF inhibitors, it is psoriasis with a reliable, easily assessable clinical endpoint [Psoriasis Area and Severity Index (PASI)]. Future of biosimilar development might focus more on this 'sensitivity' aspect of psoriasis.[49-51]

BIOSIMILARS FOR PSORIASIS: CLINICAL STUDIES TO DETERMINE SIMILARITY

International Psoriasis Consortium (IPC) has defined biosimilarity in psoriasis biosimilars on a clinical level recently. The amount and the type of clinical data generated in clinical studies involving biosimilars will inherently be less than the clinical data obtained for originator biologics. Owing to the regulatory emphasis on extrapolation eventuating in cost reduction, utilizing biosimilars in practice for diseases where little or no clinical data exist is a reality that clinicians must learn to accept. The IPC has suggested psoriasis as a future model for TNF blocker testing owing to (a) high effect sizes in clinical trials (b) lack of co-intervention (c) commonality of the disease (d) ease of conduct of trials with an easily reproducible outcome endpoint (PASI score). IPC also suggested that a biosimilar trial should also be at least as long as the primary end point in the reference product's pivotal trials, and be based on the same safety measures collected during these original trials. For example, TNF blocker biosimilar trials should include safety outcomes such as deaths, malignancies, opportunistic infections, reactivation of tuberculosis and hepatitis B virus, major adverse cardiac events, and injection site reactions. In many cases, to demonstrate clinical equivalence on efficacy and safety of the biosimilar and the reference biologic adequately powered, randomized, parallel group, preferably double-blinded, comparative clinical trials are needed.[52-54]

CONCLUSION

The principles of establishing biosimilarity are to demonstrate structural and functional similarity to a reference product using the most discriminatory analytical methods. These data are supported where necessary by focused clinical evaluation using conditions that are adequately sensitive to evaluate real risks that cannot be addressed solely by analytical data. Unanswered questions remain, particularly regarding extrapolation of indications, switching and interchangeability, naming and traceability, and long-term safety of biosimilars. Even after licensing, biosimilars (owing to the batch to batch variability inherent to biopharmaceuticals) must be subjected to intense postmarketing surveillance and pharmacovigilance. Further studies, including postmarketing surveillance using data acquired from registries, are needed to give healthcare providers confidence to accept these biosimilar agents into their armamentarium. The tighter regulation of intended copies and biomimics must be ensured to avoid safety issues which might blight the development of genuine biosimilar agents. The appropriately regulated and rationally extrapolated biosimilar development milieu will go a long way in reducing healthcare costs in the therapy of inflammatory diseases and can augment health policy decision making. Despite the increasing number of countries that have adopted biosimilar guidelines, there are clear differences in local requirements in terms of weight of evidence and data interpretation, labeling and naming of biosimilars. Such divergent regulatory decisions on the biosimilarity exercise do not assist in solving the trepidation that exists at the level of healthcare professionals and patients about biosimilars. There is a need for a global harmonization exercise for deciding upon the determinants of the concept of biosimilarity and for standardizing the regulatory requirements of biosimilars (Table 3.3).

Table 3.3: Problem areas in biosimilar products.

Consistent demonstration of pharmaceutical quality and quality assurance of the manufacturing process by biosimilar firm

Ensuring batch to batch product consistency

Lack of data on substitution, switching, interchangeability and subsequent adverse events/immunogenicity

Extrapolation of data from index disease to other indications

Intense postmarketing surveillance for safety issues: Pharma company, the primary stakeholder as opposed to practitioner driven registries

Problems with inconsistent nomenclature

Trial design complexity in demonstration of equivalence and interchangeability

Inter-regulator variations in licensing for extrapolation based on in vitro assays

Practitioner and patient apprehension regarding efficacy and safety of biosimilars

Grant of license by regulator subject to a post-authorization safety surveillance commitment.

▌ REFERENCES

1. Simoens S. Biosimilar medicines and cost-effectiveness. Clinico Economics and outcomes research: CEOR. 2011;3:29-36.
2. Schneider CK, Kalinke U. Toward biosimilar monoclonal antibodies. Nature biotechnology. 2008;;26(9):908-85.
3. European Medicines Agency. Guidelines on similar biological medicinal products. [online], Available from www.ema.europa.eu/docs/en_GB/document_library/Scientific_guideline/2014/10/WC500176768.pdf [Accessed in 2014].
4. U.S. Senate. Biologics Price Competition and Innovation Act of 2009. 2009;703:3590-686.
5. Food and Drug Administration. Guidance for Industry on Biosimilars: Q & As Regarding Implementation of the BPCI Act of 2009: Questions and Answers Part I. 2012. Available from http://www.fda.gov/Drugs/GuidanceComplianceRegulatoryInformation/Guidances/ucm259809 [Accessed in May, 2017]
6. U.S. Food and Drug Administration. Draft guidance on biosimilar product development. Available from http://www.fda.gov/Drugs/DevelopmentApprovalProcess/HowDrugsareDevelopedandApproved/ApprovalApplications/TherapeuticBiologicApplications/Biosimilars/default.htm [Accessed in October, 2012]
7. European Medicines Agency, Committee for Medicinal Products for Human Use. Guideline on similar biological medicinal products containing biotechnology-derived proteins as active substance: quality issues. 2005. Available from http://www.ema.europaeu/pdfs/human/biosimilar/4934805en.pdf [Accessed in October, 2012].
8. ICH Guideline topic QE5: Comparability of Biotechnological/Biological Products Subject to Changes in their Manufacturing Process. Available from http://www.ich.org/products/guidelines/quality/article/quality-guidelines.html [Accessed in October,2012].

9. Schellekens H. Biosimilar therapeutics: what do we need to consider? NDT Plus. 2009;2(1):i27-i36.
10. Wadhwa M, Thorpe R. The challenges of immunogenicity in developing biosimilar products. IDrugs. 2009;12(7):440-4.
11. European Medicines Agency. European public assessment reports. 2015. Available from http://www.ema.europa.eu/ema/index.jsp?curl=pages/medicines/landing/epar_search.jsp&mid=WC0b01ac058001d124 [Accessed in May, 2017].
12. O'Connor A, Rogge M. Nonclinical development of a biosimilar: the current landscape. Bioanalysis. 2013;5:537-44.
13. Schiestl M, Stangler T, Torella C, et al. Acceptable changes in quality attributes of glycosylated biopharmaceuticals. Nat Biotechnol. 2011;29:310-2.
14. Calvo B, Zuniga L. Therapeutic monoclonal antibodies: strategies and challenges for biosimilars development. Curr Med Chem. 2012;19:4445-50.
15. Blauvelt A, Cohen AD, Puig L, et al. Biosimilars for psoriasis: preclinical analytical assessment to determine similarity. Br J Dermatol. 2016;174:282-6
16. US Department of Health & Human Services. The Affordable Care Act. HHS. gov/HealthCare. Available from http://www.hhs.gov/healthcare/rights/law/index.html [Accessed in May, 2017]
17. ACR Committee on Rheumatologic Care. ACR Position Statements—Biosimilars. American College of Rheumatology. 2015. Available from http://www.rheumatology.org/Practice/Clinical/Position/Biosimilars_02_2015/.pdf [Accessed in May, 2017]
18. Tóthfalusi L, Endrényi L, Chow SC. Statistical and regulatory considerations in assessments of interchangeability of biological drug products. Eur J Health Econ. 2014;15(1):S5-11.
19. Anderson S, Hauck WW. Consideration of individual bioequivalence. J Pharmacokinet Biopharm. 1990;18(3):259-73.
20. Castañeda-Hernandez G, Szekanecz Z, Mysler E, et al. Biopharmaceuticals for rheumatic diseases in Latin America, Europe, Russia, and India: innovators, biosimilars, and intended copies. Joint Bone Spine. 2014;81(6):471-7.
21. Barile-Fabris LA, Irazoque-Palazuelos F, Vasquez RH, et al. Incidence of adverse events in patients treated with intended copies of biologic therapeutic agents in Colombia and Mexico. Arthritis Rheumatol. 2014;66,S662.
22. Braun J, Baraliakos X, Kudrin A, et al. Striking discrepancy in the development of anti-drug antibodies (ADA) in patients with rheumatoid arthritis (RA) and ankylosing spondylitis (AS) in response to infliximab (INF) and its biosimilar CTP13. Arthritis Rheumatol. 2014;66:3538-9.
23. Udata C, Yin D, Cai C, et al. Immunogenicity assessment of PF06438179, a potential biosimilar to infliximab, in healthy volunteers. Ann. Rheum. 2015;74(2):702.
24. Mok CC, Van der Kleij D, Wolbink GJ. Drug levels, anti-drug antibodies, and clinical efficacy of the anti-TNF α biologics in rheumatic diseases. Clin. Rheumatol. 2013;32:1429-35.
25. European Medicines Agency, Committee for Medicinal Products for Human Use. Guideline on immunogenicity assessment of biotechnology derived therapeutic proteins. Available from https://www.ema.europa.eu/ema/index.jsp?curl_pages/regulation/general/general_content_000408.jsp&murl_menus/regulations/regulations.jsp&mid_WC0b01ac058002958c [Accessed in October, 2012].

26. Ben-Horin S, Yavzori M, Benhar I, et al. Cross-immunogenicity: antibodies to infliximab in Remicade-treated patients with IBD similarly recognise the biosimilar Remsima. Gut. 2015;65(7):1132-8.

27. Minghetti P, Rocco P, Cilurzo F, et al. The regulatory framework of biosimilars in the European Union. Drug Dis Today. 2012;17(1):63-70.

28. European Medicines Agency. Pharmacovigilance guidelines. Available from http://www.ema.europa.eu/ema/indexjsp?curl_pages/regulation/document_ listing/document_listing_000199.jsp&murl_menus/regulations/regulations. jsp&mid_WC0b01ac05800250b3 [Accessed in May, 2017]

29. World Health Organization. 55th Consultation on International Nonproprietary Names for Pharmaceutical Substances, Geneva. 2012. Available from www.who. int/medicines/services/inn/55th_Executive_Summary.pdf [Accessed in May, 2017]

30. Pineda C, Caballero-Uribe CV, de Oliveira MG, et al. Recommendations on how to ensure the safety and effectiveness of biosimilars in Latin America: a point of view. Clin Rheumatol. 2015;34:635-40.

31. European Biopharmaceutical Enterprises. Tell me the whole story: the role of product labelling in building user confidence in biosimilars in Europe. Gen Biosimil Initiative J (GaBI J). 2014;3:188-92.

32. Weise M, Kurki P, Wolff-Holz E, et al. Biosimilars: the science of extrapolation. Blood. 2014;124:3191-6.

33. Committee for Medicinal Products for Human Use. Guideline on similar biological medicinal products containing biotechnology-derived proteins as active substance: nonclinical and clinical issues. European Medicines Agency. 2006. Available from: http://www. ema. europa. eu/docs/en_GB/document_ library/Scientific_guideline/2015/01. WC500003920. pdf May, 2017.

34. US Department of Health & Human Services. Biosimilars: questions and answers regarding implementation of the Biologics Price Competition and Innovation Act of 2009. US Food and Drug Administration. 2012. Available from [Accessed in May, 2017]

35. Danese S, Gomollon F. ECCO position statement: The use of biosimilar medicines in the treatment of inflammatory bowel disease (IBD). J. Crohns Colitis. 2013;7:586-9.

36. Fiorino G, Danese S. The biosimilar road in inflammatory bowel disease: the right way? Best Pract Res Clin Gastroenterol. 2014;28:465-71.

37. Strober BE, Armour K, Romiti R, et al. Biopharmaceuticals and biosimilars in psoriasis: what the dermatologist needs to know. J Am Acad Dermatol. 2012;66(2):317-322.

38. American College of Rheumatology. Position statement. Biosimilars. 2011. Available from http://www.rheumatology.org/Practice/Clinical/Position/ Position_Statements. [Accessed in May, 2017]

39. Minghetti P, Rocco P, Del Veccio L, et al. Biosimilars and regulatory authorities. Nephron Clin Pract. 2011;117(1):c1-c7.

40. World Health Organization. Guidelines on evaluation of similar biotherapeutic products (SBPs). 2009. Available from http://www.who.int/biologicals/areas/ biological_therapeutics/BIOTHERAPEUTICS_ FOR_WEB_22APRIL2010.pdf. [Accessed in May, 2017]

41. Dörner T, Kay J. Biosimilars in rheumatology: current perspectives and lessons learnt. Nat. Rev. Rheumatol. 2015;11:713-24.

42. Health Canada. Inflectra. Drugs and Health Products. 2015. Available from http://www.hc-sc.gc.ca/dhp-mps/prodpharma/sbd-smd/drugmed/sbd_smd_2014_inflectra_159493-eng.php [Accessed in May, 2017]

43. Scott BJ, Klein AV, Wang J. Biosimilar monoclonal antibodies: A canadian regulatory perspective on the assessment of clinically relevant differences and indication extrapolation. J Clin Pharmacol. 2014;55(3):S123-32.

44. Hazlewood, GS, Rezaie A, Borman M, et al. Comparative effectiveness of immunosuppressants and biologics for inducing and maintaining remission in Crohn's disease: a network meta-analysis. Gastroenterology. 2015;148:344-54.

45. Government of India. Guidelines on similar biologics: regulatory requirements for Marketing Authorization in India. 2012. Available from http://www.cdsco.nic.in/Bio.Similar.Guideline.pdf [Accessed in May, 2017]

46. Bandyopadhyay S, Mahajan M, Mehta T, et al. Physicochemical and functional characterization of a biosimilar adalimumab ZRC3197. Biosimilars. 2015;5:1-18.

47. Zydus Cadila. Zydus launches world's first biosimilar of Adalimumab. Zydus Cadila. 2014. Available from http://zyduscadila.com/wp-content/uploads/2015/05/PressNote09-12-14.pdf. Exemptia Prescribing Information. http://www.exemptia.com [Accessed in May, 2017]

48. Jani RH, Gupta R, Bhatia G, et al. A prospective, randomized, double-blind, multicentre, parallel-group, active controlled study to compare efficacy and safety of biosimilar adalimumab (Exemptia; ZRC-3197) and adalimumab (Humira) in patients with rheumatoid arthritis. Int J Rheumat Dis. 2015;19(11):1157-68.

49. Sandoz. Study to Demonstrate Equivalent Efficacy and to Compare Safety of Biosimilar Adalimumab (GP2017) and Humira (ADACCESS). In: ClinicalTrials.gov [Internet]. Bethesda (MD): National Library of Medicine (US). 2000 Available from http://ClinicalTrials.gov/show/NCT02016105 NLM Identifier: NCT02016105. [Accessed in May, 2014].

50. Sandoz. Study to Demonstrate Equivalent Efficacy and to Compare Safety of Biosimilar Etanercept (GP2015) and Enbrel (EGALITY). In: ClinicalTrials.gov [Internet]. Bethesda (MD): National Library of Medicine (US). 2000. Available from http://ClinicalTrials.gov/show/NCT01891864   NLM Identifier: NCT01891864. [Accessed in May, 2014].

51. Radtke MA, Augustin M. Biosimilars in psoriasis: what can we expect? J Dtsch Dermatol Ges. 2014;12:306-12.

52. Casadevall N, Thorpe R, Schellekens H. Biosimilars need comparative clinical data. Kidney Int. 2011;80(5):553.

53. Ebbers HC, Muenzberg M, Schellekens H. The safety of switching between therapeutic proteins. Expert Opin Biol Ther. 2012;12(11):1473-85.

54. Ebbers HC, Crow SA, Vulto AG, et al. Interchangeability, immunogenicity and biosimilars. Nat Biotechnol. 2012;30(12):1186-90.

Chapter

4

Pathogenesis of Psoriasis

Rajat Kandhari, Anupama Molpariya

▌ INTRODUCTION

Psoriasis is a common, chronic, inflammatory, and proliferative disorder of the skin, associated with systemic manifestations. In simplified terms, the psoriatic phenotype presents itself as a result of a complex interplay of genetic and environmental triggers (such as trauma, stress, infections, and drugs), followed by a cytokine cascade resulting in various morphological variants of psoriasis[1,2] (Fig. 4.1). Our understanding of psoriasis pathogenesis has come a long way, from psoriasis being a disease associated with abnormal proliferation and disturbed terminal differentiation with the keratinocyte at the forefront and treatments such as coal tar, anthralin, and methotrexate forming the mainstay of therapy; to an era where the T lymphocytes were considered the main culprit and were tackled by drugs such as cyclosporine, alefacept and efalizumab; this was subsequently followed by Th1 cytokines [tumor necrosis factor-alpha (TNF-α)] dominating the pathogenesis of psoriasis and molecules such as etanercept and infliximab got introduced to tackle the disorder. Today the concept of psoriasis being solely a Th1 driven disease is considered inconsistent and there is enough evidence to support the key role of the interleukin (IL)-12, IL-23, and IL-17A in the psoriatic pathogenesis. Moreover, this understanding has led to the treatment of psoriasis becoming "targeted" to certain cytokines and certain pathways leading to improved outcomes and safety.

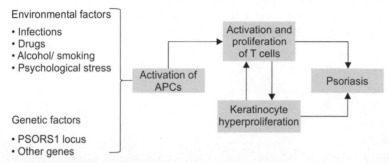

Fig. 4.1: A simplified illustration of the psoriatic pathogenesis. (APCs: Antigen-presenting cells; PSORS1: Psoriasis susceptibility 1).

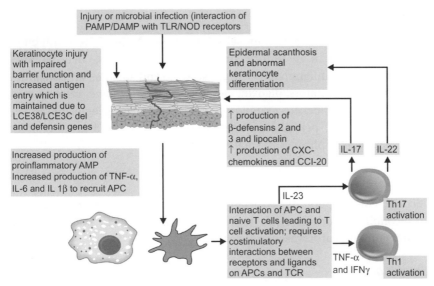

Fig. 4.2: Pathogenesis of psoriasis.[24] (APC: Antigen-presenting cell; TNF-α: Tumor necrosis factor-alpha; IFN-γ: Interferon-gamma; IL: Interleukin; TCR: T-cell receptor; DAMP: Damage-associated molecular patterns; PAMP: Pathogen-associated molecular patterns; TLR: Toll-like receptors; NOD: Nucleotide-binding oligomerization domain; CCL20: Chemokine (C-C motif) ligand 20; LCE: Late cornified envelope; Th1: Type 1 T helper cell; Th17: Type 17 T helper cell).

It is considered that various antigens activate effector T cells in the skin leading to release of inflammatory cytokines that promote further recruitment of immune cells, keratinocyte proliferation and sustained chronic inflammation (Fig. 4.2).

ETIOLOGY OF PSORIASIS

Environmental Factors

Infections

It has been proposed that certain variants of psoriasis, particularly guttate and chronic plaque psoriasis are fueled by persistent intracellular streptococcal infection.[3,4] These are not eliminated by standard antibiotic therapy but tonsillectomy appears to be effective in some patients.[5] Further, human immunodeficiency virus (HIV) infection is associated with paradoxical aggravation or worsening of psoriasis, as it causes a reduction in the T-helper cells. Suggested explanations for this occurrence include HIV-induced reduction in regulatory T cells, an increased number of memory CD8+ T cells, effects of HIV on dendritic cell populations, HIV proteins acting as superantigens or shared genetic variants between psoriasis and HIV responder status.[6]

Drugs

Drugs like antimalarials, lithium salts, interferon (INF)-α, TNF-α inhibitors and tetracyclines may induce or exacerbate psoriasis. Beta-blockers, nonsteroidal anti-inflammatory drugs (NSAIDs) and angiotensin-converting enzyme (ACE) inhibitors, digoxin, clonidine, carbamazepine, valproic acid, calcium-channel blockers, granulocyte-colony stimulating factor, potassium iodide, ampicillin, penicillin, progesterone, morphine and acetazolamide have also been implicated in smaller studies.[7]

Alcohol

Alcohol consumption is associated with moderate-to-severe psoriasis.[8] In alcoholics, psoriasis tends to be more severe, and is associated with depression and cardiovascular diseases.[9]

Smoking

It has been demonstrated that smoking increases the chances of a person developing psoriasis, psoriatic arthritis and palmoplantar pustulosis.[10,11] Moreover, the disease tends to be more severe in smokers.[10]

Other Factors

Psychological Stress

Psoriasis has been associated with depression, anxiety, and suicidal tendency and psychological stress may cause disease flares.[12,13] Meditation, weight loss and yoga leads to decreased psoriasis area severity index (PASI) scores.[14] This may be explained by the numerous neurocutaneous connections forming the brain-skin axis.[15,16] The immune-modulatory neurotransmitters may be involved in the pathogenesis of psoriasis[17] as psoriatic lesions may resolve after a sensory loss or nerve damage in the same area.[18]

Sunlight

Sun exposure generally causes improvement in psoriatic lesions but 5–20% patients may show worsening.[7] Some patients may develop psoriatic lesions over the lesions of polymorphous light eruption due to Koebner's phenomenon.[19]

Physical Trauma

Koebner's phenomenon is seen in up to 25% psoriatic patients,[20] more commonly seen in HLA-C:06:02 positive patients.[21] It is hypothesized that mechanical trauma activates innate immunity with subsequent adaptive immune activation, keratinocyte hyperproliferation and angiogenesis leading to new psoriatic lesions at the sites of trauma.[7]

Genetic Factors

Although, multiple genes are involved in determining susceptibility to psoriasis, "psoriasis susceptibility 1" or PSORS1 loci at major histocompatibility complex (MHC) region on chromosome 6p21.3 is the only locus strongly overrepresented in all patients of psoriasis worldwide. PSORS1 accounts for 35–50% of the heritability of the disease and is located on the MHC region of chromosome 6 (6p21).[23] Three genes namely, HLA-Cw6, CCHCR1 (Coiled-coil alpha-helical rod protein 1) and CDSN (corneodesmosin) are present within this region. HLA-Cw6 encodes a class I MHC protein involved in antigen presentation, CCHCR1 encodes coiled-coil alpha-helical rod protein 1, which is highly expressed in psoriatic epidermis and regulates keratinocyte proliferation and CDSN encodes corneodesmosin, a late differentiation epidermal glycoprotein overexpressed in the granular and cornified layers of the epidermis involved in keratinocyte adhesion.[1,2]

Moreover, HLA-Cw6 is carried by up to 60% of patients with early onset (type I psoriasis) and even more frequently in patients with the guttate variant. HLA-Cw6 positive patients may exhibit an earlier onset of disease, extensive plaques, nail involvement, recurrent clinical course, greater psychosocial impact and are more likely to experience remission with pregnancy and more likely to experience Koebner's phenomenon.

Several genome-wide scans have reported other loci (PSORS2-10).[22,23] A few non-MHC susceptibility loci have also been identified, but they may be of limited value in disease prediction as they confer a low-risk towards disease development.[24]

Psoriasis demonstrates a genetic spectrum, wherein one end of the spectrum is represented by the rare families in which changes in a single gene may be sufficient to cause the disease (monogenic), whereas at the other end exists the more common form in which an obvious family history may be lacking and it is likely that changes in multiple genes, interacting both with each other and the environment are required for disease expression (polygenic).[25]

Furthermore, the involvement of genetic factors contributing to the disease has been demonstrated by a higher rate of disease prevalence in cases with a positive family history [26,27] and the increase in the lifetime risk of psoriasis if both parents of an individual are affected.[28] Higher concordance rate of 72% among monozygotic twins compared to 22% among dizygotic twins has also been seen.[29] The development and severity of psoriasis have also been linked to the sex of the contributing parent, wherein men are more likely than women to transmit psoriasis to the offspring.[30] An earlier age of onset was seen when the disease was inherited from the father, consistent with 'genetic anticipation'.[30]

PATHOGENETIC PATHWAY

There are multiple molecular processes occurring simultaneously to produce the basic pathological and phenotypic features of psoriatic lesions. No single cause has been identified and it is accepted that genetic and environmental factors act together to produce immune dysregulation in the presence of a defective skin barrier.[24]

Role of Damage-Associated Molecular Patterns (DAMP)/ Pathogen-Associated Molecular Patterns (PAMP) and Maturation of Antigen-Presenting Cells

Whenever there is microbial or mechanical insult, damage-associated molecular patterns (DAMP) and pathogen-associated molecular patterns (PAMP) interact with their receptors, such as toll-like receptors (TLRs) and nucleotide-binding oligomerization domain (NOD)-like receptors (NLRs), causing activation of keratinocytes and the epidermal innate immune system and thus, increased secretion of antimicrobial proteins/peptides (AMPs).[24] This interaction also leads to the liberation of potent chemoattractants and inflammatory cytokines such as TNF-α, IL-8 and IL-1β.

In a genetically predisposed individual:

- Exposure to PAMP leads to a heightened inflammatory response and defective skin barrier repair with increased expression of keratins 6 and 17 and the late cornified envelope 3 (LCE3) family. This aberrant skin repair allows a sustained exposure to PAMPs which are engulfed by antigen-presenting cells (APCs) like Langerhans and dendritic cells.
- Subsequent to the environmental triggers, there is the release of heat-shock proteins and under the influence of aforementioned cytokines, the APCs undergo a process of maturation involving upregulation of C-C chemokine receptor type 7 (CCR7), B7 molecules and intercellular adhesion molecule 1 (ICAM-1).

These mature APCs are then ready to interact with the naïve T cells in the neighboring lymph nodes resulting in T cell activation.

Migration of the APCs to the Local Lymph Nodes and the "Immunological Synapse"

Once the APCs attain maturity they find their way via the afferent lymphatics to the nearby draining lymph nodes to interact with the naïve T cells. This process requires interaction between the MHC antigens on APCs

Table 4.1: The immunological synapse.

Signal	Interaction
Primary	• T cell receptor (TCR) and MHC I/II interaction • ICAM-1 and LFA-1 interaction—maintains adhesion between the T cell and the APC
Secondary/Co-stimulatory	• B7-CD28 interactions leads to positive activation signals to T cells • LFA-3/CD2 • CD40/CD40L • Upregulates the transcription of cytokines involved in T cell activation—IL-2, TNF-α, INF- γ, and GM-CSF
Third set of signals	• IL-2 (made by activated T cells) bind to IL-2R surface receptor and regulates mitotic activation of the T cell • IL-12 (made by mature Langerhans cells) bind to IL-12R surface receptors on the activated T cell leading to differentiation of T cells into type 1 effectors.

(TCR: T cell receptor; MHC: Major histocompatibility complex; ICAM-1: Intercellular adhesion molecule 1; LFA-1: Lymphocyte function antigen 1; LFA-3: Lymphocyte function antigen 3; CD2: Cluster of differentiation 2; CD40/CD40L: Cluster of differentiation 40/cluster of differentiation 40 ligand; IL-2: Interleukin 2; IL-2R: Interleukin 2 receptor; APC: Antigen-presenting cell; TNF-α: Tumor necrosis factor-alpha; IFN-γ: Interferon-gamma; GM-CSF: Granulocyte-macrophage colony-stimulating factor; IL-12R: Interleukin 12 receptor).

with the T-cell receptors (TCRs). In addition, co-stimulatory interactions between receptors and ligands on APCs and TCRs are important. These include interaction of lymphocyte function antigen (LFA)-3 and cluster of differentiation 2 (CD2), between ICAM-1 and LFA-1, and between B7 and CD28[31] (Table 4.1).

The interaction between the APC and naïve T cells results in activation of naïve T cells to pathogenic T cells. This is facilitated by the presence of polymorphisms in IL-23 genes and HLA-Cw6. Once the T cells are activated, both CD4+ (include Th1 and Th17 cells) and CD8+ T cells infiltrate the skin and secrete Th1 and Th17 cytokines which activate the keratinocytes (Fig. 4.3).

Maturation of T-cells and Migration into the Inflamed Skin

The IL-12 released by the mature Langerhans cells bind to IL-12R cell surface receptors on the activated T cell leading to differentiation of T cells into type 1 effector cells. The maturation of the T cells results in expression of new surface proteins, namely the cutaneous lymphocyte-associated antigen (CLA) which enables the T cells to exit the blood vessels and migrate to

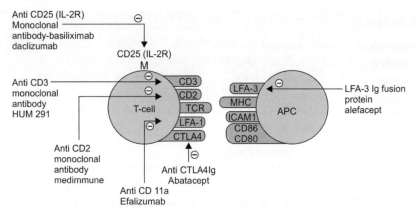

Fig. 4.3: Inhibition of T-cell activation and co-stimulation.

the skin. This is mediated by the interaction between the CLA on the T cell and E-selectin on the endothelial cells. IFN-gamma (IFN-γ) and TNF-α (released from antigen-activated T cells) induce chemokine expression from endothelial cells and keratinocytes and this chemokine gradient enhances trafficking of the T cells to the epidermis. The entry of the T cells into the epidermis is mediated by the ICAM-1 on the keratinocytes and LFA-1 on the T cells. Further, α3β7 integrin (on Tc1) binds to E-cadherin on keratinocytes, which is increased in the psoriatic epidermis facilitating transport of T cells into the epidermis and resulting in an injury response program and release of various cytokines which serve as signals for chronic epidermal hyperplasia.

Role of Keratinocytes (KCs)[32]

While the T cells have been at the forefront of the complex psoriasis patho-genesis, the keratinocyte plays an important and supportive role as well.

Role in T cell Trafficking

The keratinocytes under the influence of IFN-γ express ICAM-1 which interacts with the LFA-1 on the T cells, as mentioned above allowing entry of the T cells into the epidermis.

Further, keratinocytes release cytokines and result in the production of a chemokine gradient which is responsible for adhesion of leukocytes to endothelial cells and their trafficking into the epidermis.

Role in Neutrophil Accumulation

Keratinocytes release IL-8, a cytokine which is responsible for the attraction and accumulation of neutrophils in the epidermis, forming the characteristic "Munro's microabscess" associated with the psoriatic pathology.

Role in Angiogenesis[33-35]

There is considerable evidence to demonstrate the role of vascular endothelial growth factor (VEGF) driving the angiogenesis associated with psoriasis. The psoriatic epidermis has greater angiogenic activity compared with the skin of normal subjects, uninvolved, and treated psoriatic skin. Keratinocytes in the lesional skin are a major source of pro-angiogenic cytokines in psoriasis.

- VEGF
- Endothelial cell stimulating angiogenesis factor (ESAF)
- Thymidine phosphorylase (PDECGE/TP)
- TNF-α
- TGF-α
- Platelet-derived epidermal growth factor (PDGF)

Vascular endothelial growth factor has been demonstrated to be overexpressed in basal keratinocytes and result in chronic skin inflammation and tortuous capillaries. Moreover, serum-VEGF levels have been correlated with the disease severity.[36-38]

Further, VEGF increases the expression of vascular endothelial growth factor receptor (VEGFR) in keratinocytes and the keratinocytes, in turn regulates VEGF expression, giving support to the claim that VEGF has a role in keratinocyte proliferation.[39,40]

It is clear from the above discussion that the initiation of psoriatic pathogenesis is a complex cross talk between the T cells and the keratinocytes and the cytokines released by them leading to the phenotype of psoriasis.

At this stage it was thought that the Th1 cells and the cytokines released by them, particularly TNF-α seem to be driving the psoriatic pathogenesis, but it was in 2008 that there was a rising interest in the IL-23/Th17 axis in psoriasis and research shifted to the role of Th17 cells and their role in this complex disease.

Role of Th17 Cells and IL-23[41,42]

Following evidence points towards the involvement of Th17 cells and IL-23 in the pathogenesis of psoriasis:

- Elevated levels of IL-23 and Th17-related cytokines were observed in cutaneous lesions and serum of psoriatic patients
- Association of interleukin 23 receptor (IL23R) gene variants with psoriasis
- Evidence of a functional role of Th17 cells in autoimmunity and its significance with the comorbidities has been observed.

The development and maintenance of Th17 cells have been linked to IL-23.[41,42] IL-23, a heterodimer composed of p19 and p40 subunits, is produced by dendritic cells, macrophages, and keratinocytes. IL-23 when binds to the IL23R results in a Jak2-mediated phosphorylation of tyrosine residues located in the intracellular domain of the IL23R subunit. The phosphorylated tyrosine residues serve as a docking site for signal transducer and activator of transcription (STAT)-3 (molecules, which in turn get translocated to the nucleus of the Th17 cells resulting in transcription of pro-inflammatory cytokines (IL-17A, IL-17F, IL-22, IL-26). These cytokines, in turn, stimulate epidermal hyperplasia, acanthosis and hyperkeratosis. The activated keratinocytes further produce IL-23, which mediate a cross talk with Th17 lymphocytes. Moreover, Th17 cells induce keratinocytes to produce IL-8 and AMPs for recruitment of neutrophils, cathelicidin for activation of plasmacytoid dendritic cells (pDCs) and VEGF with resulting angiogenesis.[43]

In view of the aforementioned changes, one may speculate that the concept of psoriasis as a Th1 driven disease is inconsistent with evidence obtained since the discovery of Th17 cells which appear to play a key role in the maintenance of psoriasis (see Fig. 4.2).

Role of the Skin Barrier

Psoriasis is characterized by a compromised barrier function which leads to alteration of the innate and adaptive immunity. As discussed above, psoriasis is linked with genes specifically present on epidermal cells namely CDSN genes, β-defensin cluster genes and LCE3B and 3C genes.[44]

Abnormal Keratinization

Abnormal keratinization presents with an increased expression of early differentiation markers (such as CDSN and small proline-rich proteins, cystatin A and transglutaminase 1) and decreased expression of late differentiation markers (such as loricrin and filaggrin). This abnormal barrier leads to increased transepidermal water loss (TEWL), which is directly proportional to the clinical severity.[24]

Antimicrobial Proteins

The two major groups of AMPs, defensins and cathelicidins provide a chemical barrier to infection or injury. Psoriatic lesions are characterized by increased levels of human β-defensin-2.[45] High defensin levels possess potent pro-inflammatory activity. Similarly, cathelicidin LL-37 is also overexpressed in psoriatic skin.[46]

Abnormal Barrier Repair

The LCE gene cluster, composed of six groups (LCE1–6, with a total of 18 members) is a part of the epidermal differentiation complex and its deletion has been linked with psoriasis.[47] Increased expression of LCE3 gene and reduced expression of other LCE genes is seen in psoriatic plaques.[48] This may lead to incomplete barrier repair after minor trauma, which in turn causes penetration of various antigens and induces an inflammatory response.

Role of Adaptive and Innate Immunity

The psoriasis pathogenesis depicts a balance between the innate and acquired immune systems. The imbalance in the adaptive immune system is characterized by a skewed Th1 response.[49-51] Further, chemokines produced by keratinocytes in the epidermis act on both the innate and acquired immune systems, stimulating dendritic cells, neutrophils, and other innate mediators as well as T cells.[32] The role of the immune systems and their cells have been highlighted (Table 4.2).[52-64]

Table 4.2: Immune systems, cytokines, and their probable roles in the psoriatic pathogenesis.

Role of adaptive immunity Cell types	Cytokine production	Probable role
CD 4+ cells		
Th1 cells	INF-γ	Keratinocyte hyper-proliferation, concomitant inflammation and dermal proliferation of small vessels.[52,53]
Th17 cells	IL-17, IL-21, IL-22, IL-6	Responsible for increased AMP levels, keratinocyte hyperproliferation, neutrophil chemotaxis and angiogenesis
Th22 cells	IL-22	Mediates keratinocyte proliferation and epidermal hyperplasia
Regulatory T cells (Fox P3+ Treg)	IL-17	Role in keratinocyte hyperproliferation, skin inflammation and immune response amplification
CD 8 + Cells	IL-17, IL-22, INF-γ and TNF-α	CD8+ T cells with assistance from the CD4+ T cells play a role in induction and maintenance of the disease. The cytokines released result in keratinocyte hyperproliferation and skin inflammation, with TNF-α playing a role in dendritic cell maturation.[53]

Contd...

Contd...

γδ T cells	IL-17, IL-22, TNF-α	γδ T cells may act in an amplification loop for IL-17 synthesis and provide a possible mechanism mediating autoimmune inflammation. Further the cytokines play a role in keratinocyte hyperproliferation
Role of innate immunity		
Cell types	*Cytokines*	*Probable role*
mDCs	TNF-α, IL-23, and IL-20	Psoriatic skin contains a highly increased number of CD11c+ mDCs in the dermis.[58] They contribute to autoantigen presentation and activation of T cells in situ[59]
pDCs	Type 1 interferons.[46]	Play a role in initiating the psoriatic pathogenesis
LCs		They act as APCs which stimulate naïve T cells[24,55]
Keratinocytes	IL-6, IL-8, TGF-α, TGF-β, and IL-1	Act as APCs and play a crucial role in the entry of T cells into the epidermis, upregulation of adhesion molecules, keratinocyte hyperproliferation and skin inflammation
NK cells[62]	INF-γ, TNF-α, and IL-17	Co-express TCR and NK lineage markers and represent a component of innate immunity. Plays a role in immune-regulatory functions and an intermediary role between innate and acquired immune system, resulting in keratinocyte hyperproliferation and skin inflammation

Contd...

Contd...

Macrophages	TNF-α	They serve as APCs, regulate epidermal proliferation and differentiation and influence T cell proliferation.[63]
Neutrophils	IL-8	These are the effector cells of innate immunity, which produce IL-8, S100 proteins and proteases which act on keratinocytes to induce inflammatory genes or increase their proliferation[32]
Mast cells	Proteases, histamine, prostaglandins, leukotrienes, chemokines, MHC class II molecules	Believed to play an immune-regulatory role in psoriasis[64] as they are able to promote as well as suppress inflammation • Act as antigen-presenting cells • Recruit cells of immune system • Suppress inflammation and keratinocyte growth

(APC: Antigen-presenting cell; CD: Cluster of differentiation; TNF-α: Tumor necrosis factor-alpha; IFN-γ: Interferon-gamma; TGF-α: Transforming growth factor alpha; TGF-β: Transforming growth factor beta; MHC: Major histocompatibility complex; DCs: Dendritic cells; pDCs: Plasmacytoid DCs; mDCs: Dermal myeloid DCs; LCs: Langerhans cells; NK cells: Natural killer cells; TCR: T cell receptor).

▌REFERENCES

1. Griffiths CE, Barker JN. Pathogenesis and clinical features of psoriasis. Lancet. 2007;370(9583):263-71.
2. Monteleone G, Pallone F, Macdonald TT, et al. Psoriasis: from pathogenesis to novel therapeutic approaches. Clin Sci (Lond). 2011;120(1):1-11.
3. Sigurdardottir SL, Thorleifsdottir RH, Valdimarsson H, et al. The role of the palatine tonsils in the pathogenesis and treatment of psoriasis. Br J Dermatol. 2013;168(2):237-42.
4. Valdimarsson H, Thorleifsdottir RH, Sigurdardottir S, et al. Psoriasis—as an autoimmune disease caused by molecular mimicry. Trends Immunol. 2009;30(10):494-501.
5. Thorleifsdottir RH, Sigurdardottir SL, Sigurgeirsson B, et al. Improvement of psoriasis after tonsillectomy is associated with a decrease in the frequency of

circulating T cells that recognize streptococcal determinants and homologous skin determinants. J Immunol. 2012;188(10):5160-5.

6. Chen H, Hayashi G, Lai OY, et al. Psoriasis patients are enriched for genetic variants that protect against HIV-1 disease. PLOS Genetics. 2012;8(2):e1002514.

7. Burden A, Kirby B. Psoriasis and related disorders. In: Griffiths CEM, Barker J, Bleiker T, Chalmers R, Creamer D (Eds). Rook's Textbook of Dermatology, 9th edition. London: Blackwell Science Ltd, 2004:p.35.1-35.48.

8. Naldi L, Parazzini F, Brevi A, et al. Family history, smoking habits, alcohol consumption and risk of psoriasis. Br J Dermatol. 1992;127(3):212-17.

9. Tobin AM and Kirby B. Psoriasis: An opportunity to identify cardiovascular risk. Br J Dermatol. 2009;161(3):719.

10. Tobin AM, Veale DJ, Fitzgerald O, et al. Cardiovascular disease and risk factors in patients with psoriasis and psoriatic arthritis. J Rheumatol. 2010;37(7): 1386-94.

11. Higgins E. Alcohol, smoking and psoriasis. Clin Exp Dermatol. 2000;25(2):107-10.

12. Fortune DG, Richards HL, Griffiths CE. Psychologic factors in psoriasis: consequences, mechanisms and interventions. Dermatol Clin. 2005;23(4):681-94.

13. Meyer N, Paul C, Feneron D, et al. Psoriasis: an epidemiological evaluation of disease burden in 590 patients. J Eur Acad Dermatol Venereol. 2010;24(9): 1075-82.

14. Bostoen J, Bracke S, De Keyser S, et al. An educational programme for patients with psoriasis and atopic dermatitis: A prospective randomized controlled trial. Br J Dermatol. 2012;167(5):1025-31.

15. Roosterman D, Goerge T, Schneider SW, et al. Neuronal control of skin function: The skin as a neuroimmunoendocrine organ. Physiol Rev. 2006;86(4):1309-79.

16. Jiang WY, Raychaudhuri SP, Farber EM. Double-labeled immunofluorescence study of cutaneous nerves in psoriasis. Int J Dermatol. 1998;37(8):572-4.

17. Raychaudhuri SP, Raychaudhuri SK. Role of NGF and neurogenic inflammation in the pathogenesis of psoriasis. Prog Brain Res. 2004;146:433-7.

18. Joseph T, Kurian J, Warwick DJ, et al. Unilateral remission of psoriasis following traumatic nerve palsy. Br J Dermatol. 2005;152(1):176-98.

19. Ros AM, Eklund G. Photosensitive psoriasis. J Am Acad Dermatol. 1987;17(5 pt 1):752-8.

20. Weiss G, Shemer A, Trau H. The Koebner phenomenon: Review of the literature. J Eur Acad Dermatol Venereol. 2002;16(3):241-8.

21. Gudjonsson JE, Karason A, Antonsdottir AA, et al. HLA-Cw6-positive and HLA-Cw6-negative patients with psoriasis vulgaris have distinct clinical features. J Invest Dermatol. 2002; 118(2):362-5.

22. Capon F, Munro M, Barker J, et al. Searching for the major histocompatibility complex psoriasis susceptibility gene. J Invest Dermatol. 2002;118(5):745-51.

23. Capon F, Trembath RC, Barker JN. An update on the genetics of psoriasis. Dermatol Clin. 2004;22(4):339-47.

24. Mahajan R and Handa S. Pathophysiology of psoriasis. Indian J Venereol Leprol. 2013;79, Suppl S1:1-9.

25. Barker JN. Genetic aspects of psoriasis. Clin Exp Dermatol. 2001;26(4):321-5.

26. Nanda A, Kaur S, Kaur I, et al. Childhood psoriasis: An epidemiologic survey of 112 patients. Pediatr Dermatol. 1990;7(1):19-21.

27. al-Fouzan AS, Nanda A. A survey of childhood psoriasis in Kuwait. Pediatr Dermatol. 1994;11(2):116-9.

28. Swanbeck G, Inerot A, Martinsson T, et al. A population genetic study of psoriasis. Br J Dermatol. 1994;131(1):32-9.
29. Brandrup F, Hauge M, Henningsen J, et al. Psoriasis in an unselected series of twins. Arch Dermatol. 1978;114(6):874-8.
30. Burden AD, Javed S, Bailey M, et al. Genetics of psoriasis: Paternal inheritance and a locus on chromosome 6p. J Invest Dermatol. 1998;110(6):958-60.
31. Lebwohl M. Psoriasis. Lancet. 2003;361(9364):1197-204.
32. Lowes MA, Bowcock AM, Krueger JG. Pathogenesis and therapy of psoriasis. Nature. 2007;445(7130):866-73.
33. Heidenreich R, Röcken, M, Ghoreschi K. Angiogenesis drives psoriasis pathogenesis. Int J Exp Pathol. 2009;90(3):232-48.
34. Canavese M, Altruda F, Ruzicka, T et al. Vascular endothelial growth factor (VEGF) in the pathogenesis of psoriasis—A possible target for novel therapies? J of dermatol sci Jun; 58(3):171-6.
35. Marina ME, Roman II, Constantin AM, et al. VEGF involvement in psoriasis. Clujul Medical. 2015;88(3):247.
36. Creamer D, Allen MH, Groves RW, et al. Circulating vascular permeability factor/vascular endothelial growth factor in erythroderma. Lancet. 1996;348(9034):1101.
37. Bhushan M, McLaughlin B, Weiss JB, et al. Levels of endothelial cell stimulating angiogenesis factor and vascular endothelial growth factor are elevated in psoriasis. Br J Dermatol. 1999;141(6):1054-60.
38. Nielsen HJ, Christensen IJ, Svendsen MN, et al. Elevated plasma levels of vascular endothelial growth factor and plasminogen activator inhibitor-1 decrease during improvement of psoriasis. Inflamm Res. 2002;51(11):563-7.
39. Bachelez H. Immunopathogenesis of psoriasis: recent insights on the role of adaptive and innate immunity. J Autoimmun. 2005;25(Suppl):69-73.
40. Sabat R, Philipp S, Hoflich C, et al. Immunopathogenesis of psoriasis. Exp Dermatol. 2007; 16(10):779-98.
41. Blauvelt A. T-helper 17 cells in psoriatic plaques and additional genetic links between IL-23 and psoriasis. J Invest Dermatol. 2008;128(5):1064-7.
42. Bettelli E, Carrier Y, Gao W, et al. Reciprocal developmental pathways for the generation of pathogenic effector TH17 and regulatory T cells. Nature. 2006; 441(7090): 235-8.
43. Di Cesare A, Di Meglio P, Nestle FO. The IL-23/Th17 axis in the immunopathogenesis of psoriasis. J Invest Dermatol. 2009;129(6):1339-50.
44. Sano S. Psoriasis as a barrier disease. Dermatologica Sinica. 2015;33(2):64-9.
45. Jansen PA, Rodijk-Olthuis D, Hollox EJ, et al. Beta-defensin-2 protein is a serum biomarker for disease activity in psoriasis and reaches biologically relevant concentrations in lesional skin. PLoS One. 2009;4(3):e4725.
46. Lee E, Trepicchio WL, Oestreicher JL, et al. Increased expression of interleukin-23 p19 and p40 in lesional skin of patients with psoriasis vulgaris. J Exp Med. 2004; 199(1):125-30.
47. Bergboer JG, Tjabringa GS, Kamsteeg M, et al. Psoriasis risk genes of the late cornified envelope-3 group are distinctly expressed compared with genes of other LCE groups. Am J Pathol. 2011;178(4):1470-7.
48. Nair RP, Duffin KC, Helms C, et al. Genome-wide scan reveals association of psoriasis with IL-23 and NF-kappa B pathways. Nat Genet. 2009;41(2):199-204.
49. Uyemura K, Yamamura M, Fivenson DF, et al. The cytokine network in lesional and lesion-free psoriatic skin is characterized by a T-helper type 1 cell-mediated response. J Invest Dermatol. 1993;101(5):701-5.

50. Schlaak JF, Buslau M, Jochum W, et al. T cells involved in psoriasis vulgaris belong to the Th1 subset. J Invest Dermatol. 1994;102(2):145-9.
51. Vanaki E, Ataei M, Sanati MH, et al. Expression patterns of Th1/Th2 transcription factors in patients with guttate psoriasis. Acta Microbiol Immunol Hung. 2013; 60(2):163-74.
52. Ghoreschi K, Mrowietz U, Röcken M. A molecule solves psoriasis? Systemic therapies for psoriasis inducing interleukin 4 and Th2 responses. J Mol Med. 2003;81:471-80.
53. Jadali Z, Eslami MB. T cell immune responses in psoriasis. Iran J Allergy Asthma Immunol. 2014;13(4):220-30.
54. Ghoreschi K, Laurence A, Yang XP, et al. T helper 17 cell heterogeneity and pathogenicity in autoimmune disease. Trends Immunol. 2011;32(9):395-401.
55. Fujita H, Nograles KE, Kikuchi, et al. Human Langerhans cells induce distinct IL-22-producing CD4+ T cells lacking IL-17 production. T Proc Natl Acad Sci USA. 2009;106(51):21795-800.
56. Sugiyama H, Gyulai R, Toichi E, et al. Dysfunctional blood and target tissue CD4+CD25 high regulatory T cells in psoriasis: mechanism underlying unrestrained pathogenic effector T cell proliferation. J Immunol. 2005;174(1):164-73.
57. Cai Y, Shen X, Ding C, et al. Pivotal role of dermal IL-17-producing γδ T cells in skin inflammation. Immunity. 2011;35(4):596-610.
58. Lowes MA, Chamian F, Abello MV, et al. Increase in TNF-alpha and inducible nitric oxide synthase-expressing dendritic cells in psoriasis and reduction with efalizumab (anti-CD11a). Proc Natl Acad Sci USA. 2005;102(52):19057-62.
59. Nestle FO, Turka LA, Nickoloff BJ. Characterization of dermal dendritic cells in psoriasis. Autostimulation of T lymphocytes and induction of Th1 type cytokines. J Clin Invest. 1994;94(1):202-9.
60. Wollenberg A, Wagner M, Gunther S, et al. Plasmacytoid dendritic cells: A new cutaneous dendritic cell subset with distinct role in inflammatory skin diseases. J Invest. Dermatol. 2002;119(5):1096-102.
61. Peternel S, Kastelan M. Immunopathogenesis of psoriasis: Focus on natural killer Tcells. J Eur Acad Dermatol Venereol. 2009;23(10):1123-7.
62. Clark RA, Kupper TS. Misbehaving macrophages in the pathogenesis of psoriasis. J Clin Invest. 2006;116(8):2084-7.
63. Harvima IT, Nilsson G, Suttle MM, et al. Is there a role for mast cells in psoriasis? Arch Dermatol Res. 2008;300(9):461-78.
64. Cai Y, Fleming C, Yan J. "New insights of T cells in the pathogenesis of psoriasis." Cell Molr Immunol. 2012;9(4):302-9.

Santanu Banerjee

▌ INTRODUCTION

Etanercept is a fully human soluble recombinant tumor necrosis factor-α (TNF-α) receptor antagonist and is a dimeric fusion protein composed of the extracellular portion of two 75-kilodalton (kDa) TNF receptors joined to Fc portion of an IgG1. Etanercept was developed at Immunex and in late 1998 released it for commercial use, soon after the release of infliximab. It was first approved by Food and Drug Administration (FDA) in 1998 for rheumatoid arthritis, psoriatic arthritis in 2002, moderate-to-severe plaque psoriasis in 2004 and pediatric psoriasis in 2016.[1]

▌ PHARMACOLOGY

Etanercept is a dimeric fusion protein consists of soluble TNF-α receptor fused to Fc portion of human IgG. It binds and neutralizes both TNF-α and tumor necrosis factor-β (TNF-β), binding to both soluble and receptor bound TNF-α. Since, it is dimeric in nature the affinity of etanercept to TNF-α is 1000 times greater than the natural monomeric cellular receptor whereas the Fc region of IgG1 gives it a stability.

It has molecular weight of 150 kDa, half-life of 4.8 days and absolute bioavailability after subcutaneous etanercept is 58%.

Mechanism of Action

Tumor necrosis factor-α (TNF-α) is a naturally occurring cytokine which binds to two different receptors and initiates a cascade of cellular signals which results in production and release of inflammatory cytokines and recruitment of a host of inflammatory cells. Elevated TNF-α levels are found both in affected skin and serum of patients with psoriasis. The disease severity and remission is directly proportional to the serum levels of TNF-α.[2]

Two distinct TNF receptors (TNFRs) exist naturally as monomeric molecules on cell surfaces and in soluble forms, a 55-kDa protein (p55) and a 75-kDa protein (p75). Biological activity of TNF is dependent upon binding to either cell surface TNFR or the soluble form. Etanercept is a dimeric soluble form of the p75 TNFR that can bind competitively to TNF molecules with an affinity of 50–1000 times more than its natural receptors.

Etanercept inhibits binding of TNF-α and TNF-β to cell surface TNFRs, thus rendering TNF biologically inactive. TNF inhibition downregulates multiple inflammatory pathway. It results in apoptosis of dendritic cells in psoriatic plaques and reduced expression of nuclear factor-κB (NF-κB).[3]

USES

FDA approved indications
- Chronic plaque psoriasis
- Psoriatic arthritis.

Off label Indications
- Aphthous stomatitis
- Behcet's disease
- Pyoderma gangrenosum
- Bullous pemphigoid
- Pemphigus vulgaris
- Cicatricial pemphigoid
- Granuloma annulare
- Sarcoidosis
- Dermatomyositis
- Relapsing polychondritis
- Scleroderma
- Graft versus host disease
- Hidradenitis suppurativa
- Multicentric reticulohistiocytosis
- Synovitis-acne-pustulosis-hyperostosis-osteomyelitis (SAPHO) syndrome
- Pityriasis rubra pilaris.

PSORIASIS

Etanercept was first approved by FDA in 2004 for the treatment of chronic plaque psoriasis. It has been used in different dosing schedule in different studies, commonest being 50 mg subcutaneously twice a week for 12 weeks followed by 50 mg weekly. This has been explained in Table 5.1.

Combination Therapy

To augment the effect of biologics and reduce the cost associated with its usage, it can be used in combination therapy with conventional systemic therapy.

Etanercept and Methotrexate

To improve efficacy etanercept can be combined with methotrexate. On combining methotrexate (7.5–15 mg weekly) to etanercept 50 mg twice a

Table 5.1: Efficacy of etanercept in psoriasis.

Dose	PASI-50	PASI-75	Reference
50 mg twice a week	64.2%	49% (after 12 weeks)	Leonardi CL (2003)[1]
25 mg twice a week	52.6%	34%	
25 mg once a week	40.9%	14%	
25 mg twice weekly	–	26% (12 weeks)	Mease PJ (2000)[4]
50 mg twice a week	–	49% (12 weeks)	Papp KA (2005)[5]
		After 12 weeks, dose was reduced to 25 mg twice a week. At the end of 24 weeks, there was no reduction in efficacy of etanercept.	

(PASI-50: Psoriasis area and severity index-50; PASI-75: Psoriasis area and severity index-75).

week, 70.2% patients achieved psoriasis area and severity index (PASI)-75 after 12 weeks as compared to 54.3% patients on monotherapy with etanercept. PASI-50 and PASI-90 was achieved in 92.4% and 34% respectively in patient on combination therapy as compared to 83.8% and 23.1% in patients on monotherapy. Nonserious adverse events were slightly higher in combination group as compared to monotherapy.[6]

Etanercept and Acitretin

The combination therapy has a potential benefit of giving protection against skin cancer by acitretin and also helps in reducing the dose of etanercept to once weekly when combined with acitretin in the dose of 0.4 mg/kg.[7]

Etanercept and Narrow-band Ultraviolet B

Etanercept 50 mg once a week on combining with narrow-band ultraviolet B (NB-UVB) three times a week, results in PASI-75, 90, and 100 in 81.8%, 57.6%, and 24.6% patients respectively after 12 weeks.[8] Etanercept 25 mg twice a week has been combined with NB-UVB and was found to be very effective. Due to theoretical risk of increasing risk of malignancy with this combination, this combination should be limited to shortest period of time.[9]

Continuous vs Intermittent Therapy

Etanercept should be used continuously for sustained clinical benefit, however patient may need to discontinue therapy for some reason. In a study conducted by Gordon et al. psoriasis returns gradually after 3 months of stopping etanercept and re-treatment with etanercept is as effective as initial treatment. An open label trial by Moore et al. using etanercept continuously or intermittently concluded that continuous therapy is more effective.[10,11]

Adherence

Adherence is important for biologics treatment. A retrospective analysis conducted by Esposito et al. on survival rate of anti-TNF-α treatment revealed that global adherence was 72.9% after 28.9 months of therapy. Etanercept showed longest survival (mean 51.4 months), as compared to infliximab (36.8 months) and adalimumab (34.7 months). Main reason for discontinuation were inefficacy or adverse events.[12]

▌PSORIATIC ARTHRITIS

It was approved by FDA for management of psoriatic arthritis in 2002. Etanercept in dose of 25 mg twice a week, resulted in ACR20 (20 percent improvement) in 59% patients at the end of 12 weeks. Results were sustained till 48 weeks and it also inhibited radiographic progression.[13] Dose of 50 mg twice a week and once a week were compared in an randomised controlled trial (RCT) by Sterry et al. There is no significant difference in patient with psoriatic arthritis treated with once a week or twice a week dose. However, patient with psoriasis clears much better with twice weekly regime for 12 weeks. In patient with psoriatic arthritis without or minimal psoriasis, 50 mg once a week is an adequate treatment.[14]

Availability

- *Trade name:* Enbrel
- *Marketed by:* Amgen, Wyeth, Takeda
- *Biosimilars/intended copies:* Intacept (Intas pharmaceuticals), Etacept (Cipla).

Preparation

- Single use prefilled 25 mg and 50 mg syringe.
- Preservative free lyophilized powder containing 25 mg/vial, reconstituted with 1 mL of bacteriostatic water supplied along with the vial.

Storage

At 2–8 °C should not be frozen. It should be allowed to return to room temperature before injecting, to reduce the discomfort.

Administration

Site: Thigh, abdomen, and upper arm. Rotate injection site at least 1 inch from last injection site. Do not inject into a tender, bruised skin.

Pretreatment Evaluation

Clinical

- Rule out infections like tuberculosis (TB), cardiac failure, and demyelinating disease.

Investigations

- Complete hemogram
- Urine routine and microscopic examination
- *Liver function tests:* including hepatitis B virus (HBV) and hepatitis C virus (HCV) panel
- Renal function test
- Chest X-ray, Mantoux test, interferon gamma release assay (IGRA) test for TB
- Human immunodeficiency virus (HIV)
- Antinuclear antibody (ANA).

Monitoring during Etanercept Therapy

- Fortnightly for one month, monthly for 3 months and three monthly afterwards
- Hemogram and liver function test (LFT) with enzymes
- Chest X-ray and IGRA annually.

Adverse Effects

- *Injection site reaction*: It is usually mild-to-moderate with erythema, itching, pain, and swelling and does not necessitate discontinuation of treatment and subsides within 3–5 days.
- *Infections*: Minor infections like nasopharyngitis are most common. Risk of serious infections is less as compared to infliximab and adalimumab. Serious infections occur most commonly within 6 months of initiation of treatment. Risk of developing TB is lowest with etanercept as compared to adalimumab and infliximab. Median time for reactivation of tuberculosis with etanercept is 13 months.[15]
- *Malignancies*: Overall risk of malignancies is not increased. There may be an increased risk of non-melanoma skin cancer [basal cell carcinoma (BCC), squamous cell carcinoma (SCC)] in patient receiving anti-TNF α therapy. Risk of lymphoma is not increased.
- *Immunogenicity*: 5–6% of patients develops antidrug antibodies; however these are non-neutralizing antibodies. Seropositive status does not reduce the efficacy of drug and rates of adverse event are similar irrespective of seropositive status.[16] Antinuclear antibodies can develop

in patients on anti-TNFα therapy in almost 15% patients. Development of ANA is more common in patients on infliximab than etanercept; however development of lupus erythematosus is very rare.

- *Cardiovascular side effects*: It can exacerbate preexisting heart failure and is contraindicated in patients with severe heart failure [NYHA (New York Heart Association) III or IV]. Systematic review found no increase in major adverse cardiac event in patients on anti-TNFα therapy.[17]
- *Neurological side effects*: New onset or exacerbation of preexisting demyelinating diseases.
- *Hepatotoxicity*: Hepatotoxicity associated with etanercept is extremely rare and patients who developed hepatotoxicity to infliximab and adalimumab have been successfully treated with etanercept.

Contraindications

- Known hypersensitivity
- Patients with active serious infections warranting systemic antibiotic therapy
- Pregnancy
- *Cardiovascular disease*: Congestive heart failure (NYHA III or IV)
- *Neurological disorders*: Contraindicated in patients with demyelinating diseases such as multiple sclerosis or with first degree relative with such disease.
- *Malignancy*: Anti-TNF treatment should be avoided in patients with a current or previous history of malignancy, unless there is a high likelihood of cure or the malignancy was diagnosed and treated more than 10 years ago.
- Any concurrent administration of interleukin 1 receptor antagonist
- *Tuberculosis*: Patient with active TB should not be given etanercept. Those with latent tuberculosis should be treated with single drug or two drug anti-tubercular treatment before initiating etanercept. Etanercept can be started two months after starting treatment.

▌SPECIAL SITUATIONS

Pregnancy and Lactation

It is a category B drug. Etanercept concentration in umbilical cord serum was low when mother was exposed during pregnancy, suggesting low transplacental transmission. Breast milk concentration is very low and it is undetectable in child's serum.[18] Registry data published by Hyrich et al. included 32 patients who were exposed to anti-TNF-α therapy during pregnancy. 91% patients elected to continue pregnancy and out of these 76% delivered healthy child and 24% had first-trimester abortions. There is no evidence of maternal harm or major congenital malformations. Although they are likely to be safe in pregnancy but it is to be used with caution.[19]

Pediatric Population

In November 2016, FDA approved etanercept for management of psoriasis in pediatric population (4–17 years), making it first biologic to be approved for management of pediatric psoriasis. It is FDA approved for management of juvenile idiopathic arthritis (JIA) in children older than 2 years. Dose to be used is 0.8 mg/kg/week, maximum being 50 mg/week. Etanercept is safe, effective and has sustained benefit up to 5 years in management of psoriasis.[20,21]

Hepatitis B and C Infection

Etanercept can cause reactivation of hepatitis B and infection. All patients should be screened for hepatitis B before administering etanercept and in chronic hepatitis B carrier, it should be given along with antiviral therapy. Transaminases should be monitored during entire therapy.

Anti-TNF-α therapy is safe in patients with chronic HCV infection; however close monitoring of transaminases and viral load is indicated in these patients.[22,23]

HIV Infection

There is limited experience for use of etanercept in HIV positive patients. Existing literature suggests that etanercept can be safely used in HIV seropositive patients, even without concomitant antiretroviral therapy. However, CD4 count and viral load should be closely monitored in this scenario and antiretroviral therapy should be used concomitantly.[24,25]

▌CONCLUSION

Etanercept is one of the most widely used biologic and has excellent safety records. It can be used in special population. It can be used intermittently or continuously without loss of efficacy and can be combined with conventional therapy.

▌REFERENCES

1. Leonardi CL, Powers JL, Matheson RT, et al. Etanercept as monotherapy in patients with psoriasis. N Engl J Med. 2003;349(21):2014-22.
2. Krueger JG. The immunologic basis for the treatment of psoriasis with new biologic agents. J Am Acad Dermatol. 2002;46(1):1-23.
3. Keystone EC. Safety of biologic therapies–an update. J Rheumatol. 2005;74:8-12.

4. Mease PJ, Goffe BS, Metz J, et al. Etanercept in the treatment of psoriatic arthritis and psoriasis: a randomised trial. The Lancet. 2000;356(9227):385-90.

5. Papp KA, Tyring S, Lahfa M, et al. A global phase III randomized controlled trial of etanercept in psoriasis: safety, efficacy, and effect of dose reduction. Br J Dermatol. 2005;152(6):1304-12.

6. Gottlieb AB, Langley RG, Strober BE, et al. A randomized, double-blind, placebo-controlled study to evaluate the addition of methotrexate to etanercept in patients with moderate to severe plaque psoriasis. Br J Dermatol. 2012;167(3):649-57.

7. Smith EC, Riddle C, Menter MA, et al. Combining systemic retinoids with biologic agents for moderate to severe psoriasis. Int J Dermatol. 2008;47(5):514-8.

8. De Simone C, D'Agostino M, Capizzi R, et al. Combined treatment with etanercept 50 mg once weekly and narrow-band ultraviolet B phototherapy in chronic plaque psoriasis. Eur J Dermatol. 2011;21(4):568-72.

9. Gambichler T, Tigges C, Scola N, et al. Etanercept plus narrowband ultraviolet B phototherapy of psoriasis is more effective than etanercept monotherapy at 6 weeks. Br J Dermatol. 2011;164(6):1383-6.

10. Moore A, Gordon KB, Kang S, et al. A randomized, open-label trial of continuous versus interrupted etanercept therapy in the treatment of psoriasis. J Am Acad Dermatol. 2007;56(4):598-603.

11. Gordon KB, Gottlieb AB, Leonardi CL, et al. Clinical response in psoriasis patients discontinued from and then reinitiated on etanercept therapy. J Dermatolog Treat. 2006;17(1):9-17.

12. Esposito M, Gisondi P, Cassano N, et al. Survival rate of antitumour necrosis factor-α treatments for psoriasis in routine dermatological practice: a multicentre observational study. Br J Dermatol. 2013;169(3):666-72.

13. Mease PJ, Goffe BS, Metz J, et al. Etanercept in the treatment of psoriatic arthritis and psoriasis: a randomised trial. The Lancet. 2000;356(9227):385-90.

14. Sterry W, Ortonne JP, Kirkham B, et al. Comparison of two etanercept regimens for treatment of psoriasis and psoriatic arthritis: PRESTA randomised double blind multicentre trial. BMJ. 2010;340:c147.

15. Girolomoni G, Altomare G, Ayala F, et al. Safety of anti-TNF α agents in the treatment of psoriasis and psoriatic arthritis. Immunopharmacol and immunotoxicol. 2012;34(4):548-60.

16. Dore RK, Mathews S, Schechtman J, et al. The immunogenicity, safety, and efficacy of etanercept liquid administered once weekly in patients with rheumatoid arthritis. Clin Exp Rheumatol. 2007;25(1):40-6.

17. Ryan C, Leonardi CL, Krueger JG, et al. Association between biologic therapies for chronic plaque psoriasis and cardiovascular events: a meta-analysis of randomized controlled trials. JAMA. 2011;306(8):864-71.

18. Berthelsen BG, Fjeldsøe-Nielsen H, Nielsen CT, et al. Etanercept concentrations in maternal serum, umbilical cord serum, breast milk and child serum during breastfeeding. Rheumatology. 2010;49(11):2225-7.

19. Hyrich KL, Symmons DP, Watson KD, et al. Pregnancy outcome in women who were exposed to anti–tumor necrosis factor agents: results from a national population register. Arthritis Rheum. 2006;54(8):2701-2.

20. Bellodi Schmidt F, Shah KN. Biologic response modifiers and pediatric psoriasis. Pediatr Dermatol. 2015;32(3):303-20.

21. Paller AS, Siegfried EC, Pariser DM, et al. Long-term safety and efficacy of etanercept in children and adolescents with plaque psoriasis. J Am Acad Dermatol. 2016;74(2):280-7.

22. Calabrese LH, Zein N, Vassilopoulos D. Safety of antitumour necrosis factor (anti-TNF) therapy in patients with chronic viral infections: hepatitis C, hepatitis B, and HIV infection. Ann Rheum Dis. 2004;63(Suppl 2):ii18-24.

23. Roux CH, Brocq O, Breuil V, et al. Safety of anti-TNF-α therapy in rheumatoid arthritis and spondylarthropathies with concurrent B or C chronic hepatitis. Rheumatology. 2006;45(10):1294-7.

24. Gallitano SM, McDermott L, Brar K, et al. Use of tumor necrosis factor (TNF) inhibitors in patients with HIV/AIDS. J Am Acad Dermatol. 2016;74(5):974-80.

25. Liang SJ, Zheng QY, Yang YL, et al. Use of etanercept to treat rheumatoid arthritis in an HIV-positive patient: a case-based review. Rheumatol Int. 2017;37(7): 1207-12.

Chapter

6

Infliximab

Sehdev Singh, Shekhar Neema

INTRODUCTION

Infliximab is chimeric (25% mouse and 75% human) monoclonal antibody against tumor necrosis factor-alpha (TNF-α). It was approved for treatment of Crohn's disease in 1998 and was subsequently approved for ulcerative colitis, rheumatoid arthritis, psoriatic arthritis (PsA) and chronic plaque psoriasis.

PHARMACOLOGY

Infliximab is an immunoglobulin G (IgG)-1 monoclonal antibody which neutralizes both soluble and receptor bound TNF-α, it does not neutralize TNF-β. It being a protein, it is not metabolized by cytochrome P450 enzymes. Because of this advantage, the development of different toxic or inactive metabolites following genetic polymorphisms of P450 isoenzymes and the consequent variability in metabolism are reduced. In comparison to the small molecules, the likelihood of complex drug interactions are less.

CHARACTERISTICS

Molecular weight: 150 kDa
Half-life: 7 days in 5 mg/kg group, 9 days in 10 mg/kg group
Distribution in vascular compartment and metabolized by proteolysis.

USES

Food and Drug Administration-approved Indications

- Chronic plaque psoriasis
- Psoriatic arthritis

Off-label Indications

- Hidradenitis suppurativa
- Synovitis, acne, pustulosis, hyperostosis and osteitis (SAPHO) syndrome
- *Neutrophilic dermatoses:* Pyoderma gangrenosum, Behcet's disease
- Systemic vasculitis

Table 6.1: Efficacy of infliximab in chronic plaque psoriasis.

Dose	PASI-75	PASI-90	Reference
5 mg/Kg	80% (after 10 weeks)	57% (after 10 weeks)	EXPRESS (2005)[1]
	• PASI-75 and -90 was sustained till week 50. • In this study, patient also showed significant improvement in nail psoriasis. Improvement in nail psoriasis and severity index in 42% patients.		
3 mg/Kg	72% (after 10 weeks)		Gottlieb AB (2004)[2]
	• Improvement was observed as early as 2 weeks		

- *Granulomatous dermatoses:* Sarcoidosis, granuloma annulare
- *Connective tissue diseases:* Dermatomyositis, scleroderma, systemic lupus erythematosus (SLE)
- Graft-versus-host disease (GVHD), toxic epidermal necrolysis (TEN), Reiter's disease, pityriasis rubra pilaris (PRP).

Psoriasis

Infliximab was approved for management of chronic plaque psoriasis by Food and Drug Administration (FDA) in September 2006. It is administered in dose of 3–5 mg/Kg on 0, 2, 6 weeks and thereafter every 8 weeks. Improvement is assessed by psoriasis area and severity index (PASI) and 75% improvement in PASI from baseline (PASI 75) is a standard measure of efficacy of the drug used for treatment of psoriasis (Table 6.1).

- *Continuous therapy or intermittent therapy:* Intermittent therapy or as and when infusion is more practical in our scenario where economic constraints prevail over best possible options. Menter et al. published data in 2004 on continuous and intermittent therapy of infliximab in 3 mg/Kg and 5 mg/Kg group. PASI-75 response was better maintained in continuous therapy group (5 mg/Kg—89.6%, 3 mg/Kg—80.6%) as compared to intermittent group (5 mg/Kg—76.4%, 3 mg/Kg—72.4%). Development of anti-drug antibody (ADA) is associated with infusion reaction and loss of response. ADAs were detected in 35.8% and 41.5% patients in 5 mg/Kg in continuous and intermittent group and 51.5% and 46.2% in 3 mg/Kg in continuous and intermittent group.[3] Another study was conducted by Reich et al. (RESTORE2) in which patients were randomized to receive 5 mg/Kg infliximab as continuous or intermittent therapy. Study was terminated because of high incidence of infusion reaction in intermittent group.[4]
- *Adherence:* Adherence is very important for treatment success. Apart from economic considerations, there are various other factors like

safety and efficacy which result in treatment discontinuation in real world. Etanercept showed longest survival (1,565 days), followed by infliximab (1,120 days) and adalimumab (1,056 days) in a retrospective study. Most common cause for drug discontinuation was lack of efficacy. Discontinuation due to adverse effect was highest with infliximab followed by adalimumab and etanercept.[5]

Psoriatic Arthritis

Psoriatic arthritis develops in almost 30% patients with psoriasis. Infliximab was approved by FDA for treatment of PsA in 2005. PsA treatment is assessed by American College of Rheumatology (ACR) criteria. ACR 20, ACR 50 and ACR 70 signifies more than 20%, 50% and 70% improvement, respectively. Treatment with infliximab at 5 mg/kg resulted in ACR 20, ACR 50 and ACR 70 in 65%, 46% and 29% at the end of 16 weeks. This improvement was sustained till week 50 [infliximab multinational psoriatic arthritis controlled trial (IMPACT) study].[6] Another study which was conducted with larger sample size (IMPACT II) had similar effect in improvement of PsA. It also showed improvement in enthesopathy, quality of life and delayed radiographic progression of PsA.[7]

Off-label Indications

- *Hidradenitis suppurativa*:
  - Infliximab has been used successfully for management of hidradenitis suppurativa not responding to topical and systemic antibiotics.
  - Dose: 5 mg/kg on 0, 2, 6 weeks results in almost 50% improvement after 8 weeks of initial infusion in 26% patients. There is moderate to marked improvement in induration, sinus discharge and pain in 3–7 days after every infusion.[8]
  - Adalimumab is FDA approved for the treatment of hidradenitis suppurativa. Dose used is 160 mg subcutaneous on day 0, 80 mg on day 15 followed by 40 mg weekly starting on day 29.[9]
- *Neutrophilic dermatoses*: It can be used for management of pyoderma gangrenosum not responding to prednisolone and other immunosuppressive agents. It has also been used for management of sight threatening uveitis in Behcet's disease.[10,11]
- *Systemic vasculitis*: It can be used as salvage therapy in management of refractory systemic vasculitides like Wegener's granulomatosis and microscopic polyangiitis.[12]
- *Granulomatous dermatoses*: Refractory sarcoidosis has been treated with infliximab. However, tuberculosis needs to be ruled out objectively before administering infliximab as it increases the risk of reactivation of latent tuberculosis. Infliximab has also been used for management of

recalcitrant granuloma annulare, which does not respond to first-line therapy.[13,14]

- *Connective tissue diseases*
  - Dermatomyositis: It can be used for management of dermatomyositis refractory to treatment like corticosteroids, methotrexate, cyclosporine, intravenous immunoglobulin, azathioprine and cyclophosphamide.[15,16]
- *Miscellaneous*
  - *Graft-versus-host disease*: Infliximab has been used for management of acute GVHD not responding to steroids. However, phase III study showed no benefit from addition of infliximab to steroids in management of early acute GVHD.[17]
  - *Toxic epidermal necrolysis:* Single dose infliximab 5 mg/kg early in disease has resulted in rapid improvement in TEN in many case reports. However, the risk of infection remains high with use of this modality for treatment of TEN.[18]
  - *Reiter's syndrome*: Infliximab can be used for management of cutaneous and joint manifestation of Reiter's syndrome, not responding to steroids and methotrexate.[19]
  - *Pityriasis rubra pilaris*: It can be used successfully for management of type 1 adult PRP not responding to acitretin, methotrexate and cyclosporine or as first-line therapy for management of PRP.[20]

▌ADMINISTRATION

- Available as 100 mg lyophilized powder in 20 mL vial.
- Lyophilized powder is stored in refrigerator and reconstituted with 10 mL sterile water.
- Administered as intravenous infusion at the dose of 3–5 mg/kg at 0, 2, 6 weeks and 8 weekly thereafter.
- Total dose required after reconstitution is mixed in 250 mL normal saline and infused over not less than 2 hours and ideally over 4 hours.
- Infusion should be started within 3 hours of reconstitution.
- Premedication with hydrocortisone, pheniramine and paracetamol should be done to reduce the risk and severity of infusion reactions.

Tests to be Done Prior to Administration

- Complete blood count (CBC)
- Liver function test (LFT)
- Blood urea, serum creatinine
- Hepatitis B surface antigen, anti-hepatitis C virus immunoglobulin M

- *Rule out active and latent tuberculosis:*
  - History of past tuberculosis, history of contact with active case of tuberculosis
  - History of fever, weight loss, night sweats
  - Chest X-ray PA view
  - Purified protein derivative (PPD) or interferon-gamma release assays (IGRA)
- Antinuclear antibody (ANA).

MONITORING DURING INFLIXIMAB THERAPY

Patients who are on infliximab should be closely monitored for infusion-related reactions and development of any infection, especially tuberculosis. Patients have high-risk of development of extrapulmonary or disseminated tuberculosis and should be asked for history of weight loss, fever and night sweats during each visit.

- CBC, LFT--before every infusion
- Chest X-ray PA view, IGRA—annually.

ADVERSE EFFECTS

- *Infusion reaction:*
  - Defined as reaction occurring during infusion or within 1 hour after infusion. It is the commonest adverse reaction seen in approximately 20% patients.
  - Fever and chills are commonest symptoms of infusion reaction, other rare symptoms being cardiopulmonary symptoms (chest pain, hypotension, dyspnea), pruritus and urticaria.
  - Serious infusion reactions are seen in less than 1% of patients and includes anaphylaxis, convulsions and hypotension.
  - Patient who develop antidrug antibodies have higher risk of infusion reaction. Concomitant immunosuppressive medication reduces the severity of infusion reaction.
  - Patient who are on long-term maintenance therapy have less risk of development of infusion reaction as compared to patients who are on intermittent therapy.
- *Antidrug antibodies:*
  - Anti-infliximab antibodies develop in almost 40% patients within 1 year of therapy.
  - Development of antidrug antibodies are associated with loss of efficacy. Concomitant use of immunosuppressive therapy such as methotrexate, cyclosporine, azathioprine, etc. can reduce the formation of antidrug antibodies and addition of an immunomodulator can restore clinical response with anti-TNF-α blockers.[21,22]

- *Infections*
  - *Tuberculosis*: Increased risk of reactivation of latent tuberculosis by almost 20 times and also of extrapulmonary and disseminated tuberculosis.[23]
  - *Invasive fungal infections*: Increased risk of development of disseminated candidiasis, histoplasmosis and invasive aspergillosis.[24]
  - *Hepatitis B infection*: Patient with chronic carrier state due to hepatitis B, when administered infliximab can lead to reactivation of hepatitis B and liver failure.[25]
- *Malignancy*: There has been concern that anti-TNF α drugs can lead to increase in risk of development of malignancies. However, meta-analyses and literature evaluation does not either refute or verify the risk of development of malignancies resulting from use of anti-TNF-α blockers.[26]
- *Congestive heart failure*: It can cause worsening of heart failure. Contraindicated in patients with New York Heart Association (NYHA) class III or IV failure.[27]
- *Demyelinating diseases*: There are various reports of diseases like multiple sclerosis (MS), optic neuritis and Guillain–Barré syndrome developing in patients who were administered infliximab. Use of TNF-α blockers can lead to worsening of MS. It can also lead to unmasking of MS in patient with family history of demyelinating disorders.[28]
- *Hepatotoxicity*: Anti-TNF-α drugs are an uncommon cause of drug-induced liver injury (DILI). It can result in both hepatocellular as well as cholestatic type of DILI; however hepatocellular injury is more common. Infliximab is more common cause of DILI out of etanercept, adalimumab and infliximab. Majority of cases of DILI are autoimmune type with positive ANA and anti-smooth muscle antibody.[29]
- *Autoimmunity*: ANA and anti-double stranded DNA positivity can be seen in almost 60% and 10% patients on infliximab, respectively. However, development of clinical SLE is very rare.
- *Serum sickness type reaction*: Since infliximab is a chimeric protein, it can result in serum sickness type of reaction, especially when it is used intermittently. Patient presents with fever, severe joint pains and myalgia 3–10 days after infliximab infusion and these symptoms cannot be explained by an alternative diagnosis.[30]
- *Induction of psoriasis by infliximab*: Use of anti-TNF-α drugs can lead to paradoxical induction of psoriasis in patients with inflammatory bowel disease.[31]

CONTRAINDICATIONS

- *Absolute*: Hypersensitivity to murine proteins, active infections
- *Relative*: Congestive heart failure, family history of demyelinating disease.

SPECIAL SITUATIONS

- *Pregnancy and lactation:* It is pregnancy category B drug and has been safely used even intentionally during pregnancy without fetal harm. However, infliximab passes through placenta and live vaccines should be avoided in neonates whose mother have been given infliximab during pregnancy.[32]
- *Children:* Approved for use in children more than 6 years old in Crohn's disease and ulcerative colitis. Can also be used in psoriasis in children if clinically indicated.
- *Latent tuberculosis:* Infliximab should not be used in patient with latent tuberculosis (PPD or IGRA positive), because of high-risk of reactivation of tuberculosis. Patient should be treated with isoniazid monotherapy for 6–9 months or isoniazid-rifampicin for 3–4 months. Infliximab therapy can be initiated once treatment for latent tuberculosis infection has been completed for at least 2 months.
- *Hepatitis B and Hepatitis C infection:* Infliximab can lead to flare of hepatitis in patients with chronic hepatitis B carrier state. It should be used cautiously in patient with chronic carrier state, in consultation with hepatologist. Regular monitoring of aminotransferases and prophylactic antiviral therapy should be used if indicated.

  Patients with chronic hepatitis C generally do not develop acute flare due to use of infliximab, however caution during use of infliximab in patient with chronic hepatitis C carrier is important.[33]
- *Human immunodeficiency infection:* Infliximab should not be used in patients who are HIV positive. However, in patient in whom it is clinically indicated it can be used along with antiretroviral therapy.[34]
- *Immunization:* Live vaccines should be avoided while patient is on infliximab therapy. Patient should be immunized against hepatitis B, pneumococcus and influenza prior to initiation of therapy.

CONCLUSION

Infliximab is a cost-effective option for management of psoriasis or PsA, especially when rapid control of the disease is required. Use of infliximab requires screening for infections particularly latent tuberculosis infection and monitoring during infusion. While contemplating infliximab use, patient should be primed for continuous therapy rather than as when required.

REFERENCES

1. Reich K, Nestle FO, Papp K, et al. Infliximab induction and maintenance therapy for moderate-to-severe psoriasis: a phase III, multicentre, double-blind trial. Lancet. 2005;366(9494):1367-74.

2. Gottlieb AB, Evans R, Li S, et al. Infliximab induction therapy for patients with severe plaque-type psoriasis: a randomized, double-blind, placebo-controlled trial. J Am Acad Dermatol. 2004;51(4):534-42.

3. Menter A, Feldman SR, Weinstein GD, et al. A randomized comparison of continuous vs. intermittent infliximab maintenance regimens over 1 year in the treatment of moderate-to-severe plaque psoriasis. J Am Acad Dermatol. 2007;56(1):31-e1.

4. Reich K, Wozel G, Zheng H, et al. Efficacy and safety of infliximab as continuous or intermittent therapy in patients with moderate-to-severe plaque psoriasis: results of a randomized, long-term extension trial (RESTORE2). Br J Dermatol. 2013;168(6):1325-34.

5. Esposito M, Gisondi P, Cassano N, et al. Survival rate of antitumour necrosis factor-α treatments for psoriasis in routine dermatological practice: a multicentre observational study. Br J Dermatol. 2013;169(3):666-72.

6. Antoni CE, Kavanaugh A, Kirkham B, et al. Sustained benefits of infliximab therapy for dermatologic and articular manifestations of psoriatic arthritis: results from the infliximab multinational psoriatic arthritis controlled trial (IMPACT). Arthritis Rheum. 2005;52(4):1227-36.

7. Antoni C, Krueger GG, de Vlam K, et al. Infliximab improves signs and symptoms of psoriatic arthritis: results of the IMPACT 2 trial. Ann Rheum Dis. 2005;64(8):1150-7.

8. Grant A, Gonzalez T, Montgomery MO, et al. Infliximab therapy for patients with moderate to severe hidradenitis suppurativa: a randomized, double-blind, placebo-controlled crossover trial. J Am Acad Dermatol. 2010;62(2):205-17.

9. van Rappard DC, Leenarts MF, Meijerink-van 't Oost L, et al. Comparing treatment outcome of infliximab and adalimumab in patients with severe hidradenitis suppurativa. J Dermatolog Treat. 2012;23(4):284-9.

10. Hubbard VG, Friedmann AC, Goldsmith P. Systemic pyoderma gangrenosum responding to infliximab and adalimumab. Br J Dermatol. 2005;152(5):1059-61.

11. Sfikakis PP, Theodossiadis PG, Katsiari CG, et al. Effect of infliximab on sight-threatening panuveitis in Behcet's disease. Lancet. 2001;358(9278):295-6.

12. Josselin L, Mahr A, Cohen P, et al. Infliximab efficacy and safety against refractory systemic necrotising vasculitides: long-term follow-up of 15 patients. Ann Rheum Dis. 2008;67(9):1343-6.

13. Doty JD, Mazur JE, Judson MA. Treatment of sarcoidosis with infliximab. Chest. 2005;127(3):1064-71.

14. Amy de la Breteque M, Saussine A, Rybojad M, et al. Infliximab in recalcitrant granuloma annulare. Int J Dermatol. 2016;55(2):220-2.

15. Riley P, McCann LJ, Maillard SM, et al. Effectiveness of infliximab in the treatment of refractory juvenile dermatomyositis with calcinosis. Rheumatology. 2008;47(6):877-80.

16. Dold S, Justiniano ME, Marquez J, et al. Treatment of early and refractory dermatomyositis with infliximab: a report of two cases. Clin Rheumatol. 2007;26(7):1186-8.

17. Couriel DR, Saliba R, de Lima M, et al. A phase III study of infliximab and corticosteroids for the initial treatment of acute graft-versus-host disease. Biol Blood Marrow Transplant. 2009;15(12):1555-62.

18. Hunger RE, Hunziker T, Buettiker U, et al. Rapid resolution of toxic epidermal necrolysis with anti-TNF-Alpha treatment. J Allergy Clin Immunol. 2005;116(4): 923-4.

19. Gill H, Majithia V. Successful use of infliximab in the treatment of Reiter's syndrome: a case report and discussion. Clin Rheumatol. 2008;27(1):121-3.
20. Petrof G, Almaani N, Archer CB, et al. A systematic review of the literature on the treatment of pityriasis rubra pilaris type 1 with TNF-antagonists. J Eur Acad Dermatol Venereol. 2013;27(1):e131-5.
21. Wolbink GJ, Vis M, Lems W, et al. Development of antiinfliximab antibodies and relationship to clinical response in patients with rheumatoid arthritis. Arthritis Rheumatol. 2006;54(3):711-5.
22. Ben–Horin S, Waterman M, Kopylov U, et al. Addition of an immunomodulator to infliximab therapy eliminates antidrug antibodies in serum and restores clinical response of patients with inflammatory bowel disease. Clin Gastroenterol Hepatol. 2013;11(4):444-7.
23. Carmona L, Gómez-Reino JJ, Rodríguez-Valverde V, et al. Effectiveness of recommendations to prevent reactivation of latent tuberculosis infection in patients treated with tumor necrosis factor antagonists. Arthritis Rheum. 2005; 52(6):1766-72.
24. Filler SG, Yeaman MR, Sheppard DC. Tumor necrosis factor inhibition and invasive fungal infections. Clin Infect Dis. 2005;41(Supplement 3):S208-12.
25. Esteve M, Saro C, Gonzalez-Huix F, et al. Chronic hepatitis B reactivation following infliximab therapy in Crohn's disease patients: need for primary prophylaxis. Gut. 2004;53(9):1363-5.
26. Askling J, Fahrbach K, Nordstrom B, et al. Cancer risk with tumor necrosis factor alpha (TNF) inhibitors: meta-analysis of randomized controlled trials of adalimumab, etanercept, and infliximab using patient level data. Pharmacoepidemiol Drug Saf. 2011;20(2):119-30.
27. Heslinga SC, Sijl AM, De Boer K, et al. Tumor necrosis factor blocking therapy and congestive heart failure in patients with inflammatory rheumatic disorders: a systematic review. Curr Med Chem. 2015;22(16):1892-902.
28. Bradshaw MJ, Mobley BC, Zwerner JP, et al. Autopsy-proven demyelination associated with infliximab treatment. Neurol Neuroimmunol Neuroinflamm. 2016;3(2):e205.
29. French JB, Bonacini M, Ghabril M, et al. Hepatotoxicity associated with the use of anti-TNF-α agents. Drug Saf. 2016;39(3):199-208.
30. Lichtenstein L, Ron Y, Kivity S, et al. Infliximab-related infusion reactions: systematic review. J Crohns Colitis. 2015;9(9):806-15.
31. Barthel C, Biedermann L, Frei P, et al. Induction or exacerbation of psoriasis in patients with Crohn's disease under treatment with anti-TNF antibodies. Digestion. 2014;89(3):209-15.
32. Mahadevan U, Kane S, Sandborn WJ, et al. Intentional infliximab use during pregnancy for induction or maintenance of remission in Crohn's disease. Aliment Pharmacol Ther. 2005;21(6):733-8.
33. Nathan DM, Angus PW, Gibson PR. Hepatitis B and C virus infections and anti-tumor necrosis factor-α therapy: Guidelines for clinical approach. J Gastroenterol Hepatol. 2006;21(9):1366-71.
34. Gaylis N. Infliximab in the treatment of an HIV positive patient with Reiter's syndrome. J Rheumatol. 2003;30(2):407-11.

INTRODUCTION

Adalimumab is a recombinant, fully human monoclonal IgG1 antibody against tumor necrosis factor-alpha (TNF-α). It is produced by recombinant technology from Chinese hamster ovary (CHO) cells specific for human TNF. It functions by specifically binding to TNF-α and obstructs its interaction with the p55 and p75 cell surface TNF receptors.

MECHANISM OF ACTION

Intracellular signaling mediated by TNF occurs through interactions with cell bound TNF receptors. These receptors are present on almost all the cells. The two distinct but structurally similar TNF receptors are designated p55 and p75. These receptors form dimer on the cell surface, where they bind a trimeric TNF molecule, thus initiating signal transduction. Adalimumab binds specifically to TNF-α and blocks its interaction with the p55 and p75 cell surface TNF receptors.

PHARMACOLOGY

- After subcutaneous administration, serum concentration reaches its peak after 5 days
- Average bioavailability–64%
- Mean terminal phase half-life is approximately two week with a single dose of adalimumab.

Therapeutic Indications

FDA approved:
- Rheumatoid arthritis
- Juvenile idiopathic arthritis
- Crohn's disease and ulcerative colitis
- Ankylosing spondylitis
- Psoriatic arthritis
- Chronic plaque psoriasis
- Hidradenitis suppurativa
- Uveitis

Off-label indications:
- Nail psoriasis
- *Neutrophilic dermatoses:* Behçet's disease, pyoderma gangrenosum
- PAPA syndrome (pyogenic arthritis, pyoderma gangrenosum and acne) and PASH syndrome (pyoderma gangrenosum, acne and hidradenitis suppurativa)
- Cutaneous vasculitis
- Granulomatous dermatoses

CHRONIC PLAQUE PSORIASIS

Adalimumab was FDA approved for the management of chronic plaque psoriasis in 2008. Efficacy of adalimumab for management of chronic plaque psoriasis is explained in Table 7.1.

Table 7.1: Efficacy of adalimumab for management of chronic plaque psoriasis.

Dose	Schedule	Outcome	Reference
80 mg–Day 0 40 mg week 1 and every other week	52-week randomized, placebo controlled trial 16 weeks: Blinded, 17 weeks onwards – open label extension	Week 16–71% patients achieved PASI-75, 45% PASI-90 and 20% PASI-100 Week 33–52– Patients who achieved PASI-75 at week 33, lost PASI response by week 52 on stopping adalimumab	Menter A et al.[1]
80 mg–Day 0, 40 mg EOW	Randomized controlled comparative study of adalimumab with methotrexate	Week 16–79.6% patients with adalimumab and 35.5% patients in methotrexate group achieved PASI-75 PASI-100-16.7% and 7.3% in adalimumab and Mtx group respectively	Saurat JH et al.[2]
	Dose of methotrexate used was not fixed. It was given in 7.5 mg/week on week 0, 10 mg on week 2 and 15 mg at week 4. Patients who did not achieve PASI-50 by week 8 and week 12, dose was increased to 20 mg and 25 mg per week respectively		
40 mg every week or every other week	Randomized double-blind placebo controlled study Follow up–60 weeks	12 weeks–PASI 75 in 53% patients taking adalimumab EOW 80% in weekly adalimumab group Response sustained till 60-weeks	Gordon KB et al.[3]

(PASI: Psoriasis area and severity index, EOW: End of the week, Mtx: Methotrexate).

- **Re-treatment:** Majority of the patients who discontinue therapy relapse, median time to relapse is 141 days. Re-treatment results in satisfactory response in majority of the patients. Patients who respond early and have higher Psoriasis Area and Severity Index (PASI) reduction, maintain remission for longer period of time off therapy.[4]

PALMOPLANTAR PSORIASIS

Adalimumab has been used for the management of psoriasis involving hands and feet. Randomized placebo-controlled trial conducted by Leonardi et al. included 75 patients with plaque psoriasis involving hands and feet and 25 placebo. Dose of adalimumab used was 40 mg subcutaneously at week 0, followed by 40 mg every other week starting at week 1. Results revealed that 31% of patients treated with adalimumab were clear or almost clear from disease at the end of 16 weeks compared with 4% of placebo. The outcome for palmoplantar involvement was measured by erythema, scaling, induration, fissuring score (ESIF). ESIF-75 was achieved in 29% patients as compared to 4% in placebo.[5]

NAIL PSORIASIS

In March 2017, FDA approved addition of moderate to severe fingernail psoriasis data to adalimumab prescribing information, making it first biologic to have fingernail psoriasis data in prescribing information for chronic plaque psoriasis. 26 weeks, multi-centric, phase 3 placebo-controlled trial for adalimumab in nail psoriasis was conducted by Elewski et al. in 2016. Adalimumab was administered in a dose of 40 mg every other week. Severity of nail psoriasis was measured by modified nail psoriasis severity index (m-NAPSI) and physician global assessment (PGA). At 26 weeks, 46.6% in adalimumab group achieved m-NAPSI-75 compared to 3.4% in placebo group. 48.9% patients achieved PGA 0/1 compared to 6.9% in placebo group.[6]

PSORIATIC ARTHRITIS

Adalimumab was FDA approved for the management of psoriatic arthritis in 2005. The outcome measures used in psoriatic arthritis are ACR 20 and modified total sharp score of structural damage of joints. Efficacy of adalimumab in management of psoriatic arthritis is discussed in Table 7.2.

Table 7.2: Efficacy of adalimumab in management of psoriatic arthritis.

Dose	Schedule	Outcome	Reference
40 mg every other week	24-weeks randomized, double-blind, placebo-controlled trial Efficacy endpoints was ACR-20 at week 12 and change in sharp score at week 24	Week 12 and 24–ACR-20 response rate of 58% in adalimumab group vs 14% in placebo group ACR-50 and ACR-70 response seen in 36% and 17% patients respectively Week 24–Significant improvement in sharp score	Mease PJ et al.[7] (ADEPT trial)
	• ACR-20, 50 and 70 responses were same in patients receiving adalimumab alone and adalimumab in combination with methotrexate • Open label extension till 48 weeks–ACR-20, ACR-50 and ACR-70 response seen in 56%, 44% and 30% patients respectively. It was safe and well-tolerated till 48-weeks. A 2-year follow-up of this trial was also published demonstrating safety and efficacy of long term adalimumab.		
40 mg every other week	12-weeks, adalimumab for psoriatic arthritis in patients who have failed disease modifying antirheumatic drug therapy.	12-weeks–ACR-20 in 39% of treated patient	Van den Bosch F et al.[8]

(ACR: American college of rheumatology improvement, ADEPT: Abnormal Doppler enteral prescription).

HIDRADENITIS SUPPURATIVA

Adalimumab was FDA approved for the management of hidradenitis suppurativa (HS) in Sep 2015. Efficacy of adalimumab in management of HS is discussed in Table 7.3.

DOSES AND METHODS OF ADMINISTRATION

• *Psoriatic arthritis:* 40 mg administered every other week
• *Plaque psoriasis:* 80 mg on day 1 followed by 40 mg every other week, starting week one.
• *Hidradenitis Suppurativa (HS):*
  ▪ 160 mg on day 1, 80 mg on day 15.
  ▪ 40 mg on day 29 then every week.

Table 7.3: Efficacy of adalimumab in management of HS.

Dose	Schedule	Outcome	Reference
80 mg baseline followed by 40 mg subcutaneously every other week	Placebo-controlled trial (n-21), 15 adalimumab and 6 placebo Treatment for 12-weeks and follow-up for 12-weeks	Significant reduction in Sartorius score at end of 6 weeks and 24 weeks. No significant change after 12-weeks during follow-up period	Miller I et al.[9]
Week 0–160 mg Week 2–80 mg Week 4 onwards-40 mg weekly	Placebo-controlled trial Period 1–till week 12 Period 2–Re-randomization and continue for 24-weeks Assessment based on HiSCR	Week 12– PIONEER I–41.8% vs 26% (placebo) PIONEER II-58.9% vs 27.6% (placebo)	Kimball AB et al.[10]

(HiSCR: Hidradenitis suppurative clinical response).

CONTRAINDICATIONS

Adalimumab, sterile solution for injection is contraindicated in the following conditions:

- Hypersensitivity to the active substance or to any of the excipients
- Moderate to severe heart failure
- Active tuberculosis or other severe infections such as sepsis and opportunistic infections
- Along with live vaccines.

SPECIAL WARNING AND PRECAUTIONS FOR USE

Infection

- Patients should be treated with adalimumab after active infection including chronic or localized infections are controlled.
- Complete diagnostic evaluation when patients develop a new infection while being treated with adalimumab.
- Serious infection like sepsis, pyelonephritis, pneumonia, and opportunistic fungal infections like histoplasmosis may develop.

Tuberculosis

- Active or latent tuberculosis infection should be ruled out by history, clinical examination, chest X-ray, purified protein derivative (PPD) or interferon gamma release assay (IGRA) tests.
- Adalimumab should not be used in patients with active tuberculosis and treatment for latent tuberculosis infection should be started before adalimumab therapy is started.

Hepatitis B Reactivation

Reactivation of hepatitis B can occur in chronic carriers. Hepatologist should be consulted in patients who are hepatitis B surface antigen positive, before initiating adalimumab.

Neurological Event

Adalimumab is associated with exacerbation or new onset of central or peripheral nervous system demyelinating disorders such as multiple sclerosis and Guillain-Barré syndrome.

Allergic Reactions

Anaphylaxis and allergic reactions are rare. It should be discontinued if serious allergic reactions such as anaphylaxis, allergic rash, fixed drug reaction, nonspecified drug reaction or urticaria are observed in patients.

Malignancy

There has been concern regarding increase in risk of development of malignancies in patients taking TNF-α blocker. However, meta-analysis does not support or refute this concern.

Hematologic Reactions

Pancytopenia, bicytopenia or thrombocytopenia has rarely been reported.

Vaccinations

Live vaccines are contraindicated in patients on adalimumab.

Congestive Heart Failure

Increased mortality and worsening congestive heart disease have been reported in patients treated with TNF-antagonists including adalimumab. It is contraindicated in New York Heart Association (NYHA) class III or IV congestive heart failure (CHF).

Autoimmunity

- Anti-drug antibodies (ADA) develop in almost 30% of patients after three years of treatment. Patient with ADA have lower adalimumab level and lower chances of clinical remission.[11]
- Concomitant methotrexate use reduces the immunogenicity of adalimumab.
- ANA positivity and lupus-like syndrome can also develop rarely.

Concurrent Administration with Anakinra

Serious infections have been reported with concurrent use of anakinra with etanercept. Therefore, adalimumab is not recommended to be used with anakinra.

SPECIAL SITUATIONS

Pediatric Population

Adalimumab has been approved by European Medical Agency for the management of moderate to severe psoriasis in children older than 4 years in 2015. While etanercept is food and drug administration (USFDA) approved for the management of pediatric psoriasis, adalimumab is not USFDA approved yet.

A Phase III randomized double-blind study was conducted by Kim Papp et al. in 114 children with severe psoriasis. Adalimumab was used in the dose of 0.8 mg/Kg (max 40 mg), 0.4 mg/Kg (max 20 mg) every other week and methotrexate in the dose of 0.1-0.4 mg/Kg/week. 58% of patients in adalimumab 0.8 mg/kg group achieved PASI-75.[12]

Elderly Population

Adalimumab has been used in patients older than 65 years and found to be safe and effective. Risk of infection is higher in this population and one should be careful about infections and particular emphasis should be placed on immunization.[13]

Surgery

Rheumatoid arthritis patients on biologics undergo orthopedic procedure because of the disease itself. Similar situation can arise in patients with psoriatic arthritis or psoriasis patients requiring elective surgical procedure for unrelated illness. The risk of infections and complications appear to be higher in patients on adalimumab and it should be stopped prior to the surgery. However, data regarding complications are conflicting and there are studies which showed no significant difference in complications in patients on TNF-α blockers. The long half-life of adalimumab should be considered prior to planning a surgery and the patients should be monitored for infections.[14]

Pregnancy

Adalimumab is pregnancy category B drug. TNF-α blockers are not teratogenic drugs and have been used safely in many patients with successful pregnancy outcome. These drugs cross placenta and cord blood levels are higher than maternal serum. These drugs should ideally be stopped prior to conception in view of absence of robust safety data in pregnancy and tendency to cross placenta. In case one needs to continue these drugs in pregnancy to control the disease, immunosuppression in neonate is a major concern and one needs to stop these drugs prior to delivery. Adalimumab should be discontinued at 26–28 weeks of pregnancy.[15]

Lactation

Concentration of TNF-α blockers in breast milk of women taking these drugs were either undetectable or significantly lower than maternal serum. These drugs appear to be safe in lactation, however due to unavailability of large studies; it is not advisable to be used during lactation.[16]

TESTS TO BE DONE PRIOR TO ADMINISTRATION

- Complete blood count
- Liver function test
- Blood urea, Serum creatinine
- Hepatitis B surface antigen, Anti-hepatitis C virus (HCV) -IgM
- *Rule out active and latent tuberculosis:*
  - History of past tuberculosis, history of contact with active case of tuberculosis
  - History of fever, weight loss, and night sweats
  - Chest X-ray posteroanterior (PA) view
  - PPD or IGRA
- Antinuclear antibodies (ANA)

MONITORING DURING ADALIMUMAB THERAPY

Patients who are on adalimumab should be closely monitored for development of any infection specially tuberculosis. Three monthly complete blood count and liver function test and yearly chest X-ray is advisable.

REFERENCES

1. Menter A, Tyring SK, Gordon K, et al. Adalimumab therapy for moderate to severe psoriasis: a randomized, controlled phase III trial. Journal of the American Academy of Dermatology. 2008;58(1):106-15.
2. Saurat JH, Stingl G, Dubertret L, et al. Efficacy and safety results from the randomized controlled comparative study of adalimumab vs. methotrexate vs. placebo in patients with psoriasis (CHAMPION). British Journal of Dermatology. 2008;158(3):558-66.
3. Gordon KB, Langley RG, Leonardi C, et al. Clinical response to adalimumab treatment in patients with moderate to severe psoriasis: double-blind, randomized controlled trial and open-label extension study. Journal of the American Academy of Dermatology. 2006;55(4):598-606.
4. Papp K, Crowley J, Ortonne JP, et al. Adalimumab for moderate to severe chronic plaque psoriasis: efficacy and safety of retreatment and disease recurrence following withdrawal from therapy. British Journal of Dermatology. 2011;164(2):434-41.
5. Leonardi C, Langley RG, Papp K, et al. Adalimumab for Treatment of Moderate to Severe Chronic Plaque Psoriasis of the Hands and Feet Efficacy and Safety Results From REACH, a Randomized, Placebo-Controlled, Double-blind Trial. Arch Dermatol. 2011;147(4):429-36.
6. Elewski BE, Rich PA, Okun MM, et al. Adalimumab for nail psoriasis: efficacy and safety from the first 26 weeks of a Phase-3, randomized, placebo-controlled trial. J Am Acad Dermatol. 2016; 30:65.
7. Mease PJ, Gladman DD, Ritchlin CT, et al. Adalimumab for the treatment of patients with moderately to severely active psoriatic arthritis: results of a double-blind, randomized, placebo-controlled trial. Arthritis & Rheumatology. 2005;52(10):3279-89.
8. Van den Bosch F, Manger B, Goupille P, et al. Effectiveness of adalimumab in treating patients with active psoriatic arthritis and predictors of good clinical responses for arthritis, skin and nail lesions. Annals of the rheumatic diseases. 2010;69(2):394-9.
9. Miller I, Lynggaard CD, Lophaven S, et al. A double-blind placebo-controlled randomized trial of adalimumab in the treatment of hidradenitis suppurativa. British J Derm. 2011;165(2):391-8.
10. Kimball AB, Okun MM, Williams DA, et al. Two phase 3 trials of adalimumab for hidradenitis suppurativa. N Engl J Med. 2016;375(5):422-34.
11. Bartelds GM, Krieckaert CL, Nurmohamed MT, et al. Development of antidrug antibodies against adalimumab and association with disease activity and treatment failure during long-term follow-up. Jama. 2011;305(14):1460-8.
12. Papp K, Thaçi D, Marcoux D, et al. Efficacy and safety of adalimumab every other week versus methotrexate once weekly in children and adolescents with severe chronic plaque psoriasis: a randomised, double-blind, phase 3 trial. The Lancet. 2017;390(89):40-9.
13. Esposito M, Giunta A, Mazzotta A, et al. Efficacy and safety of subcutaneous anti-tumor necrosis factor-alpha agents, etanercept and adalimumab, in elderly patients affected by psoriasis and psoriatic arthritis: an observational long-term study. Dermatology. 2012;225(4):312-9.

14. Ruyssen-Witrand A, Gossec L, Salliot C, et al. Complication rates of 127 surgical procedures performed in rheumatic patients receiving tumor necrosis factor alpha blockers. Clin Exp Rheumatol. 2007;25(3):430-6.

15. Soh MC, MacKillop L. Biologics in pregnancy–for the obstetrician. The Obstetrician & Gynaecologist. 2016;18(1):25-32.

16. Krause ML, Amin S, Makol A. Use of DMARDs and biologics during pregnancy and lactation in rheumatoid arthritis: what the rheumatologist needs to know. Therapeutic advances in musculoskeletal disease. 2014;6(5):169-84.

Chapter 8

IL-17 Blockers: Secukinumab

SG Parasramani, Jisha Pillai

INTRODUCTION

Secukinumab is a recombinant fully human immunoglobulin G1 (IgG1)/κ monoclonal antibody that selectively targets interleukin (IL)-17A, which is a key pathogenic cytokine in psoriasis, acting directly on keratinocytes to stimulate the secretion of proinflammatory mediators.[1] In 2010, a proof of concept study was carried out by Hueber et al. which demonstrated the efficacy of secukinumab in the treatment of chronic plaque-type psoriasis, rheumatoid arthritis, and chronic noninfectious uveitis.[1]

The importance of IL-17A in psoriasis pathogenesis has been validated by the clinical efficacy of secukinumab in pivotal 52-week phase III trials; secukinumab was shown to be superior to placebo and to etanercept in achieving a strong and sustained response with a favorable safety profile.[2] Secukinumab was directly compared in the CLEAR trial with ustekinumab and was found to be superior in efficacy and also had a favorable safety profile.[3]

PHARMACOLOGY

- Secukinumab is a recombinant fully human monoclonal antibody that selectively binds to and neutralizes the proinflammatory cytokine IL-17A.
- It is of the IgG1/κ-class produced in Chinese hamster ovary (CHO) cells.
- It works by targeting IL-17A and inhibits its interaction with the IL-17 receptor, which is expressed on various cell types including keratinocytes. Its molecular weight is 150 kDa.[4]
- Following a single subcutaneous dose of either 150 mg or 300 mg in plaque psoriasis patients, secukinumab reached peak serum concentrations of 13.7 ± 4.8 µg/mL or 27.3 ± 9.5 µg/mL, respectively, between 5 days and 6 days post dose.[4]
- Average absolute bioavailability: 73%.[5]
- The mean elimination half-life was estimated to be 27 days (22–31 days) in plaque psoriasis patients.[4]
- It is filtered by the kidney only to a very small degree, thereby only very small amounts of antibody are excreted in the urine. Human IgG1 monoclonal antibodies are metabolized similarly to endogenous IgG via intracellular catabolism.[4]

USES

Food and Drug Administration-approved Indications

- Moderate-to-severe plaque psoriasis in adults who are candidates for systemic therapy
- Psoriatic arthritis
- Ankylosing spondylitis[6]
- Rheumatoid arthritis
- Nail psoriasis
- Palmoplantar psoriasis.

Off-label Indications

- Pustular psoriasis
- Chronic noninfectious uveitis.[7]

Psoriasis

On 20th November 2014, secukinumab was approved in adult patients having moderate-to-severe plaque psoriasis who are candidates for systemic therapy. This is the first instance of a biologic product having been approved for first-line treatment of moderate-to-severe psoriasis by the European Medicines Agency (EMA). On 21st January 2015, secukinumab was also approved by the United States Food and Drug Administration for the treatment of moderate-to-severe plaque psoriasis in adult patients who are candidates for systemic therapy or phototherapy.[8]

Clinical response [i.e. a 50% reduction in the mean Psoriasis Area and Severity Index (PASI) PASI score] occurred more rapidly with each secukinumab dose (median, 3.0 weeks with 300 mg and 3.9 weeks with 150 mg) than with etanercept (median, 7.0 weeks) (Table 8.1).

PASI 75 was maintained over 52 weeks in 80% of the patients with the 300 mg dose of secukinumab and in 60% of the patients taking 150 mg dose. PASI 90 was maintained over 52 weeks in 70% of the patients with the 300 mg dose of secukinumab and in 50% of the patients taking 150 mg dose.

PASI 75 was seen over 2-year period in 88.2% patients with 300 mg dose and 75.5% patients who received secukinumab continuously.

On withdrawal of secukinumab relapse occurred within 12 weeks in patients who received 150 mg of secukinumab and within 18 weeks in those patients who received 300 mg of the dose.

Patients who discontinue secukinumab for 3 months will require readministration of complete five induction doses before starting maintenance therapy of secukinumab. On restarting therapy with 300 mg secukinumab, 94.8%, 70.3% and 38.4% patients achieved PASI 75, PASI 90

Table 8.1: Clinical response to secukinumab in studies.

Dose	Schedule	Outcome	References
300 mg or 150 mg subcutaneous on week 0, 1, 2, 3, 4 and then every 4 weeks	Randomized double blind placebo controlled trial *Follow-up period*: 52 weeks Efficacy assessment at week 12 and 52	*Week 12*: Psoriasis Area and Severity Index (PASI) 75 of 81.6% and 71.6% in 300 mg and 150 mg group, respectively PASI 90: 59.2% and 39.1% PASI 100: 28.6% and 12.8%	ERASURE[2]
300 mg or 150 mg subcutaneous on week 0, 1, 2, 3, 4 and then every 4 weeks Etanercept 50 mg twice weekly till week 12	Randomized double blind placebo controlled with an active control (Etanercept) Efficacy assessment at week 12 and 52	*Week 12*: 300 mg—PASI 75–77.1% PASI 90: 54.2% PASI 100: 24.1% 150 mg—PASI 75–67% PASI 90: 41.9% PASI 100: 14.4% Etanercept PASI 75: 44% PASI 90: 20.7% PASI 100: 4.3%	FIXTURE[2]

and PASI 100 response, respectively. However, many experts believe that secukinumab can be administered in maintenance dose after discontinuation (unpublished observation).

Secukinumab treatment sustained high response rates over 3 years. PASI 75, PASI 90 and PASI 100 response was seen in 83%, 63.8% and 42.6% of patients receiving secukinumab 300 mg dose through year 3. PASI 75, PASI 90 and PASI 100 response was seen in 62.4%, 36.8% and 17.9% of patients receiving secukinumab 150 mg dose through year 3.[9]

In the CLEAR study, secukinumab showed superiority over ustekinumab while in the FIXTURE study superiority of secukinumab over etanercept was demonstrated.[10]

Psoriatic Arthritis

Secukinumab 300 mg and 150 mg significantly improved joint and skin symptoms in patients with PsA, with associated improvements in physical function and skin-related quality of life.[11] Improvements in signs and symptoms of PsA were demonstrated with secukinumab 300 mg and 150 mg in both the concomitant methotrexate (MTX) and without MTX subgroups.[12]

ACR20 response rates at week 24 were significantly higher in the group receiving secukinumab at doses of 150 mg (50.0%) and 75 mg (50.5%) than in those receiving placebo (17.3%). Secondary end points, including the ACR50 response and joint structural damage, were significantly better in the secukinumab groups than in the placebo group.[13]

Nail Psoriasis

In the TRANSFIGURE study,[14] secukinumab 300 mg and secukinumab 150 mg resulted in superior efficacy to placebo as measured by Nail Psoriasis Severity Index (NAPSI) percent change at Week 16. NAPSI percent change was-45.4% for secukinumab 300 mg, −38.9% for secukinumab 150 mg, and −11.2% for placebo. With regard to secondary endpoints, the responses for PASI 75 and modified Investigator Global Assessment (IGA) score of clear or almost clear were significantly higher for both secukinumab 300 mg (PASI 75: 87.1% and IGA 0/1: 74.0%) and secukinumab 150 mg (PASI 75: 77.0% and IGA 0/1: 68.3%), compared to placebo (PASI 75: 5.1% and IGA 0/1 3.1%). PASI 90 responses were seen in 72.5% patients receiving secukinumab 300 mg dose, 54.0% patients receiving secukinumab 150 mg while in patients on placebo PASI 90 was seen in 1.7% of patients.

Palmoplantar Psoriasis

In the GESTURE study[15] at week 16, the percentage of subjects who achieved clear or almost clear palms and soles (or ppIGA 0/1) with secukinumab 300 mg and 150 mg was 33.3% and 22.1%, respectively, compared to placebo which was 1.5%.

Palmoplantar Psoriasis Area and Severity Index (pp PASI) significantly reduced with secukinumab 300 mg (−54.5%) and 150 mg (−35.3%) compared with placebo (−4.0%).

Dermatology Life Quality Index (DLQI) 0/1 responses from subjects in the secukinumab groups were also significantly higher compared with placebo at week 16 and pain and function of palms and soles was markedly improved with secukinumab as measured by the palmoplantar.

Quality-of-life instrument—secukinumab 300 mg consistently showed the best outcomes. The safety profile was favorable and similar to previous studies.

▌ADMINISTRATION

The powder is a white solid lyophilisate in a 6 mL glass vial. Lyophilized powder is stored in refrigerator and reconstituted with 1 mL sterile water for injection.

Dosage

The recommended dose is 300 mg by subcutaneous injection with initial dosing at weeks 0, 1, 2, 3 and 4, followed by monthly maintenance dosing 4 weekly. Each 300 mg dose is given as two subcutaneous injections of 150 mg over the anterolateral aspect of the thigh.

Dose in psoriatic arthritis is 150 mg on week 0, 1, 2, 3, 4 and 4 weekly thereafter.

Tests to be Done Prior to Administration

- Complete blood count (CBC)
- Liver function test (LFT)
- Blood urea, serum creatinine
- Hepatitis B surface antigen, anti-hepatitis C virus immunoglobulin M, human immunodeficiency virus (HIV)
- Rule out active and latent tuberculosis:
  - History of past tuberculosis, history of contact with active case of tuberculosis
  - History of fever, weight loss, night sweats
  - Chest X-ray PA view
  - Purified protein derivative (PPD) or interferon-gamma release assays (IGRA), if required
- Antinuclear antibody (ANA)
- Routine urine and stool examination
- Fasting and post prandial blood sugar
- Electrocardiography (ECG)
- Abdominal sonography
- Urinary pregnancy test (UPT) in females.

▊ MONITORING DURING SECUKINUMAB THERAPY

Patients who are on secukinumab should be closely monitored for development of candidial infection especially if the patient has diabetes. Check for oral thrush, balanoposthitis, and vulvovaginitis on every visit.
- CBC after induction phase and every 12 weeks thereafter for neutropenia
- Chest X-ray PA view, IGRA—annually.

▊ ADVERSE EFFECTS

- Anti-secukinumab antibodies were detected in four patients after the start of secukinumab treatment in the FIXTURE study (0.4% of the 980 secukinumab treated patients tested). No patient had neutralizing antibodies. In the ERASURE study, anti-secukinumab antibodies that developed during treatment were detected in 2 of 702 (0.3%) secukinumab-treated patients tested.[2]
- *Injection site reactions*: Seven patients (0.7%) in the combined secukinumab groups versus 36 patients (11.1%) in the etanercept group experienced injection-site reactions during the entire study.[2]
- *Infections*:[2] No serious infections were reported which warranted stoppage of the therapy.
  - *Upper respiratory tract infections*:[2] Nasopharyngitis, rhinorrhea, cough.

- ▪ *Candidiasis:*[2] IL-17A plays a key role in host mucocutaneous microbial surveillance.[14] All *Candida* infections in patients treated with secukinumab were mucocutaneous, mild or moderate in severity, responded to standard oral or topical treatment, and did not lead to discontinuation of secukinumab.[16]
  - ▪ Oral herpes.[17]
- *Gastrointestinal*: Diarrhea[2]
- Headache[2]
- *Others:*[18] Pruritis, hypertension, arthralgia, back pain
- *Neutropenia*: Neutropenia is an important adverse effect that can occur with IL-17A blockers. IL-17A stimulates granulopoiesis and neutrophil trafficking.[19] Rich et al.[20] found Grade 1 or 2 neutropenia in 19 secukinumab patients and 1 placebo patient in the 12-week induction phase and in 30 secukinumab patients in the maintenance phase (weeks 12–32). Dosing was not interrupted or held as no clinically significant adverse events were associated with the development of neutropenia. The incidence of Grade 3 neutropenia in patients receiving secukinumab was 0.5% compared with 0.1% in patients receiving placebo. No cases of Grade 4 neutropenia was observed with secukinumab.[2] The neutropenia resolved during the course of the study in all cases.[20]
- Hypersensitivity, urticaria and angioedema were reported in a very small percentage of patients in the pool of four placebo-controlled phase III trials.[4]

CONTRAINDICATIONS FOR SECUKINUMAB

- Severe hypersensitivity reactions to the active substance or to any of the excipients.
- If an anaphylactic or other serious allergic reaction occurs, administration of secukinumab should be discontinued immediately and appropriate therapy initiated.
- In clinical studies, urticaria and one case of anaphylactic reaction to secukinumab were observed.

SPECIAL SITUATIONS

- *Pregnancy:*
  - ▪ *Pregnancy and lactation*: Secukinumab is pregnancy category B. There is no data regarding use of this biologic in pregnancy. Animal studies do not indicate direct or indirect harmful effects with respect to pregnancy, embryonic/fetal development, parturition or postnatal development. Animal reproduction studies are not always predictive of human response hence it is not used in pregnancy unless; the benefits clearly outweigh the potential risks.[4]

Secukinumab passes through placenta and live vaccines should be avoided in neonates whose mother have been given secukinumab during pregnancy.[4]

- *Breastfeeding:* It is not known whether secukinumab is excreted in human milk. Because immunoglobulins are excreted in human milk, caution should be exercised when secukinumab is administered to a woman who is breastfeeding.[4]
- *Fertility:* The effect of secukinumab on human fertility has not been evaluated. Animal studies do not indicate direct or indirect harmful effects with respect to fertility.[4]
- *Vaccinations:* Live vaccines should not be given concurrently with secukinumab.[21] However, inactivated or non-live vaccinations may be administered. In a study, after *meningococcal* and inactivated *influenza* vaccinations, a similar proportion of patients treated with secukinumab and patients treated with placebo were able to mount an adequate immune response of at least a 4-fold increase in antibody titers to *meningococcal* and *influenza* vaccines.[21] The data suggest that secukinumab does not suppress the humoral immune response to the *meningococcal* or *influenza* vaccines.[21]

Live or live attenuated vaccines are contraindicated less than 2 weeks before, during, and for 6 months after discontinuation of biologic therapy. Recommended vaccines are inactivated vaccines which should be administered 2 weeks before starting therapy to ensure optimal immune responses.

- *Inflammatory bowel disease:* Patients with active Crohn's disease and ulcerative colitis should not receive secukinumab or with caution. They can experience exacerbation or flare up of their disease with secukinumab.[22]
- *Tuberculosis:* Secukinumab should not be used in patients with active and latent tuberculosis (PPD or IGRA positive). Patients should be enquired for past history of tuberculosis, family history and recent contact with a tuberculosis patient or visit to an endemic area where tuberculosis is prevalent. No cases of reactivation of latent tuberculosis was seen in any of the 10 psoriasis studies. Study inclusion criteria allowed patients with latent tuberculosis to be randomized, provided that antituberculosis treatment, implemented according to local clinical practice, was ongoing or had been completed before randomization.[23]
- *Malignant or unspecified tumors:* During the first 12 weeks, the incidence of malignant or unspecified tumors was comparable in the secukinumab 300 mg, 150 mg, and placebo groups; none was reported with etanercept. Over the entire 52 weeks, exposure-adjusted incidence rate (IR) of malignant or unspecified tumors was comparable in the secukinumab 300 mg, 150 mg, and etanercept groups (0.77, 0.97, and 0.68, respectively). The majority of tumors were nonmelanoma skin

cancers (NMSCs), including basal cell carcinoma (BCC) and squamous cell carcinoma. Most NMSCs were BCC in patients who had undergone previous treatment with phototherapy. No lymphoma was reported.[23]

- *Adjudicated major adverse cardiovascular events:* During the first 12 weeks, adjudicated major adverse cardiovascular events (MACEs) were reported in subjects receiving secukinumab 300 mg (0.26%) and placebo (0.10%). During the entire 52 weeks, the exposure-adjusted IR of adjudicated MACEs was comparable in subjects receiving secukinumab 300 mg (0.42 per 100 subject-years), 150 mg (0.35), and etanercept (0.34) despite higher cardiovascular risk factors in secukinumab groups at baseline. All subjects with MACE had previous or active cardiovascular disease or risk factors (e.g. hypertension, smoking, obesity, dyslipidemia, or diabetes).[23]
- *Hepatitis B, hepatitis C and HIV coinfection:* There is no data on the use of secukinumab in patients with HIV, hepatitis B and C infection. No cases of overdose have been reported in clinical studies.

TIPS

- Secukinumab should not be used as and when required. If the drug has been discontinued for 3 months then induction phase of five weekly doses should be repeated to attain the minimum inhibitory concentration levels. If cost is a factor then instead of 300 mg monthly dose in the maintenance phase, 150 mg of the drug can be used.
- Secukinumab is not combined with MTX as incidence of neutralizing antibodies is very low and also secukinumab alone achieves PASI 90 and PASI 100 response.
- In case of nonresponders to secukinumab 300 mg dose can be given once every 2 weeks (optimize study) or 3 weeks as maintenance dose or even intravenous secukinumab can be given (stature study).[24]

REFERENCES

1. Hueber W, Patel DD, Dryja T, et al. Effects of AIN457, a fully human antibody to interleukin-17A, on psoriasis, rheumatoid arthritis, and uveitis. Sci Transl Med. 2010;2:52-72.
2. Langley RG, Elewski BE, Lebwohl M, et al. Secukinumab in plaque psoriasis–results of two phase 3 trials. N Engl J Med. 2014;371(4):326-38.
3. Nestle FO, Kaplan DH, Barker J. Psoriasis. N Engl J Med. 2009;361:496-509.
4. Novartis Pharmaceuticals Corporation. (2015). Highlights of Prescribing Information [online] Available from http://www.pharma.us.novartis.com/product/pi/pdf/cosentyx.pdf. [Accessed December 2017].
5. Wang W, Wang EQ, Balthasar JP. Monoclonal antibody pharmacokinetics and pharmacodynamics. Clin Pharmacol Ther. 2008;84(5):548-58.

6. Baraliakos X, Borah B, Braun J, et al. Long-term effects of secukinumab on MRI findings in relation to clinical efficacy in subjects with active ankylosing spondylitis: an observational study. Ann Rheum Dis. 2016;75(2):408-12.
7. Letko E, Yeh S, Foster CS, et al. Efficacy and safety of intravenous secukinumab in noninfectious uveitis requiring steroid-sparing immunosuppressive therapy. Ophthalmology. 2015;122(5):939-48.
8. Lopez-Ferrer A, Vilarrasa E, Puig L. Secukinumab (AIN457) for the treatment of psoriasis. Expert Rev Clin Immunol. 2015;11(11):1177-88.
9. Bissonnette R, Luger T, Thaçi D, et al. Secukinumab maintains high levels of efficacy through 3 years of treatment: results from an extension to a phase 3 study (SCULPTURE) Presented at the 24th Annual Congress of the European Academy of Dermatology and Venereology. Copenhagen, Denmark: European Academy of Dermatology and Venereology; 2015.
10. Thaci D, Blauvelt A, Reich K, et al. Secukinumab is superior to ustekinumab in clearing skin of subjects with moderate to severe plaque psoriasis: CLEAR, a randomized controlled trial. J Am Acad Dermatol. 2015;73(3):400-9.
11. McInnes IB, Mease PJ, Kirkham B, et al. Secukinumab, a human anti-interleukin-17A monoclonal antibody, in patients with psoriatic arthritis (FUTURE 2): a randomised, double-blind, placebo-controlled, phase 3 trial. Lancet. 2015;386:1137-46.
12. Gottlieb AB, McInnes I, Mease P, et al. Secukinumab improves signs and symptoms of psoriatic arthritis: Results of phase 3 FUTURE 2 study stratified by concomitant methotrexate use. J Am Acad Dermatol. 2016;74(5):AB270.
13. Mease P, McInnes IB, Kirkham B, et al. Secukinumab inhibition of interleukin-17A in patients with psoriatic arthritis. Philip J. N Engl J Med. 2015;373(14): 1329-39.
14. Reich K, Arenberger P, Mrowietz U, et al. Secukinumab shows high and sustained efficacy in nail psoriasis: Week 80 results from the TRANSFIGURE study. J Am Acad Dermatol. 2017;76(6):AB232.
15. Gottlieb A, Sullivan J, van Doorn M, et al. Secukinumab shows significant efficacy in palmoplantar psoriasis: Results from GESTURE, a randomized controlled trial. J Am Acad Dermatol. 2017;76(1):70-80.
16. Huang W, Na L, Fidel PL, et al. Requirement of interleukin 17A for systemic anti-*Candida albicans* host defense in mice. J Infect Dis. 2004;190(3):624-31.
17. Blauvelt A. Safety of secukinumab in the treatment of psoriasis. Expert Opin Drug Saf. 2016;15(10):1413-20.
18. International Federation of Psoriasis Associations. 4th World Psoriasis and Psoriatic Arthritis Conference. Stockholm, Sweden: International Federation of Psoriasis Associations; 2015.
19. Ley K, Smith E, Stark MA. IL-17A-producing neutrophil-regulatory Tn lymphocytes. Immunol Res. 2006;34(3):229-42.
20. Rich P, Sigurgeirsson B, Thaci D, et al. Secukinumab induction and maintenance therapy in moderate-to-severe plaque psoriasis: a randomized, double-blind, placebo-controlled, phase II regimen-finding study. Br J Dermatol. 2013; 168(2):402-11.
21. Chioato A, Noseda E, Stevens M, et al. Treatment with the interleukin-17A-blocking antibody secukinumab does not interfere with the efficacy of influenza and meningococcal vaccinations in healthy subjects: results of an open-label, parallel-group, randomized single-center study. Clin Vaccine Immunol. 2012;19(10):1597-1602.

22. Hueber W, Sands BE, Lewitzky S, et al. Secukinumab, a human anti-IL-17A monoclonal antibody, for moderate to severe Crohn's disease: unexpected results of a randomised, double-blind placebo-controlled trial. GUT. 2012;61(12):1693-700.

23. van de Kerkhof PC, Griffiths CE, Reich K, et al. Secukinumab long-term safety experience: A pooled analysis of 10 phase II and III clinical studies in patients with moderate to severe plaque psoriasis. J Am Acad Dermatol. 2016;75(1): 83-98.

24. Thaçi D, Humeniuk J, Frambach Y, et al. Secukinumab in psoriasis: randomized, controlled phase 3 trial results assessing the potential to improve treatment response in partial responders (STATURE). Br J Dermatol. 2015;173(3):777-87.

Chapter 9

Anti-CD6 Monoclonal Antibody: Itolizumab

Krupashankar DS, Swaroop HS

▊ INTRODUCTION

Itolizumab is a humanized anti-CD6 monoclonal antibody. It was approved in India by DCGI (Drug Controller General of India) in 2012 for the treatment of moderate-to-severe chronic plaque psoriasis. Till date Itolizumab is the only Indian research biologic available in India.

▊ PHARMACOLOGY

Itolizumab is a humanized recombinant anti-CD6 monoclonal antibody (mAB) of immunoglobulin G1 (IgG1) isotype which binds to domain of CD6. It contains two heavy chains with 449 amino acids and two light chains with 214 amino acids with a molecular weight of 148 kDa.[1] The initial anti-CD6 mAB was a murine antibody iorT1. It was immunogenic in nature due to its murine origin. With progresses in genetic engineering, the murine content was replaced by human counterparts. The resulting antibody retained the same CD6 affinity of iorT1, with improved side effect profile.[2] Molecular structure of CD6 is shown in Figure 9.1.

Mechanism of Action

Itolizumab is a humanized monoclonal antibody that recognizes the membrane-distal domain scavenger receptor cysteine-rich (SRCR1) (D1) of CD6, which modulates T lymphocyte activation and proliferation. Itolizumab binds to D1 of CD6, thereby it reduces the interaction of D3 of CD6 to activated leukocyte cell adhesion molecule (ALCAM), which helps in differentiation of T-helper cells into T-helper 1 cells (Th1) and T-helper 17 cells (Th17). Hence, it is an upstream inhibitor. It blocks intracellular mitogen-activated protein kinase (MAPK) and signal transducer and activator of transcription-3 (STAT-3) signaling pathways, thereby it blocks the secretion of pro-inflammatory cytokines (including tumor necrosis factor-α, interferon-γ and interleukin-6) and T cell proliferation. Itolizumab is an immunomodulator, it does not cause T cell depletion and whenever depletion occurs, it is transient in nature.[3] Mechanism of action of Itolizumab is illustrated in Figure 9.2.

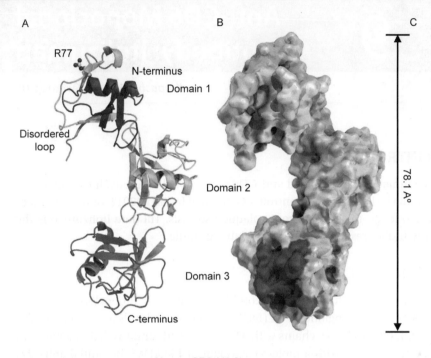

Fig. 9.1: Molecular structure of CD6 with its three domains.[4] (A) Loop structure of CD6, (B) Three-dimensional structure of CD6, (C) Total length of CD6.

Downregulation of both Downstream and Upstream Mediators in Psoriasis

Gupta et al.[5] reported a case report of recalcitrant psoriasis patient successfully treated with cyclosporine for first 15 days followed with Itolizumab, where the patient achieved psoriasis area and severity index (PASI) 90 in 12 weeks and maintained a remission of PASI 90 up to 15 months. The rationale behind this case report is to downregulate both upstream and downstream mediators in psoriasis pathogenesis.

In recalcitrant psoriasis, Th17 skewing of naive T cells leads to the local production of IL-17 ligand, keratinocytes in turn are stimulated by these IL-17 ligands leading to an aberrant differentiation and elevated production of pro-inflammatory factors. These keratinocyte-derived factors in turn stimulate further IL-17 producing cells, this establish a self-sustaining inflammatory feedback loop at keratinocytes. This in turn leads to recalcitrant psoriasis.

Cyclosporine, which is a calcineurin inhibitor, within 2 weeks of commencing treatment with cyclosporine lead to suppression of Th17 activation, in turn leads to decreased IL-17, IL-22 and downstream genes including beta-defensin-2 (DEFB-2), lipocalin-2 (LCN2), chemokine (C-X-C

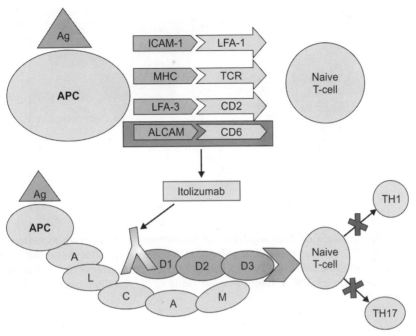

Fig. 9.2: Mechanism of action of itolizumab. (Ag: Antigen; APC: Antigen-presenting cell; TH1: T helper 1 cell; TH17: T helper 17 cell; ICAM: Intercellular adhesion molecule; MHC: Major histocompatibility complex; LFA-1: Lymphocyte function-associated antigen 1; LFA-3: Lymphocyte function-associated antigen 3; TCR: T-cell receptor; ALCAM: Activated lymphocyte cell adhesion molecule; CD2: Cluster of differentiation 2, CD6: Cluster of differentiation 6.

motif) ligand 1 (CXCL1) and chemokine (C-C motif) ligand 20 (CCL20). This might abolish self-sustaining inflammatory feedback loop. Itolizumab which is an anti-CD6 monoclonal antibody, which causes downregulation of priming and activation of T cells to Th1 and Th17 cells, subsequently leads to downregulation of downstream mediators like TNF-α, IL-17, and IL-23. Continuing inflammatory process is blocked at epidermis. This leads to the normalization of the skin architecture and long-term remission of lesions in psoriasis. However, this hypothesis has been proved only in one patient, hence larger randomized controlled studies are required to corroborate these results and to standardize the relevant guidelines.[6,7] Illustration of downstream and upstream mediators in psoriasis as shown in Figure 9.3.

▌LITERATURE SEARCH

Itolizumab phase 2 and 3 studies were randomized, multicentric, placebo controlled studies, which determined the efficacy of Itolizumab and rest of the efficacy data is from individual case reports and series, which is mentioned in Table 9.1.

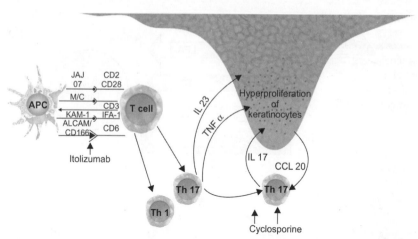

Fig. 9.3: Illustration of downregulation of downstream and upstream mediators in psoriasis. (APC: Antigen-presenting cell; ALCAM: Activated lymphocyte cell adhesion molecule; TH1: T helper 1 cell; TH17: T helper 17 cell; CD6: Cluster of differentiation 6; IL-23: Interleukin-23; TNF-α: Tumor necrosis factor-α; CCL-20: Chemokine (C-C motif) ligand 20).

Table 9.1: Summary of efficacy studies of itolizumab.[8-10]				
Study name	*Indication*	*Dosing schedule*	*Results*	*ADR*
Phase 2 study	Plaque psoriasis	1.6 mg/kg body weight, once every 2 weeks for 12 weeks, followed with once in month for next 12 week	PASI-75 scores at 12 weeks: 45%	Chills and rigors
Phase 3	Plaque psoriasis	1.6 mg/kg body weight, once every 2 weeks for 12 weeks, followed with once in month for next 12 week	PASI-75 at 45.5% at 28 weeks PASI-90 at 21.6% at 28 weeks 52.5% of patients maintained drug free remission at 52 weeks	Infusion related reactions Upper respiratory tract infections, pyrexia
Nott et al. case series of 5 patients	Plaque psoriasis	1.6 mg/kg body weight, once every 2 weeks for 12 weeks, followed with once in month for next 12 week	All 5 patients achieved PASI-75 at 8 weeks	None reported

Contd...

Contd...

Study name	Indication	Dosing schedule	Results	ADR
Anchala et al. case series of 20 patients	Plaque psoriasis	1.6 mg/kg body weight, once every 2 weeks for 12 weeks, followed with once in month for next 12 week	18 patients achieved PASI-75 at 24 weeks	None reported
Pai et al. case series of 5 patients	Plaque psoriasis with psoriatic arthritis	1.6 mg/kg body weight, once every 2 weeks for 12 weeks, followed with once in month for next 12 week	All 5 patients achieved PASI-75 at 24 weeks. Significant improvement in psoriatic arthropathy in one patient	None reported
Singh V case series of 7 patients	Plaque psoriasis	1.6 mg/kg body weight, once every 2 weeks for 12 weeks, followed with once in month for next 12 week	All 7 patients achieved PASI-75 at 24 weeks.	None reported
Singh V case report	Pustular psoriasis	1.6 mg/kg body weight, once every 2 weeks for 12 weeks, followed with once in month for next 12 week	PASI-90 achieved at 24 weeks	None reported
Parasramani case series of 10 patients	Plaque psoriasis	1.6 mg/kg body weight, once every 2 weeks for 12 weeks, followed with once in month for next 12 week	7 patients achieved >PASI 75 at 24 weeks and 3 patients achieved PASI-90 at 24 weeks	None reported
Gupta et al.	Plaque psoriasis	Cyclosporine 200 mg for first 15 days followed with itolizumab regime	Patient achieved PASI-90 at 12 weeks and sustained remission for 15 months	None reported

(PASI-75: Psoriasis area and severity index-75; PASI-90: Psoriasis area and severity index-90; ADR: Adverse drug reaction).

INDICATIONS

Drug Controller General of India (DCGI) approved: Moderate-to-severe chronic plaque psoriasis.
Off-label: Psoriatic arthritis.

CONTRAINDICATIONS

Itolizumab should not be administered to patients having history of severe allergy or known hypersensitivity reaction to any component of Itolizumab or any murine proteins. Additionally, Itolizumab is contraindicated in patients with any active serious infection and latent tuberculosis.

SIDE EFFECTS

The adverse effects of Itolizumab is listed as per system-wise in Table 9.2.

CHECKLIST

History of any serious infections or tuberculosis or immune-comprised conditions to be ruled out.

Table 9.2: Adverse effects of itolizumab.

System	Adverse drug reactions
Acute infusion reactions	Nausea, flushing, urticaria, cough, hypersensitivity, pruritus, rash, wheezing, dyspnea, dizziness, headache and hypertension
Gastrointestinal	Diarrhea, toothache, vomiting, gastritis, gastrointestinal inflammation
Infections and infestations	Abscess, folliculitis, gastroenteritis, lymphadenitis, lymph node tuberculosis, oral herpes, pyrexia, urinary tract infection, rhinitis, tooth abscess
Metabolism and nutrition disorders	Dehydration, hepatic steatosis, hypertriglyceridemia
Musculoskeletal	Musculoskeletal pain, pain in extremity, arthralgia, and back pain
Nervous system	Headache, peripheral neuropathy, cerebrovascular accident
Psychiatric disorder	Adjustment disorder with anxiety
Respiratory disorders	Cough, oropharyngeal pain, rhinorrhea

Investigations

- Complete blood count
- Screening for tuberculosis (TB) (Clinical)—Signs and symptoms of TB to be evaluated.
- Mantoux test and chest X-ray to rule out TB before starting the therapy.

Vaccinations

It is recommended that live/attenuated vaccines should not be given concurrently with Itolizumab. The patient's vaccination record and the need for immunization prior to receiving Itolizumab should be carefully investigated. Caution is advised in the administration of live vaccines to infants born to female patients treated with Itolizumab during pregnancy, since Itolizumab may cross the placenta.

Dosing

The recommended dosage of Itolizumab for the treatment of plaque psoriasis is 1.6 mg/kg given as intravenous infusion once every 2 weeks for first 12 weeks, followed by 1.6 mg/kg once in 4 weeks up to 24 weeks.

Maintenance Regimens

Once in 3 months post the 24 weeks of the therapy is advisable.

Special Population

Pregnancy

As with other IgG antibodies, Itolizumab may cross the placenta during pregnancy. It is not known whether Itolizumab can cause fetal harm when administered to a pregnant woman, or whether it can affect reproductive capacity or fertility.

Lactation

It is not known whether Itolizumab is excreted in human milk or absorbed systemically after ingestion. Because many drugs and immunoglobulin are excreted in human milk, and because of the potential for serious adverse reactions in nursing infants from Itolizumab, a decision should be made whether to discontinue nursing or to discontinue the drug, taking into account the importance of the drug to the mother.

Monitoring of a Patient on Biologic

Patients on Itolizumab should be closely monitored for development of any infection specially TB. Patient should be asked for history of weight loss, fever and night sweats during each visit to rule out any extra pulmonary tuberculosis.

REFERENCES

1. India: Biocon, Inc (2013). Alzumab™ (Itolizumab) solution for IV infusion [prescribing information]. [online] Available from http://www.biocon.com/docs/prescribing_information/immunotherapy/Alzumab_pi.pdf. [Accessed May, 2017].
2. Alonso-Ramirez R, Loisel S, Buors C, et al. Rationale for targeting CD6 as a treatment for autoimmune diseases. Arthritis. 2010;2010:130646.
3. Nair P, Melarkode R, Rajkumar D, et al. CD6 synergistic co-stimulation promoting pro-inflammatory response is modulated without interfering with the activated leucocyte cell adhesion molecule interaction. Clin Exp Immunol. 2010;162:116-130.
4. Chappell PE, Garner LI, Yan J, et al. Structures of CD6 and Its Ligand CD166 Give Insight into Their Interaction. Structure. 2015;23(8):1426-36.
5. Gupta A, Sharma YK, Deo K, et al. Severe recalcitrant psoriasis treated with itolizumab, a novel anti-CD6 monoclonal antibody. Indian J Dermatol Venereol Leprol. 2016;82(4):459-61.
6. Alonso R, Huerta V, DE Leon et al. Towards the definition of a chimpanzee and human conserved CD6 domain 1 epitope recognized by T1 monoclonal antibody. Hybridoma (Larchmt). 2008;27(4):291-301.
7. Haider AS, Lowes AM, Farnias MS et al. Identification of cellular pathways of "type 1," Th 17 T cells and TNF alpha and inducible nitric oxide synthase-producing dendritic cells in autoimmune inflammation through pharmacogenomics study of cyclosporine A in psoriasis. J Immunol. 2008;180(3):1913-20.
8. Doral S, Uprety S and Suresh SH. Itolizumab, a novel anti-CD6 monoclonal antibody: a safe and efficacious biologic agent for management of psoriasis. Expert Opin Biol Ther. 2017:395-402.
9. Parthasaradhi A. Safety and Efficacy of Itolizumab in the Treatment of Psoriasis: A Case Series of 20 Patients. J Clin Diagn Res. 2016;10(11):WD01-WD03.
10. Singh V. Clinical Outcome of a Novel Anti-CD6 Biologic Itolizumab in Patients of Psoriasis with Comorbid Conditions. Dermatol Res Pract. 2016;2016:1316326.

Newer Biologics

Abir Saraswat, Anupam Das

▌ INTRODUCTION

Biologics have emerged as very powerful and popular molecules for managing innumerable dermatological conditions. Though the invention and use of biologics in dermatology date back to a few decades ago, there has always been a rising need for the development of newer biologics with better pharmacological properties, receptor specific actions and better safety profile. In this chapter, we have briefly discussed the upcoming and newer biologics, either approved recently for their use in dermatological conditions or which are awaiting approval and would be available for use soon. We have focused on atopic dermatitis, psoriasis and pyoderma gangrenosum.

▌ ATOPIC DERMATITIS

Nemolizumab (CIM331)

Mechanism of Action

It is a humanized monoclonal antibody against interleukin (IL)-31 receptor A. It binds to the specific receptor and inhibits the signaling of IL-31; thus, controlling the pruritus.[1-3]

Observations

- *Nemoto et al.:* A single subcutaneous dose of nemolizumab reduced pruritus, improved the quality of sleep and reduced the need for using topical steroids in moderate-to-severe atopic dermatitis in adults.[4]
- *Ruzicka et al.:* Nemolizumab, at all monthly doses, improved the pruritus in adults with moderate-to-severe atopic dermatitis. More modest improvements in Eczema Area and Severity Index (EASI) score and body surface area were achieved. Conclusions regarding the adverse events (nasopharyngeal infections, headache, myalgia, etc.) could not be made on account of the small sample size, but peripheral edema was seen only in study patients, but not in the placebo group.[5]

Dupilumab

Mechanism of Action

It is a fully humanized monoclonal antibody directed against the IL-4 α receptor subunit and effectively blocks signaling from both IL-4 and IL-13.[6,7]

Observations

- *Beck et al.:* Patients with moderate-to-severe atopic dermatitis whose symptoms were not controlled with topical glucocorticoids and calcineurin inhibitors, were included in multiple clinical trials. In the 4-week monotherapy trials, the new biologic resulted in rapid, significant and dose-dependent improvements in Investigator's Global Assessment Score, percentage reduction in the affected body surface area, EASI, score on the 5-D pruritus scale, score on the pruritus numerical rating scale and reduction in levels of thymus- and activation-regulated chemokine (TARC) and immunoglobulin E (IgE). The results of the 12-week study of dupilumab monotherapy trial reproduced the results of the previous trials conducted for 4 weeks. In the combination trials (dupilumab and topical steroids) for 4 weeks, 100% of the patients in the dupilumab group showed statistically significant improvement in comparison to the group receiving placebo and topical steroids. There was a dose-dependent decrease in K16 (marker of keratinocyte proliferation and innate immunity). Nasopharyngitis and headache were the commonest side effects associated with dupilumab, but these were not dose-limiting.[8]
- *Thaci et al.:* Subcutaneous dupilumab was associated with significant improvement in EASI and Investigator's Global Assessment Score in adults with moderate-to-severe atopic dermatitis, without any significant safety and tolerability concerns. Dose regimens of 300 mg dupilumab once weekly and 300 mg once in alternate weeks, provided the best results and these dose regimens are now being assessed in phase 3 studies.[9]
- *Simpson et al.:* Subcutaneous dupilumab produced rapid and sustained patient-reported and clinically-relevant improvements (pruritus numeric rating scale; patient-reported sleep item on Scoring AD scale; Patient-oriented eczema measure; hospital anxiety and depression scale; dermatology life quality index and 5-dimension 3-level EuroQol). The group receiving two 300-mg dose regimens showed the best results.[10]
- *Simpson et al.:* In two phase 3 trials comparing dupilumab and placebo, dupilumab improved the pruritus, symptoms of anxiety and depression, and quality of life as compared with placebo.[11]
- *Blauvelt et al.:* In a large 1-year phase 3 trial comparing dupilumab and topical corticosteroids with placebo and topical corticosteroids,

39% patients on dupilumab achieved an Investigator's Global Assessment Score of 0 or 1 versus 12% on placebo. Almost three times as many patients on dupilumab achieved a 75% reduction in EASI compared to placebo. Adverse events, including serious adverse events, were similar across drug versus placebo groups.[12]

Lebrikizumab

Mechanism of Action

It is a humanized antibody against soluble IL-13, preventing downstream signaling that activates type 2 IgE mediated inflammation.[13]

Observations

- *Simpson EL et al.*: In a 12-week dose ranging study done on 211 patients with atopic dermatitis, a 50% reduction in EASI was achieved in 82.4% patients versus 62.9% with placebo (p <0.05). No serious adverse events were reported in this short study.[14]

Pitrakinra

Mechanism of Action

It is a 15-kDa human recombinant protein of wild-type human IL-4.

The drug has been applied both as a subcutaneous injection and as an inhalation in asthma. Further studies are required for commenting on its effectiveness in atopic eczema.

Tralokinumab

Mechanism of Action

It targets IL-13 and is being investigated for atopic dermatitis (Phase 2b).

▌PSORIASIS

Ustekinumab

Mechanism of Action

It is a humanized monoclonal antibody against the p40 subunit of IL-23 and IL-12. The p40 subunit binds to the IL-12Rß1 subunit. However, ustekinumab blocks the interaction of p40 with the IL-12Rß1 receptor and thus, neutralizes IL-12 and IL-23.[15-19]

Observations

- *Krueger et al:* In a phase 2 clinical trial comparing ustekinumab and placebo, percentage of patients achieving PASI 75 and PASI 90 at 12th week and percentage of patients achieving Static Physicians Global Assessment (sPGA) of "clear" or "minimal" was significantly better in the group receiving ustekinumab. The three commonest adverse effects were upper respiratory tract infection, headache and pain, but this was not statistically significant.[20]

- *Leonardi et al. and Papp et al.:* Two phase 3 trials compared the effectiveness, safety and tolerability of ustekinumab versus placebo in psoriatic patients. The number of patients achieving PASI 75 and PASI 90 at 4th week and 12th week was significantly higher, who received ustekinumab. The cumulative data showed that patients on ustekinumab maintained PASI 75 better (for a minimum of 12 months) than those who were withdrawn from treatment at week 40.[21,22]

Besides, ustekinumab has been found to be better than etanercept, in terms of effectiveness and cost incurred.[23-25]

Briakinumab

Mechanism of Action

It is a fully humanized monoclonal antibody against the shared p40 subunit of IL-23 and IL-12.[17,26]

Observations

- *Kimball et al:* In a phase 2 clinical trial, 180 patients were tested for 36 weeks. PASI 75 was achieved at week 12 in 63% of the patients receiving 200 mg once, 93% of the patients receiving 100 mg every other week for 12 weeks, 90% of patients receiving 200 mg weekly for 4 weeks, 93% of patients receiving 200 mg every other week for 12 weeks, 90% of patients receiving 200 mg weekly for 12 weeks and 3% of patients receiving placebo.[26]

- *Gordon et al. and Papp et al:* Following the success of the trial conducted by Kimball et al., phase 3 clinical trials were conducted and it was concluded that briakinumab 100 mg (every 4 weeks) in psoriasis patients led to better improvement of lesions in comparison to those who received 100 mg every 12 weeks and of course, placebo group. Rare serious adverse events included infections, nonmelanoma skin cancers, cardiac events, etc.[27,28]

In two studies, briakinumab, etanercept and placebo were compared to determine their efficacy and safety in treating psoriasis (12 weeks). Briakinumab was found to be superior to both etanercept and placebo.[29,30]

Another study compared briakinumab to methotrexate over 52 weeks and the authors concluded that briakinumab was more efficacious than methotrexate.[31]

Tildrakizumab

Mechanism of Action

IT IS A HUMANIZED IMMUNOGLOBULIN G1 (IGG1)/X ANTIBODY TARGETED AGAINST THE P19 subunit of IL-23. A 64-week, phase 3, randomized, placebo-controlled, parallel design study is ongoing, which plans to evaluate the efficacy and safety of subcutaneous tildrakizumab in moderate-to-severe chronic plaque psoriasis. The estimated date of completion of the study is October 2019.[17,18,32]

Observation

- *Papp et al.:* A three-part, randomized, double-blind, phase 2b trial was conducted in 355 adults with chronic plaque psoriasis over a period of 52 weeks. Tildrakizumab was superior to placebo and the effects persisted for 20 weeks after cessation of therapy.[33]

Guselkumab

Mechanism of Action

Human monoclonal antibody against p19 subunit of IL-23. The United States Food and Drug Administration (FDA) has approved guselkumab for the treatment of adults with moderate-to-severe plaque psoriasis. It is administered as a 100 mg subcutaneous injection every 8 weeks, following two initial doses at weeks 0 and 4.[17,18,34]

Observations

- *VOYAGE I study*: Guselkumab was found to be superior to adalimumab and placebo and better tolerated in psoriatic patients over a period of 1 year.[35]
- *VOYAGE II study*: A phase 3, multicenter, randomized, double-blind, placebo and active comparator-controlled study is ongoing, which plans to evaluate the efficacy and safety of guselkumab versus adalimumab in moderate-to-severe plaque psoriasis, with randomized withdrawal and retreatment.[36]
- *NAVIGATE study*: A phase 3, multicenter, randomized, double-blind study has been recently completed which has evaluated the efficacy and safety of guselkumab in moderate-to-severe plaque-type psoriasis and an inadequate response to ustekinumab. The results are yet to be announced.[37]
- *Gordon et al.:* In a 52-week, phase 2, dose-ranging, randomized, double-blind, placebo-controlled, active-comparator trial, 293 patients were

recruited. Authors compared guselkumab with adalimumab in patients with moderate-to-severe plaque psoriasis. Guselkumab was found to be highly effective.[38]

- *Zhuang et al.:* In a phase 1, randomized study, a single or dose of guselkumab was administered to 47 healthy subjects and a single subcutaneous dose was administered to 24 patients with moderate-to-severe plaque type psoriasis. Guselkumab pharmacokinetic profiles were comparable between healthy subjects and patients with psoriasis. It was well-tolerated in healthy subjects and patients with psoriasis.[39]

Ixekizumab

Mechanism of Action

Humanized IgG4 monoclonal antibody that selectively binds and neutralizes IL-17.[17]

Observations

1. *Leonardi et al.:* In a phase 2, double-blind, placebo-controlled trial, 142 patients with chronic moderate-to-severe plaque psoriasis were randomized and given subcutaneous injections of ixekizumab and followed for 12 weeks. Ixekizumab was found to be efficacious in improving the clinical symptoms of psoriasis.[40]
2. *UNCOVER-1*: A multicenter study with a randomized, double-blind, placebo-controlled induction dosing period followed by a randomized maintenance dosing period and a long-term extension period is ongoing. The study plans to evaluate the efficacy and safety of ixekizumab in moderate-to-severe plaque psoriasis. The study is estimated to be completed in November 2018.[41]
3. *UNCOVER-3*: A 12-week multicenter, randomized, double-blind, placebo-controlled study is ongoing which plans to compare the efficacy and safety of ixekizumab to etanercept and placebo in moderate-to-severe plaque psoriasis. The study is estimated to be completed in August 2019.[42]
4. *Gordon et al.*: A phase 2, randomized, placebo-controlled trial conducted over 120 patients over a period of 52 weeks showed that 77% of patients responded to ixekizumab therapy and maintained clinical responses throughout the duration of treatment.[43]
5. *Langley et al.*: A phase 2 study comprising a 20-week randomized, placebo-controlled trial (RCT) period and 48 weeks of an open-label extension (OLE) period conducted over 142 patients. Ixekizumab monotherapy improved scalp psoriasis quickly in the majority of patients. Besides, more than 50% of patients with nail psoriasis experienced complete resolution of nail lesions by 48th week.[44]

Brodalumab

Mechanism of Action

Human anti-IL-17 receptor antibody, blocking the activity of IL-17A, 17E, 17A/F, and 17E.[17]

Observations

- *Papp et al.:* In this phase 2, randomized, double-blind, placebo-controlled, dose-ranging study, efficacy and safety of brodalumab was assessed in the treatment of psoriasis and it was found that brodalumab significantly improved plaque psoriasis.[45]
- Three clinical trials were being conducted which planned to evaluate the efficacy and safety of brodalumab in moderate-to-severe psoriasis but these have been terminated by the sponsor (AMAGINE 1, 2 and 3).

Apremilast

Mechanism of Action

It specifically targets phosphodiesterase 4 (PDE4) and inhibits the production of tumor necrosis factor (TNF)-α, IL-12 and IL-23. Plenty of trials have been conducted which have given results in favor of using this new drug on psoriasis.[46-50]

Tofacitinib

Mechanism of Action

It is an oral Jak (Janus kinase) inhibitor that inhibits signaling by the heterodimeric receptors associated with Jak3 and/or Jak1.[46]

Observations

- *Boy et al.:* Substantial clinical improvement was reported in a double-blind, placebo-controlled phase 1 study.[51]
- *Papp et al.:* 197 moderate-to-severe plaque psoriasis patients were studied over a period of 12 weeks in a phase 2b study and tofacitinib was found to be superior to placebo.[52]

PYODERMA GANGRENOSUM

Newer biologics such as ustekinumab, ixekizumab and brodalumab seem to be promising because of the effects of IL-17 on neutrophil migration. But, the effectiveness, safety and tolerability of these drugs in pyoderma gangrenosum are yet to be evaluated.[53]

CONCLUSION

Nemolizumab (anti-IL-31 receptor), dupilumab (IL-4α receptor) and lebrikizumab (anti IL-13) are the newest molecules for the management of atopic dermatitis. Ustekinumab and briakinumab (anti p40 subunit of IL-23 and IL-12) are increasingly being used in psoriasis. Tildrakizumab and guselkumab (anti-p19 subunit of IL-23) have interesting mechanism of action and are being tried right now for psoriasis. Secukinumab (anti-IL-17) is gaining huge popularity as an anti-psoriatic biologic. Ixekizumab is a newer biologic, with mechanism of action similar to that of secukinumab and being investigated for psoriasis. Apremilast is an oral PDE inhibitor and it looks promising in the management of psoriasis. Tofacitinib is an oral JAK (Janus kinase) inhibitor being investigated in psoriasis and it is too early to comment on its effectiveness, safety and tolerability. Ustekinumab, ixekizumab and brodalumab could be useful in pyoderma gangrenosum (attributable to the effects of IL-17 on neutrophil migration). But, the effectiveness, safety and tolerability of these drugs in pyoderma gangrenosum are yet to be evaluated and we cannot comment on the same, right now.

REFERENCES

1. Cornelissen C, Lüscher-Firzlaff J, Baron JM, et al. Signaling by IL-31 and functional consequences. Eur J Cell Biol. 2012;91:552-66.
2. Dillon SR, Sprecher C, Hammond A. et al. Interleukin 31, a cytokine produced by activated T cells, induces dermatitis in mice. Nat Immunol. 2004;5:752-60.
3. Sonkoly E, Muller A, Lauerma AI, et al. IL-31: a new link between T cells and pruritus in atopic skin inflammation. J Allergy Clin Immunol. 2006;117:411-7.
4. Nemoto O, Furue M, Nakagawa H, et al. The first trial of CIM331, a humanized anti-human IL-31 receptor A antibody, for healthy volunteers and patients with atopic dermatitis to evaluate safety, side effect profile and pharmacokinetics of a single dose in a randomised, double-blind, placebo-controlled study. Br J Dermatol. 2016;174:296-304.
5. Ruzicka T, Hanifin JM, Furue M, et al. Anti-Interleukin-31 receptor α antibody for atopic dermatitis. N Engl J Med. 2017;376:826-35.
6. Wenzel S, Ford L, Pearlman D, et al. Dupilumab in persistent asthma with elevated eosinophil levels. N Engl J Med. 2013;368:2455-66.
7. Suárez-Fariñas M, Dhingra N, Gittler J, et al. Intrinsic atopic dermatitis shows similar TH2 and higher TH17 immune activation compared with extrinsic atopic dermatitis. J Allergy Clin Immunol. 2013;132:361-70.
8. Beck LA, Thaci D, Hamilton JD, et al. Dupilumab treatment in adults with moderate-to-severe atopic dermatitis. N Engl J Med. 2014;371:130-9.
9. Thaçi D, Simpson EL, Beck LA, et al. Efficacy and safety of dupilumab in adults with moderate-to-severe atopic dermatitis inadequately controlled by topical treatments: a randomised, placebo-controlled, dose-ranging phase 2b trial. Lancet. 2016;387:40-52.

10. Simpson E, Gadkari A, Worm M, et al. Dupilumab therapy provides clinically meaningful improvement in patient-reported outcomes (PROs): A phase IIb, randomized, placebo-controlled, clinical trial in adult patients with moderate to severe atopic dermatitis (AD). J Am Acad Dermatol. 2016;75:506-15.

11. Simpson EL, Bieber T, Guttman-Yassky E, et al. Two phase 3 trials of dupilumab versus placebo in atopic dermatitis. N Engl J Med. 2016;375:2335-48.

12. Blauvelt A, de Bruin-Weller M, Gooderham M, et al. Long-term management of moderate-to-severe atopic dermatitis with dupilumab and concomitant topical corticosteroids (LIBERTY AD CHRONOS): a 1-year, randomised, double-blinded, placebo-controlled, phase 3 trial. Lancet. 2017;389(10086):2287-2303.

13. Gandhi NA, Pirozzi G, Graham NMH. Commonality of the IL-4/IL-13 pathway in atopic diseases. Expert Rev Clin Immunol. 2017;13:425-37.

14. 25th European Academy of Dermatology and Venereology (EADV) Congress. Vienna, Austria: EADV; 2016 (Unpublished Data).

15. Yeilding N, Szapary P, Brodmerkel C, et al. Development of the IL-12/23 antagonist ustekinumab in psoriasis: past, present, and future perspectives. Ann N Y Acad Sci. 2011;1222:30-9.

16. Toichi E, Torres G, McCormick TS, et al. An anti-IL-12p40 antibody down-regulates type 1 cytokines, chemokines, and IL- 12/IL-23 in psoriasis. J Immunol. 2006;177:4917-26.

17. Tausend W, Downing C, Tyring S. Systematic review of interleukin-12, interleukin-17, and interleukin-23 pathway inhibitors for the treatment of moderate-to-severe chronic plaque psoriasis: ustekinumab, briakinumab, tildrakizumab, guselkumab, secukinumab, ixekizumab, and brodalumab. J Cutan Med Surg. 2014;18:156-69.

18. Gaspari AA, Tyring S. New and emerging biologic therapies for moderate-to-severe plaque psoriasis: mechanistic rationales and recent clinical data for IL-17 and IL-23 inhibitors. Dermatol Ther. 2015;28:179-93.

19. Stinco G, Errichetti E. Erythrodermic psoriasis: current and future role of biologicals. Bio Drugs. 2015;29:91-101.

20. Krueger GG, Langley RG, Leonardi C, et al. A human interleukin- 12/23 monoclonal antibody for the treatment of psoriasis. N Engl J Med. 2007;356: 580-92.

21. Leonardi CL, Kimball AB, Papp KA, et al. Efficacy and safety of ustekinumab, a human interleukin-12/23 monoclonal antibody, in patients with psoriasis: 76-week results from a randomised, double-blind, placebo-controlled trial (PHOENIX 1). Lancet. 2008;371:1665-74.

22. Papp KA, Langley RG, Lebwohl M, et al. Efficacy and safety of ustekinumab, a human interleukin-12/23 monoclonal antibody, in patients with psoriasis: 52 week results from a randomized, double-blind, placebo-controlled trial (PHOENIX 2). Lancet. 2008;371:1675-84.

23. Griffiths CE, Strober BE, van de Kerkhof P, et al. Comparison of ustekinumab and etanercept for moderate-to-severe psoriasis. N Engl J Med. 2010;362:118-28.

24. Pan F, Brazier NC, Shear NH, et al. Cost utility analysis based on a head-to-head phase III trial comparing ustekinumab and etanercept in patients with moderate-to-severe plaque psoriasis: a Canadian perspective. Value Health. 2011;14:652-6.

25. Staidle JP, Dabade TS, Feldman SR. A pharmacoeconomic analysis of severe psoriasis therapy: a review of treatment choices and cost efficiency. Expert Opin Pharmacother. 2011;12:2041-54.

26. Kimball AB, Gordon KB, Langley RG, et al. Safety and efficacy of ABT-874, a fully human interleukin 12/23 monoclonal antibody, in the treatment of moderate to severe chronic plaque psoriasis. Arch Dermatol. 2008;144:200-7.

27. Gordon KB, Langlet RG, Gottlieb AB, et al. A phase III, randomized, controlled trial of the fully human IL-12/23 mAb briakinumab in moderate-to-severe psoriasis. J Invest Dermatol. 2012;132:304-14.

28. Papp KA, Sundaram M, Bao Y, et al. Effects of briakinumab treatment for moderate to severe psoriasis on health-related quality of life and work productivity and activity impairment: results from a randomized phase III study. J Eur Acad Dermatol Venereol. 2014;28(6):790-8.

29. Gottlieb AB, Leonardia C, Kerdel F, et al. Efficacy and safety of briakinumab vs. etanercept and placebo in patients with moderate to severe chronic plaque psoriasis. Br J Dermatol. 2011;165:652-60.

30. Strober BE, Crowley JJ, Yamauchi PS, et al. Efficacy and safety results from a phase III, randomized controlled trial comparing the safety and efficacy of briakinumab with etanercept and placebo in patients with moderate to severe chronic plaque psoriasis. Br J Dermatol. 2011;165:661-8.

31. Reich K, Langley RG, Papp KA, et al. A 52-week trial comparing briakinumab with methotrexate in patients with psoriasis. N Engl J Med. 2011;365:1586-96.

32. US National Institutes of Health. (2012). A study to evaluate the efficacy and safety of subcutaneous Tildrakizumab, followed by an optional long-term safety extension study, in participants with moderate-to-severe chronic plaque psoriasis. (Tildrakizumab-010 AM3). [online] Available from http://clinicaltrials.gov/ct2/show/NCT01722331. [Accessed December 2017]

33. Papp K, Thaçi D, Reich K. et al. Tildrakizumab (MK-3222), an anti-interleukin-23p19 monoclonal antibody, improves psoriasis in a phase IIb randomized placebo-controlled trial. Br J Dermatol. 2015;173:930-9.

34. The Pharmaceutical Journal. (2017). Psoriasis drug approved by FDA. [online] Available from http://www.pharmaceutical-journal.com/news-and-analysis/news-in brief/psoriasis-drug-approved-by-fda/20203210 article. [Accessed December 2017]

35. Blauvelt A, Papp KA, Griffiths CE, et al. Efficacy and safety of guselkumab, an anti-interleukin-23 monoclonal antibody, compared with adalimumab for the continuous treatment of patients with moderate to severe psoriasis: Results from the phase III, double-blinded, placebo- and active comparator-controlled VOYAGE 1 trial. J Am Acad Dermatol. 2017;76(3):405-17.

36. US National Institutes of Health. (2014). A study of guselkumab in the treatment of participants with moderate to severe plaque-type psoriasis with randomized withdrawal and retreatment (VOYAGE 2). [online]. Available from https://clinicaltrials.gov/ct2/show/NCT02207244. [Accessed December 2017].

37. US National Institutes of Health. (2014). A study of guselkumab in participants with moderate to severe plaque-type psoriasis and an inadequate response to ustekinumab (NAVIGATE). [online]. Available from https://clinicaltrials.gov/ct2/show/results/NCT02203032. [Accessed December 2017].

38. Gordon KB, Duffin KC, Bissonnette R, et al. A phase 2 trial of guselkumab versus adalimumab for plaque psoriasis. N Engl J Med. 2015;373:136-44.

39. Zhuang Y, Calderon C, Marciniak SJ Jr, et al. First-in-human study to assess guselkumab (anti-IL-23 mAb) pharmacokinetics/safety in healthy subjects and patients with moderate-to-severe psoriasis. Eur J Clin Pharmacol. 2016;72:1303-10.

40. Leonardi C, Matheson R, Zacharie C, et al. Anti-interleukin-17 monoclonal antibody ixekizumab in chronic plaque psoriasis. N Engl J Med. 2012;366: 1190-9.

41. US National Institutes of Health. (2014). A phase 3 study in participants with moderate to severe psoriasis (UNCOVER-1). [online] Available from https://clinicaltrials.gov/ct2/show/study/NCT01474512. [Accessed December 2017].

42. US National Institutes of Health. (2012). A study in participants with moderate to severe psoriasis (UNCOVER-3). [online] Available from https://clinicaltrials.gov/ct2/show/NCT01646177. [Accessed December 2017].

43. Gordon KB, Leonardi CL, Lebwohl M, Blauvelt A, Cameron GS, Braun D, Erickson J, Heffernan M. A 52-week, open-label study of the efficacy and safety of ixekizumab, an anti-interleukin-17A monoclonal antibody, in patients with chronic plaque psoriasis. J Am Acad Dermatol. 2014;71:1176-82.

44. Langley RG, Rich P, Menter A, et al. Improvement of scalp and nail lesions with ixekizumab in a phase 2 trial in patients with chronic plaque psoriasis. J Eur Acad Dermatol Venereol. 2015;29:1763-70.

45. Papp KA, Leonardi C, Menter A, et al. Brodalumab, an anti- interleukin-17-receptor antibody for psoriasis. N Engl J Med. 2012;366:1181-9.

46. Gan EY, Chong WS, Tey HL. Therapeutic strategies in psoriasis patients with psoriatic arthritis: focus on new agents. BioDrugs. 2013;27:359-73.

47. Gottlieb AB, Strober B, Krueger JG, et al. An open-label, single arm pilot study in patients with severe plaque-type psoriasis treated with an oral anti-inflammatory agent, apremilast. Curr Med Res Opin. 2008;24:1529-38.

48. Papp K, Zeldis J, Rohane P, et al. A phase 2 study demonstrating the efficacy and safety of the oral therapy CC-10004 in subjects with moderate to severe psoriasis [abstract no. P2614]. J Am Acad Dermatol. 2008;58:AB3.

49. Papp K, Hu A, Day R. Oral apremilast is active in the treatment of moderate to severe plaque psoriasis: results from a phase 2b, randomized, controlled study (PSOR-005) [abstract no. 273]. J Invest Dermatol. 2011;131:S46.

50. Schett G, Wollenhaupt J, Papp K. et al. Oral apremilast in the treatment of active psoriatic arthritis: results of a multicenter, randomized, double-blind, placebo-controlled study. Arthritis Rheum. 2012;64:3156-67.

51. Boy MG, Wang C, Wilkinson BE, et al. Double-blind, placebo-controlled, dose-escalation study to evaluate the pharmacological effect of CP-690,550 in patients with psoriasis. J Invest Dermatol. 2009;129:2299-302.

52. Papp KA, Menter A, Strober B, et al. Efficacy and safety of tofacitinib, an oral Janus kinase inhibitor, in the treatment of psoriasis: a phase 2b, randomized, placebo-controlled doseranging study. Br J Dermatol. 2012;167:668-77.

53. Patel F, Fitzmaurice S, Duong C, et al. Effective strategies for the management of pyoderma gangrenosum: a comprehensive review. Acta Derm Venereol. 2015;95:525-31.

Chapter
11
Anti-CD20 Monoclonal Antibody: Rituximab

Dipankar De, Muhammed Razmi T

INTRODUCTION

Rituximab is a chimeric murine/human monoclonal IgG1 kappa antibody against the CD20 antigen. It was first approved as a cancer chemotherapy agent and subsequently found useful in various autoimmune disorders.

PHARMACOLOGY

Heavy and light chain variable regions of the molecule are from a murine antibody to CD20. The murine variable regions selectively target the CD20 antigen present on the surface of B lymphocytes. Human IgG1 and kappa-chain constant regions of rituximab bind to the Fc receptors on human effector cells and decrease its immunogenicity.

CHARACTERISTICS

- Molecular weight: 145 kDa
- Half-life: 30–400 hours
- Excretion: Phagocytosis and catabolism in the reticuloendothelial system.

MECHANISM OF ACTION

The Fab portion of rituximab attaches particularly to the CD20 antigen which is expressed specifically on the cell membranes of B lymphocytes from the pre-B cell stage to the mature B cell stage. The immune effector cells such as natural killer (NK) cells bind to rituximab via Fc receptors and help in the destruction of the bound CD20+ B lymphocytes via three possible mechanisms: complement-dependent cytotoxicity, antibody-dependent cell-mediated cytolysis, and apoptosis.

PHARMACOKINETICS

The mean half-life ($t^{1/2}$) of rituximab is around 3 weeks, similar to the other IgG1 related biological agents. Moreover, levels of serum rituximab increase with multiple infusions, since lesser antigens will be available due to depletion. B cell depletion occurs within 2–3 weeks of the initial infusion of rituximab. There is sustained reduction of B cells over first 6 months until first year of treatment when the B cell numbers start returning to normal. Plasma cell numbers, being maintained owing to the absence of CD20 on their surface and overall levels of immunoglobulin do not decline drastically.

TREATMENT PROTOCOLS

There are two main protocols for rituximab administration as mentioned below:

1. Lymphoma protocol (LP): Rituximab is administered weekly at a dose of 375 mg/m^2 body surface area for 4 weeks. Most of the initial studies of rituximab followed this protocol.
2. Rheumatoid arthritis protocol (RAP): One gram each dose of rituximab is administered at an interval of 15 days. This protocol is increasingly used by the dermatologists as primary indication of rituximab in dermatology in pemphigus vulgaris which is similar to rheumatoid arthritis, both being autoimmune diseases.

   Rituximab has also been administered intralesionally, mainly for cutaneous B cell lymphomas, at a dose of 10 mg/mL, with 1 mL per lesion administered in several sessions. Rituximab has also been combined with intravenous immunoglobulin (IVIg), immunoadsorption and dexamethasone pulse therapy in autoimmune blistering diseases.

USES

Food and Drug Administration Approved Indications
- Follicular and diffuse large B cell non-Hodgkin lymphoma (NHL)
- Chronic lymphocytic leukemia (CLL)
- Rheumatoid arthritis (RA)
- Granulomatosis with polyangiitis (GPA), formerly Wegener's granulomatosis (WG)
- Microscopic polyangiitis (MPA).

Off-label Indications

Of these indications, first three indications are recognized by the food and drug administration (FDA) as "orphan designations."
- Autoimmune thrombocytopenia
- Rasmussen's encephalitis
- Pemphigus vulgaris
- Other autoimmune bullous diseases
- Systemic lupus erythematosus
- Autoimmune hemolytic anemia
- Autoimmune neuropathies

- Graft-versus-host disease
- Mixed cryoglobulinemia
- Dermatomyositis (DM) and polymyositis (PM)
- Sjogren's syndrome
- Cutaneous B cell lymphomas (intralesional)
- Lymphomatoid granulomatosis.

Dermatological Uses of Rituximab

Pemphigus Vulgaris and Pemphigus Foliaceus

Rituximab has emerged as a promising agent for pemphigus vulgaris. Most of the patients had rapid resolution of lesions within 2–3 weeks and an absolute clearance of the clinical disease was achieved within 6–8 weeks of starting the treatment.[1] Skin lesions respond faster than mucosal lesions and most patients have remained on a reduced dose of systemic immunosuppressive therapy.[1] A recent systematic review and meta-analysis[2] suggested a complete clinical remission in 76% of 578 patients with pemphigus (496 with pemphigus vulgaris and 82 with pemphigus foliaceus) after 1 cycle of rituximab. Remission was achieved at an average duration of 5.8 months and the patients remained in remission for 14.5 months with a relapse rate of 40% over a mean follow-up period of 23 months. The meta-analysis showed that in contrast to smaller doses of rituximab (less than 1,500 mg/cycle), larger doses (greater than or equal to 2,000 mg/cycle) resulted in long-lasting remission. In other parameters, different dosing regimens like LP and RAP or high-dose rituximab and low-dose rituximab showed comparable outcomes.

While some studies on autoimmune bullous disorders suggest a single cycle of rituximab (either LP or RAP) can induce a complete response, the other studies suggest a need of maintenance dosing over long periods to induce response.[3] In our clinical experience, a proportion of the patients need a repeat cycle at 12–18 months due to relapse and repeated dosing improves the clinical outcome without increasing the adverse effects. Rituximab significantly reduces the need of oral corticosteroids. After rituximab administration, most of the patients can be rapidly shifted from systemic steroids to steroid sparing agents, which are continued until complete remission.

Other Autoimmune Bullous Diseases

Rituximab has been found to be effective in the following blistering diseases also:
- *Paraneoplastic pemphigus (PNP):* The efficacy is less impressive. There are conflicting reports. Some reports[4,5] showed improvement in the oral

and cutaneous lesions, whereas others reported[6,7] minimal improvement in the mucosal lesions.

- *Bullous pemphigoid (BP):* Better alternative in cases which are refractory to the conventional treatment based on the evidence obtained from small cases series and case reports. Limited number of refractory BP patients were treated with rituximab as per LP or RAP and almost 70% had a complete remission.[1] Prior to the initiation of rituximab in BP patients, immune status, and cardiac risk should be evaluated more vigorously considering the advanced age in this patient population and an increased risk of death due to bacterial sepsis or cardiac complications.

- *Mucous membrane pemphigoid (MMP):* Rituximab is beneficial in severe cases unresponsive to the standard therapy. Reported clinical remission rate is 60%.[1] Rituximab is unlikely to improve the scarring sequelae.

- *Epidermolysis bullosa acquisita (EBA):* Rituximab is beneficial in refractory cases. Reported clinical remission rate was 70%. Ninety percent of those who achieved remission had relapse.[1]

Autoimmune Connective Tissue Diseases

B cells are implicated in the pathogenesis of autoimmune connective tissue diseases. Hence, rituximab is likely to be used increasingly in these disorders.

Dermatomyositis: Rituximab is an effective treatment option in dermatomyositis. Two pilot studies showed conflicting results on the beneficial effects of rituximab in the cutaneous manifestation of dermatomyositis. Whereas one open-label study[8] using LP demonstrated its efficacy on the skin manifestations of all the seven patients, the other open-label study[9] using RAP showed no beneficial effect on the skin manifestations of all the eight patients. Rituximab was found to be useful as an adjunctive therapy on the skin and muscle manifestations of juvenile dermatomyositis.[10]

Cutaneous lupus erythematosus (CLE): Although there are reports of beneficial effects of rituximab in CLE,[11] overall data suggests poor outcome in chronic CLE and variable outcome in subacute CLE.[12] Its use in systemic lupus has also showed controversial results. Two randomized trials found no significant benefit when rituximab was compared with the controls (who received high doses of glucocorticoids and immunosuppressives).[13,14] Latest guideline for treatment of CLE by the European Dermatology Forum (EDF) does not recommend rituximab for the management of CLE.[15]

Systemic sclerosis (SSc): The EUSTAR [European League Against Rheumatism (EULAR) Scleroderma Trials and Research group] study showed amelioration of skin fibrosis and prevention of further deterioration of lung function in rituximab treated SSc patients versus untreated matched controls, suggesting a beneficial effect of rituximab in SSc.[16] A recent review states that "on current evidence, its use could only be supported in those patients with the rapidly progressive diffused form of the disease, where trialling unproven therapies are ethically justifiable."[17]

Vasculitis: In WG with polyangiitis with moderate-to-severe involvement, rituximab in combination with systemic steroids is increasingly used for induction of remission and maintenance.[18] Rituximab was found to be superior to azathioprine or cyclophosphamide for sustained remission in antineutrophil cytoplasmic antibody (ANCA)-associated vasculitides.[18,19]

Primary cutaneous B-cell lymphoma (PCBCL): Owing to its beneficial effect in nodal B cell lymphoma, rituximab has been used in PCBCL. It was found to be effective and safe in the management of PCBCL, when used as per LP, even in combination with high-dose chemotherapy or in elderly patients. Even though recurrences were noted in those with generalized skin involvement, continuation of rituximab infusion was not indicated as these were managed effectively with other treatment measures.[20,21] Single agent rituximab therapy may be employed for PCBCL.[22] For primary cutaneous diffuse large B-cell lymphoma, leg type (PCBCL-LT), multi-agent chemotherapy should be used.[23] Intralesional rituximab at a dose of 10 mg/mL, 1 mL per lesion, 3 times a week was found to be useful.[24,25] PCBCL lesions in those patients with severe flu-like symptoms after intralesional injection respond better to rituximab.[26] Response was noted in lesions away from the intralesional site and decrease in B cell count in peripheral blood was documented suggesting systemic absorption.[3] PCBCL tends to relapse and high recurrence is noted with intralesional rituximab.[27] Rituximab was found to be useful in cutaneous lymphoid hyperplasia with documented B-cell hyperplasia.[3]

Graft-versus-host disease (GVHD): Rituximab showed promising results in the management of GVHD with improvement in the mucocutaneous and musculoskeletal manifestations.[28,29] However, when it was used as a prophylactic agent along with myeloablative conditioning regimen, it did not prevent the development of GVHD.[30]

Atopic dermatitis: Rituximab was found to be beneficial in severe atopic dermatitis in an open study of eight patients when it was used alone.[31] In another study, six refractory atopic dermatitis patients achieved an impressive clinical improvement after a "sequential switch therapy with omalizumab and rituximab."[32] However, its failure in some patients as highlighted by McDonald et al.[33] stresses on the need of more robust studies to recommend its use in severe atopic dermatitis.

GENERAL INSTRUCTIONS

- Dosage form: 100 mg/10 mL and 500 mg/50 mL solution in a nonreusable vial for injection (brands in India are Ikgdar from Emcure, MabThera from Roche, Reditux from Dr. Reddy's and Ristova from Roche. Rituxan SubQ is a subcutaneous formulation available in Canada).
- To be given as intravenous infusion and not as intravenous bolus or push.
- Can be stored at 2°C to 8°C for 24 hours (rituximab have been shown to be stable for an extra 24 hours at room temperature). Store the reconstituted solution at 2°C to 8°C as it is free of preservatives.

ADMINISTRATION

- Use aseptic precautions.
- Premedication with intravenous hydrocortisone 100 mg and pheniramine maleate 22.75 mg along with oral Paracetamol 500 mg.
- Rituximab can be reconstituted in an infusion bag with either 0.9% sodium chloride or 5% dextrose in water to a final strength of 1 mg/mL to 4 mg/mL.
- Mix the solution by gently inverting the bag (no other drugs should be added).
- The rate of the initial infusion should be 50 mg/hour.
- If there are no adverse reactions, the infusion rate can be slowly increased by 50 mg/hour every 30 minutes up to 400 mg/hour.
- Vitals are checked after every 30 minutes, before increasing the dose, in the form of blood pressure, pulse rate, respiratory rate, and temperature.
- If the initial infusion was uneventful, further infusions can be started at 100 mg/hour and be increased to a maximum infusion rate of 400 mg/hour.
- In case of immediate adverse reactions like infusion reactions, treatment should be discontinued temporarily.
- After waiting for 30 minutes, restart the infusion at a slower rate (half the flow rate).
- Hydrocortisone and antihistamines must be readministered.
- Discontinue the infusion if there is serious or life-threatening cardiac complications and manage the event as per the protocol.

Tests to be Done Prior to Administration

- *Routine investigations:* Complete blood count (CBC), liver function test, renal function test, urine for routine examination, and electrocardiogram.
- Rule out active and latent tuberculosis (LTBI) in Indian scenario

- History of past tuberculosis (TB), history of contact with active case of TB
- History of fever, weight loss, and night sweats
- Chest X-ray
- Mantoux test or interferon-gamma release assays (IGRAs)
- Rule out hepatitis infection/carrier status
  - Hepatitis B surface antigen (HBsAg) and hepatitis B core antibody (anti-HBc) [consider testing for HBc (hepatitis B core antigen) and hepatitis B surface antibody (anti-HBs)]
  - Anti-HCV IgM
- Human immunovirus infection by enzyme-linked immunosorbent assay (ELISA) method
- Urine pregnancy test
- Echocardiography
- Baseline assessment of IgG, IgM, and IgA levels.

MONITORING DURING RITUXIMAB THERAPY

Monitor CBC every 2 weeks during rituximab infusions and every 1–3 months thereafter. Periodic CD19(+) B lymphocytes monitoring may help in predicting relapses.[34] It is recommended to monitor IgG levels in elderly population and in those with a low baseline IgG.[35]

ADVERSE EFFECTS

Infusion Reactions

One of the most predictable and serious acute side effect of rituximab is a constellation of symptoms and signs that manifests within 2 hours of initial infusion. Incidence is up to 30% to 45%. Adverse effects are mild in nature, consist mainly of fever, chills, and rigors with 80% to 90% of the cases having National Cancer Institute (NCI) toxicity grade 1 or 2. Other symptoms include headache, flushing, nausea, dyspepsia, urticaria/rash, fatigue, sweating, throat irritation, rhinitis, pruritus, tachycardia, mild hypotension, dyspnea, and backache. Less than 10% of cases develop bronchospasm and/or severe hypotension. Severe (grade 3 or 4) reactions like anaphylaxis are seen in less than 5% of cases. Fever and muscle pain are not the features of anaphylaxis and such complaints represent standard infusion reaction. In most patients, standard infusion reaction is mild and brief, lacks typical symptoms of anaphylaxis and resolves completely when drug infusion is withheld. However, some typical symptoms and signs like throat tightness/change in voice, incessant cough, urticarial, and wheeze should alert clinicians to a possibility of anaphylaxis and should be managed vigorously.

Management

Mild reactions can be managed by holding the infusion for a while and restarting later at a slower rate as explained above. An additional dose of Paracetamol and diphenhydramine can be given for the reaction to subside. Anaphylaxis should be managed by subcutaneous/intramuscular epinephrine. Intramuscular route is preferred at a dose of 0.2 mg to 0.5 mg of 1 mg/mL (1:1,000) solution every 5–15 minutes until clinical improvement. Additional therapies include saline infusion, bronchodilator inhalations, and parenteral glucocorticoids. Anaphylaxis is type 1 hypersensitivity reaction and infusion reactions are due to cytokine release. Anaphylaxis cannot be prevented by premedications, but infusion reactions can. Desensitization protocol is being devised for readministering rituximab after anaphylaxis or severe type 1 hypersensitivity.[36,37]

Tumor Lysis Syndrome

It is seen in less than 0.05% patients who cannot appropriately clear the dying cells, especially in the setting of lymphomas. It is characterized by hyperuricemia, hyperkalemia, hypocalcemia, hyperphosphatemia, deranged renal function tests, and elevated lactate dehydrogenase. It usually occurs within 12–24 hours of rituximab administration.

Cardiac Complications

Recent studies have highlighted the overall cardioprotective effects of rituximab by reducing the inflammatory burden in autoimmune diseases.[38–40] However, cardiovascular toxicities have been reported in 8% of patients with rituximab infusion.[41] Patients are advised to withhold their antihypertensive medications in the morning of the rituximab infusion given the increased frequency of mild-to-moderate hypotension occurring during rituximab infusions. Based on some case reports on adverse cardiac events like myocardial infarctions, atrial fibrillation, and worsening of preexisting cardiac dysfunction, a thorough cardiac evaluation is indicated especially in those with cardiovascular risk factors.[42] The etiologies of acute events like myocarditis/arrhythmia are postulated to be due to cytokine release from dying B cells that leads to platelet activation, vasoconstriction, and plaque rupture. Cardiomyopathy may occur due to accumulation of reticulin fibers upon multiple cycles of rituximab infusion.[43] Such a scenario is unlikely in the setting of dermatological indications where only two doses of rituximab are given and repeated if required at the most once in a year. However, the patients receiving rituximab should be closely monitored for any cardiovascular signs or symptoms. Any chest pain during the infusion warrants an electrocardiography and the help of a cardiologist should be sought.[44] Adequate hydration before staring rituximab infusion and slower rate of infusion may prevent these cardiovascular adverse effects.[44]

Infections

Though a single course of rituximab will not result in significant hypogammaglobulinemia, it occurs on repeated infusions. Preexisting hypogammaglobulinemia and concomitant immunosuppressant use such as cyclophosphamide are known risk factors for rituximab induced hypogammaglobulinemia. Rheumatology literature recommends baseline assessment of IgG, IgA, and IgM levels before starting rituximab. A study[45] has shown 56% incidence of IgG hypogammaglobulinemia after rituximab infusion. IgG replacement was initiated in 4% of patients because of recurrent infections. Case reports of new infection or reactivation of varicella zoster, parvovirus B19, hepatitis B and C, cytomegalovirus (CMV), John Cunningham (JC) virus [causes progressive multifocal leukoencephalopathy (PML)], West Nile virus (WNV), and herpes simplex virus (HSV) has been documented after rituximab administration.[46] Rituximab was found to increase the incidence of infectious complications in the setting of hematological malignancies and transplant recipients. However, no increase in the incidence of opportunistic infections was apparent in the Rheumatoid arthritis (RA) patients.[47]

Late-Onset Neutropenia after Rituximab Therapy (R-LON)

Late-onset neutropenia after rituximab therapy (R-LON), typically seen several months after drug administration, was defined as otherwise unexplained grade 3–4 neutropenia after rituximab.[48] A retrospective analysis[48] found a 1 year cumulative incidence of 9%. Older age (greater than 60 years), advanced stage of lymphoma, and purine analogue or methotrexate administration were found to be significant or borderline significant risk factors for R-LON. In general, R-LON is self-limiting and rarely has significant clinical sequelae. However, treatment with granulocyte colony-stimulating factor is a good option in grade 4 R-LON patients with high-risk of infection.

Human Anti-Chimeric Antibodies (HACA)

In comparison to lymphoma patients, the occurrence of human anti-chimeric antibodies (HACA) to rituximab is higher in RA and SLE patients. This may be due to autoimmune nature of primary diseases promoting the development of anti-drug antibodies, lower dosage of rituximab used and lack of use of additional immunosuppressants in autoimmune disorders compared to lymphoma. HACA may lead to increased incidence of infusion reactions and decrease in the therapeutic efficacy of rituximab.

Other Less Common Adverse Effects

- *Serious mucocutaneous reactions:* Stevens-Johnson syndrome, vesiculo-bullous dermatitis and toxic epidermal necrolysis.
- *Serum sickness:* Should be suspected when the patient develops fever, arthralgia and characteristic urticated lesions on the palms and soles that may last days to weeks.
- No enhanced malignancy risk was reported with rituximab.

▎CONTRAINDICATIONS[3,35]

- Known anaphylaxis or IgE hypersensitivity to murine proteins or components of rituximab
- Active hepatitis B virus (HBV) infection
- Human immunodeficiency virus (HIV) infection (CD4 cell count less than 250/mL)[49]
- Severe heart failure (New York Heart Association class IV)
- Sepsis
- Pregnancy and lactation.

▎SPECIAL SITUATIONS

Pregnancy and Lactation[50]

Pregnancy category C drug: Much experience is derived from individual cases. Rituximab caused complete but transient B cell depletion in the newborn of a mother with Burkitt's lymphoma who received rituximab as a part of polychemotherapy.[51] In another lady who was inadvertently given rituximab during her first trimester of pregnancy, the course of pregnancy and its outcome was normal.[52] However, a recent review of pregnancy outcomes from the rituximab global drug safety database identified 231 cases of maternal rituximab exposure during pregnancy. Of 153 pregnancies with known outcomes, spontaneous abortion happened in 33 and elective termination was needed in 28. Of 90 live births, 22 had abnormalities at birth; four had neonatal infections and two had congenital malformations.[50] The reported miscarriage rate can be attributed to the autoimmune nature of the disease in the patients treated in addition to own teratogenic potential of rituximab and other immunosuppressants. No specific congenital malformation pattern associated with rituximab was reported and the malformation rate was comparable to the general obstetric population. Given the B cell depleting action of rituximab, the focus should be on detection of early signs of infection in the mother or in the neonate. Whether these neonates are able to mount protective immune response to vaccination warrants further studies.[53] A complete hemogram of the neonate may be ordered to detect clinically significant cytopenias, particularly when maternal exposure occurred shortly before or during gestation. Serial monitoring for leukopenias is not recommended. Contraception is recommended for 12 months after the last rituximab administration.[50] The European League Against Rheumatism (EULAR) task force advises the discontinuation of rituximab before planned pregnancy in view of insufficient data on fetal safety.[54] There are insufficient data to address the issue of safety for breastfed infants. Rituximab in low-level was documented in breast milk in a mother treated during lactation.[55] The data on paternal rituximab exposure and fetal outcome is also insufficient to draw a conclusion.

Children

Food and drug administration does not recommend rituximab in patients less than 16 years due to concerns regarding the potential for prolonged immunosuppression owing to B cell depletion in the actively developing juvenile immune system. There are reports suggesting that children with autoimmune disorders have an especially high-risk of infection and rituximab toxicities, including infusion reactions, low antimicrobial antibody titres, hypogammaglobulinemia, angioedema and fatal sepsis.[56] However, it was generally safe and effective in most of the children treated with rituximab. Nowadays, its use is increasing in children for newer indications like refractory nephrotic syndrome[57] and newer route of administration are being tried, for example intrathecal administration[58] for B cell lymphomas.

Latent Tuberculosis

Although the role of B cells in the host defense against *Mycobacterium tuberculosis* infection has been demonstrated in the previous studies,[59] active TB has not been reported from RA patients receiving rituximab therapy in clinical trials or in real-world practice. Only 3 cases of active TB were reported in a survey conducted by the Emerging Infections Network (EIN).[60] People with a positive Mantoux test or people with evidence of LTB, should be offered either 3 months of isoniazid (with pyridoxine) and rifampicin, or 6 months of isoniazid (with pyridoxine).[61] The IGRA provide a higher specificity than tuberculin skin test (TST) in detecting LTB in the BCG-vaccinated population.[60] The need of LTB screening prior to rituximab infusion is still debatable. However, some authors believe such screenings are mandatory.[47] One particular problem of performing Mantoux test in patients of active autoimmune bullous diseases who are considered for putting on rituximab is koebnerization at the local site giving a false impression of severe Mantoux test positivity.[62] In such an occurrence, histopathological examination of skin biopsy taken from the local site should be considered—in case of koebnerization, the histopathology features will be similar to that of the primary disease whereas in Mantoux positivity, the infiltrate will be comprised of lymphomononuclear cells and histiocytes.

Hepatitis B Infection[63,64]

Recently, the US FDA has issued black box warning on the risk of HBV reactivation in those who receive rituximab. Most experts believe that the risk of HBV reactivation is highest for anti-CD20 agents among immunosuppressive therapies.[65] Reactivation of HBV is diagnosed by the detection of HBV DNA in a previously HBV DNA negative patient or rise in HBV DNA by more than 2 $\log_{10}$ international units/mL (greater than or equal to 10-fold as in some studies from baseline or reverse seroconversion (previously HBsAg-negative becomes HBsAg-positive).

Screening

Risk for HBV reactivation following rituximab is particularly high in patients who are positive for HBsAg or anti-HBc. Whether or not to include anti-HBs in the screening process is still controversial. The presence of anti-HBs in unvaccinated patients could be the only marker of past HBV infection in HBsAg-negative/anti-HBc-negative patients. Reactivation of HBV is rare in such cases. However, some authors suggest "triple screening" (HBsAg, anti-HBc, and anti-HBs), because knowledge of anti-HBs status could increase vigilance during chronic therapy with high-risk biologics, such as rituximab, and may help to decide the vaccination against HBV prior to such therapy.

Based on the results of this initial screening, the following actions can be taken:

- HBsAg or anti-HBc-positive patients should have baseline HBV DNA levels measured.
- Patients who are nonimmune to HBV (anti HBs less than 10 IU/L) should be vaccinated.

Management Approach

- If HBsAg+ (chronic HBV infection): Start oral antiviral treatment
- If HBsAg-, anti-HBc+, and anti-HBs± (past HBV infection): Do HBV DNA levels at baseline, 6 months, and 12 months of last infusion; if present start oral antiviral treatment, if absent only regular monitoring is needed.
- If HBsAg-, anti-HBc-, and anti-HBs- (no previous exposure): Consider vaccination for patients at risk.
- If HBsAg-, anti-HBc-, and anti-HBs+ (history of HBV vaccination): No further action needed.

Regular monitoring for liver enzyme derangement is recommended in all of the above categories. The most recent guidelines recommend entecavir or tenofovir as antiviral agents against HBV. Prophylactic antiviral treatment was found to be superior to "on-demand" antiviral therapy in HBV reactivation. Treatment needs to be continued for at least 12 months after the last infusion of rituximab.

Hepatitis C Infection

The association between rituximab administration and hepatitis C virus (HCV) reactivation is controversial. HCV reactivation and hepatic complications reported in lymphoma patients can be attributed to the concomitant chemotherapy administered for lymphoma. Such complications were not reported in most of the rheumatology literature where rituximab was used without concomitant chemotherapy.[66] Rituximab has also been used for extrahepatic autoimmune manifestations of HCV like cryoglobulinemic vasculitis with good safety. Given the HCV-related hepatitis is also an immune phenomenon, rituximab associated HCV reactivation was not associated with adverse hepatic outcome. Coadministration of rituximab and interferon-α/ribavirin in HCV-related advanced liver disease did not increase the side effects in rheumatology patients.[67] However, increased hematological side effects were noted on concomitant administration of Rituximab-Cyclophosphamide, doxorubicin, vincristine, prednisolone (R-CHOP) plus anti-HCV treatment.[68] The presence of HCV infection is not a contraindication for rituximab administration. However, such patients are closely monitored for HCV viral load serially and should be managed under the supervision of a hepatologist.[66]

Human Immunodeficiency Virus (HIV)

The loss of humoral immunity by rituximab in addition to the underlying destruction of the cellular immune system by HIV may further increase the risk of infection. Hence, rituximab is contraindicated in HIV infection with CD4 cell count of less than $250/\mu L$.[49]

Active Severe Infection/Sepsis

Secondary bacterial infection in pemphigus is a usual scenario in dermatology practice and is a major cause of mortality. Hence, rituximab and any immunosuppressive agent should be used judiciously in this clinical setting. Active and serious infection contraindicates rituximab use and these infections should be ruled out by cultures of blood, urine, and pus. All patients with infection or bacteremia are potential candidates for sepsis. Modified version of the sequential (sepsis-related) organ failure assessment (SOFA) score called the quick SOFA (qSOFA) score helps to identify early sepsis.[69] The qSOFA score is easy to calculate at bedside and has three components each weighing one point: respiratory rate greater than or equal to 22/minute; altered mentation and systolic blood pressure less than or equal to 100 mm Hg. A score greater than or equal to 2 indicates poor prognosis due to sepsis and warrant prompt referral and further sepsis-related investigations. Other parameters like fall or rise in white cell counts, thrombocytopenia, rise in C-reactive protein (CRP), rising trend of serum lactate despite correcting dehydration, deranged organ function tests, and coagulopathy also point to sepsis. Even though nonspecific, serum procalcitonin levels more than two standard deviations above the normal value helps in a quick diagnosis of bacterial sepsis, even before getting culture reports.

Vaccinations[35,70,71]

It has been consistently seen that rituximab has the most profound impact on vaccine immunogenicity compared to other immunosuppressive agents. All the patients planned for rituximab therapy should be given all indicated vaccines like hepatitis B vaccination for at-risk population, *Pneumococcus*, tetanus toxoid vaccinations every 10 years and annual influenza vaccine. Though live vaccines are not routinely advocated in those who have been treated with rituximab recently, the risks need to be studied further. Ideally vaccination should be done before starting rituximab. If the treatment has already started, vaccines can be administered at least 6 months after the last dose and at least 4 weeks before the next course.

FUTURE TRENDS

Rituximab is increasingly used as a combination therapy with IVIg resulting in long-term disease free period in autoimmune disorders. Recent clinical trials have suggested rituximab as a first-line and monotherapy agent in pemphigus.[69,72] More studies are needed in this direction. Newer anti-CD20 biologicals have been introduced to address the issue of rituximab nonresponse. Second-generation monoclonal antibodies (e.g. ofatumumab) are humanized or fully human with unmodified Fc region, thus reducing the immunogenicity. Third-generation antibodies (e.g. obinutuzumab) have bioengineered Fc domains, thus improving the therapeutic activity especially in those who express low-affinity version of Fc receptor on B cells.

REFERENCES

1. Ahmed AR, Shetty S. The emerging role of rituximab in autoimmune blistering diseases. Am J Clin Dermatol. 2015;16:167-77.

2. Wang HH, Liu CW, Li YC, Huang YC. Efficacy of rituximab for pemphigus: A systematic review and meta-analysis of different regimens. Acta Derm Venereol. 2015;95:928-32.

3. Espana A, Ornilla E, Panizo C. Rituximab in dermatology. Actas Dermosifiliogr. 2013;104:380-92.

4. Heizmann M, Itin P, Wernli M, et al. Successful treatment of paraneoplastic pemphigus in follicular NHL with rituximab: report of a case and review of treatment for paraneoplastic pemphigus in NHL and CLL. Am J Hematol. 2001;66:142-4.

5. Qian SX, Li JY, Hong M, et al. Nonhematological autoimmunity (glomerulo-sclerosis, paraneoplastic pemphigus and paraneoplastic neurological syndrome) in a patient with chronic lymphocytic leukemia: diagnosis, prognosis and management. Leuk Res. 2009;33(3):500-5.

6. Rossum MM, Verhaegen NT, Jonkman MF, et al. Follicular non-Hodgkin's lymphoma with refractory paraneoplastic pemphigus: case report with review of novel treatment modalities. Leuk Lymphoma. 2004;45:2327-32.

7. Hoque SR, Black MM, Cliff S. Paraneoplastic pemphigus associated with CD20-positive follicular non-Hodgkin's lymphoma treated with rituximab: a third case resistant to rituximab therapy. Clin Exp Dermatol. 2007;32:172-5.

8. Levine TD. Rituximab in the treatment of dermatomyositis: an open-label pilot study. Arthritis Rheum. 2005;52:601-7.

9. Chung L, Genovese MC, Fiorentino DF. A pilot trial of rituximab in the treatment of patients with dermatomyositis. Arch Dermatol. 2007;143:763-7.

10. Cooper MA, Willingham DL, Brown DE, et al. Rituximab for the treatment of juvenile dermatomyositis: a report of four pediatric patients. Arthritis Rheum. 2007;56:3107-11.

11. Kieu V, O'Brien T, Yap LM, et al. Refractory subacute cutaneous lupus erythematosus successfully treated with rituximab. Australas J Dermatol. 2009;50:202-6.

12. Vital EM, Wittmann M, Edward S, et al. Brief report: Responses to rituximab suggest B cell-independent inflammation in cutaneous systemic lupus erythematosus. Arthritis Rheumatol. 2015;67:1586-91.

13. Merrill JT, Neuwelt CM, Wallace DJ, et al. Efficacy and safety of rituximab in moderately-to-severely active systemic lupus erythematosus: the randomized, double-blind, phase II/III systemic lupus erythematosus evaluation of rituximab trial. Arthritis Rheum. 2010;62:222-33.

14. Rovin BH, Furie R, Latinis K, et al. Efficacy and safety of rituximab in patients with active proliferative lupus nephritis: the Lupus Nephritis Assessment with Rituximab study. Arthritis Rheum. 2012;64:1215-26.

15. Kuhn A, Aberer E, Bata-Csorgo Z, et al. S2k guideline for treatment of cutaneous lupus erythematosus-guided by the European Dermatology Forum (EDF) in cooperation with the European Academy of Dermatology and Venereology (EADV). J Eur Acad Dermatol Venereol. 2017;31:389-404.

16. Jordan S, Distler JH, Maurer B, et al. Effects and safety of rituximab in systemic sclerosis: an analysis from the European Scleroderma Trial and Research (EUSTAR) group. Ann Rheum Dis. 2015;74:1188-94.

17. McQueen FM, Solanki K. Rituximab in diffuse cutaneous systemic sclerosis: should we be using it today? Rheumatology (Oxford). 2015;54:757-67.

18. Guillevin L, Pagnoux C, Karras A, et al. Rituximab versus azathioprine for maintenance in ANCA-associated vasculitis. N Engl J Med. 2014;371:1771-80.

19. Stone JH, Merkel PA, Spiera R, et al. Rituximab versus cyclophosphamide for ANCA-associated vasculitis. N Engl J Med. 2010;363:221-32.
20. Paterno G, Zizzari A, Nasso D, et al. Intravenous Administration of Rituximab in the Treatment of Primary Cutaneous B-Cell Lymphomas (PCBCLs): a retrospective study. Blood. 2014;124:5470.
21. Brandenburg A, Humme D, Terhorst D, et al. Long-term outcome of intravenous therapy with rituximab in patients with primary cutaneous B-cell lymphomas. Br J Dermatol. 2013;169:1126-32.
22. Valencak J, Weihsengruber F, Rappersberger K, et al. Rituximab monotherapy for primary cutaneous B-cell lymphoma: response and follow-up in 16 patients. Annals of Oncology. 2009;20:326-30.
23. Wilcox RA. Cutaneous B-cell lymphomas: 2016 update on diagnosis, risk-stratification, and management. Am J Hematol. 2016;91:1052-5.
24. Penate Y, Hernandez-Machin B, Perez-Mendez LI, et al. Intralesional rituximab in the treatment of indolent primary cutaneous B-cell lymphomas: an epidemiological observational multicentre study. The Spanish Working Group on Cutaneous Lymphoma. Br J Dermatol. 2012;167:174-9.
25. Fink-Puches R, Wolf IH, Zalaudek I, et al. Treatment of primary cutaneous B-cell lymphoma with rituximab. J Am Acad Dermatol. 2005;52:847-53.
26. Eberle FC, Holstein J, Scheu A, et al. Intralesional anti-CD20 antibody for low-grade primary cutaneous B-cell lymphoma: adverse reactions correlate with favorable clinical outcome. J Dtsch Dermatol Ges. 2017;15:319-23.
27. Vakeva L, Ranki A, Malkonen T. Intralesional rituximab treatment for primary cutaneous b-cell lymphoma: nine Finnish cases. Acta Derm Venereol. 2016;96:396-7.
28. Kim SJ, Lee JW, Jung CW, et al. Weekly rituximab followed by monthly rituximab treatment for steroid-refractory chronic graft-versus-host disease: results from a prospective, multicenter, phase II study. Haematologica. 2010;95:1935-42.
29. Arai S, Pidala J, Pusic I, et al. A randomized phase II crossover study of imatinib or rituximab for cutaneous sclerosis after hematopoietic cell transplantation. Clin Cancer Res. 2016;22:319-27.
30. Glass B, Hasenkamp J, Wulf G, et al. Rituximab after lymphoma-directed conditioning and allogeneic stem-cell transplantation for relapsed and refractory aggressive non-Hodgkin lymphoma (DSHNHL R3): an open-label, randomised, phase 2 trial. Lancet Oncol. 2014;15:757-66.
31. Simon D, Hosli S, Kostylina G, et al. Anti-CD20 (rituximab) treatment improves atopic eczema. J Allergy Clin Immunol. 2008;121:122-8.
32. Sanchez-Ramon S, Eguiluz-Gracia I, Rodriguez-Mazariego ME, et al. Sequential combined therapy with omalizumab and rituximab: a new approach to severe atopic dermatitis. J Investig Allergol Clin Immunol. 2013;23:190-6.
33. McDonald BS, Jones J, Rustin M. Rituximab as a treatment for severe atopic eczema: Failure to improve in three consecutive patients. Clin Exp Dermatol. 2016;41:45-7.
34. Trouvin AP, Jacquot S, Grigioni S, et al. Usefulness of monitoring of B cell depletion in rituximab-treated rheumatoid arthritis patients in order to predict clinical relapse: a prospective observational study. Clin Exp Immunol. 2015;180:11-8.
35. Buch MH, Smolen JS, Betteridge N, et al. Updated consensus statement on the use of rituximab in patients with rheumatoid arthritis. Ann Rheum Dis. 2011;70:909-20.

36. Castells MC, Tennant NM, Sloane DE, et al. Hypersensitivity reactions to chemotherapy: outcomes and safety of rapid desensitization in 413 cases. J Allergy Clin Immunol. 2008;122:574-80.

37. Amoros-Reboredo P, Sanchez-Lopez J, Bastida-Fernandez C, et al. Desensitization to rituximab in a multidisciplinary setting. Int J Clin Pharm. 2015;37:744-8.

38. Gudu T, Mazilu D, Peltea A, et al. A1.85 Can rituximab treatment in rheumatoid arthritis patients decrease cardiovascular risk? Ann Rheum Dis. 2014;73:A37-A38.

39. Provan SA, Berg IJ, Hammer HB, et al. The impact of newer biological disease modifying anti-rheumatic drugs on cardiovascular risk factors: a 12-month longitudinal study in rheumatoid arthritis patients treated with rituximab, abatacept and tociliziumab. PLoS One. 2015;10:e0130709.

40. Hsue PY, Scherzer R, Grunfeld C, et al. Depletion of B-cells with rituximab improves endothelial function and reduces inflammation among individuals with rheumatoid arthritis. J Am Heart Assoc. 2014;3:1-11.

41. Foran JM, Rohatiner AZ, Cunningham D, et al. European phase II study of rituximab (chimeric anti-CD20 monoclonal antibody) for patients with newly diagnosed mantle-cell lymphoma and previously treated mantle-cell lymphoma, immunocytoma, and small B-cell lymphocytic lymphoma. J Clin Oncol. 2000;18:317-24.

42. Passalia C, Minetto P, Arboscello E, et al. Cardiovascular adverse events complicating the administration of rituximab: report of two cases. Tumori. 2013;99:288e-92e.

43. Ng KH, Dearden C, Gruber P. Rituximab-induced Takotsubo syndrome: more cardiotoxic than it appears? BMJ Case Reports. 2015.

44. Verma SK. Updated cardiac concerns with rituximab use: a growing challenge. Indian Heart J. 2016;68(Suppl 2):S246-S8.

45. Roberts DM, Jones RB, Smith RM, et al. Rituximab-associated hypogammaglo-bulinemia: Incidence, predictors and outcomes in patients with multi-system autoimmune disease. J Autoimmun. 2015;57:60-5.

46. Gea-Banacloche JC. Rituximab-associated infections. Semin Hematol. 2010;47: 187-98.

47. Kelesidis T, Daikos G, Boumpas D, et al. Does rituximab increase the incidence of infectious complications? A narrative review. Int J Infect Dis. 2011;15:e2-e16.

48. Arai Y, Yamashita K, Mizugishi K, et al. Risk factors for late-onset neutropenia after rituximab treatment of B-cell lymphoma. Hematology. 2015;20:196-202.

49. Hertl M, Zillikens D, Borradori L, et al. Recommendations for the use of rituximab (anti-CD20 antibody) in the treatment of autoimmune bullous skin diseases. J Dtsch Dermatol Ges. 2008;6:366-73.

50. Chakravarty EF, Murray ER, Kelman A. Pregnancy outcomes after maternal exposure to rituximab. Blood. 2011;117:1499-506.

51. Friedrichs B, Tiemann M, Salwender H, et al. The effects of rituximab treatment during pregnancy on a neonate. Haematologica. 2006;91:1426-7.

52. Kimby E, Sverrisdottir A, Elinder G. Safety of rituximab therapy during the first trimester of pregnancy: a case history. Eur J Haematol. 2004;72:292-5.

53. Pendergraft WF, McGrath MM, Murphy AP, et al. Fetal outcomes after rituximab exposure in women with autoimmune vasculitis. Ann Rheum Dis. 2013;72: 2051-3.

54. Götestam Skorpen C, Hoeltzenbein M, Tincani A, et al. The EULAR points to consider for use of antirheumatic drugs before pregnancy, and during pregnancy and lactation. 2016;75:795-810.

55. Bragnes Y, Boshuizen R, de Vries A, et al. Low level of Rituximab in human breast milk in a patient treated during lactation. Rheumatology (Oxford). 2017.

56. Kincaid L, Weinstein M. Rituximab therapy for childhood pemphigus vulgaris. Pediatr Dermatol. 2016;33:e61-4.
57. Ravani P, Rossi R, Bonanni A, et al. Rituximab in children with steroid-dependent nephrotic syndrome: a multicenter, open-label, noninferiority, randomized controlled trial. J Am Soc Nephrol. 2015;26:2259-66.
58. Ceppi F, Weitzman S, Woessmann W, et al. Safety and efficacy of intrathecal rituximab in children with B cell lymphoid CD20+ malignancies: an international retrospective study. Am J Hematol. 2016;91:486-91.
59. Maglione PJ, Xu J, Chan J. B cells moderate inflammatory progression and enhance bacterial containment upon pulmonary challenge with Mycobacterium tuberculosis. J Immunol. 2007;178:7222-34.
60. Liao TL, Lin CH, Chen YM. Different risk of tuberculosis and efficacy of isoniazid prophylaxis in rheumatoid arthritis patients with biologic therapy: a nationwide retrospective cohort study in Taiwan. PLoS One. 2016;11:e0153217.
61. Hoppe LE, Kettle R, Eisenhut M, et al. Tuberculosis—diagnosis, management, prevention, and control: summary of updated NICE guidance. BMJ. 2016;352: h6747.
62. Vinay K, Kanwar A, Saikia U. Pemphigus occurring at tuberculin injection site: role of cytokines in acantholysis. Indian J Dermatol Venereol Leprol. 2013;79:539-41.
63. Kusumoto S, Tobinai K. Screening for and management of hepatitis B virus reactivation in patients treated with anti-B-cell therapy. Hematology Am Soc Hematol Educ Program. 2014;2014:576-83.
64. Koutsianas C, Thomas K, Vassilopoulos D. Hepatitis B reactivation in rheumatic diseases: screening and prevention. Rheum Dis Clin North Am. 2017;43:133-49.
65. Perrillo RP, Gish R, Falck-Ytter YT. American Gastroenterological Association Institute technical review on prevention and treatment of hepatitis B virus reactivation during immunosuppressive drug therapy. Gastroenterology. 2015;148:221-44.e3.
66. Amber KT, Kodiyan J, Bloom R, et al. The controversy of hepatitis C and rituximab: a multidisciplinary dilemma with implications for patients with pemphigus. Indian J Dermatol Venereol Leprol. 2016;82:182-3.
67. Petrarca A, Rigacci L, Caini P, et al. Safety and efficacy of rituximab in patients with hepatitis C virus-related mixed cryoglobulinemia and severe liver disease. Blood. 2010;116:335-42.
68. Musto P, Dell'Olio M, La Sala A, et al. Diffuse B-Large cell lymphomas (DBLCL) with hepatitis-C virus (HCV) infection: clinical outcome and preliminary results of a pilot study combining R-CHOP with antiviral therapy. Blood. 2005;106:2447.
69. Seymour CW, Liu VX, Iwashyna TJ, et al. Assessment of clinical criteria for sepsis: for the third international consensus definitions for sepsis and septic shock (Sepsis-3). JAMA. 2016;315:762-74.
70. Friedman MA, Winthrop KL. Vaccines and disease-modifying antirheumatic drugs: practical implications for the rheumatologist. Rheum Dis Clin North Am. 2017;43:1-13.
71. Westra J, Rondaan C, van Assen S, et al. Vaccination of patients with autoimmune inflammatory rheumatic diseases. Nat Rev Rheumatol. 2015;11:135-45.
72. Joly P, Maho-Vaillant M, Prost-Squarcioni C, et al. First-line rituximab combined with short-term prednisone versus prednisone alone for the treatment of pemphigus (Ritux 3): a prospective, multicentre, parallel-group, open-label randomised trial. Lancet. 2017;389:2031-40.

Chapter

12

Anti-IgE Monoclonal Antibody: Omalizumab

Kiran Godse

INTRODUCTION

Omalizumab is a recombinant humanized immunoglobulin G1 (IgG1) monoclonal antibody against human immunoglobulin E (IgE). It blocks the attachment of IgE to mast cells and other immune cells, and reduces serum levels of IgE, thereby preventing IgE-mediated inflammatory changes.

PHARMACOLOGY

It is derived from a murine monoclonal antibody which was humanized to produce omalizumab in its present form. The complementarity-determining regions (CDRs) form 5% of its nonhuman amino-acid residues.[1]

CHARACTERISTICS

- Route of administration—subcutaneous
- Peak serum concentration—after 7–8 days
- Half-life—around 26 days
- Elimination—via reticuloendothelial system
- Distributed in intravascular compartment.

MECHANISM OF ACTION

Omalizumab binds to free IgE with a greater affinity than IgE itself binds to the high affinity FcɛRI receptors on the basophils. It binds to IgE at the same site where it binds to FcɛRI receptor, thus reducing the availability of free IgE for binding. Omalizumab forms IgE–anti IgE complex, thereby reducing free IgE level by up to 90%. These hexamers are nonimmunogenic, have half-life of about 40 days and are cleared by reticuloendothelial system. Serum total IgE level increases after first dose due to formation of omalizumab–IgE complexes.

Omalizumab does not bind to the receptor-bound IgE nor the FcɛRI receptor. Thus, omalizumab neutralizes IgE-mediated immune response without causing basophil degranulation or cross-linking with basophil-bound IgE.

Omalizumab also promotes FcεRI receptor downregulation on basophils as the number of FcεRI receptors on basophil depends on the free serum IgE levels.

The reduced levels of IgE cause dissociation of IgE from basophils with subsequent receptor downregulation.[2]

USES

Food and Drug Administration (FDA) Approved

- *Non-dermatological use*: Bronchial asthma
- *Dermatological use*: Chronic spontaneous urticaria (CSU)

Off-label Indications

- Atopic dermatitis (AD)
- Bullous pemphigoid
- Systemic mastocytosis
- Hyperimmunoglobulin E syndrome (HIES).

Bronchial Asthma

It is approved for use in moderate-to-severe persistent asthma in adults and adolescents older than 12 years of age with a positive skin test to a perennial antigen. The body weight and pretreatment serum IgE levels determine the dose in bronchial asthma and is administered subcutaneously every 2–4 weeks.[3] In July 2016, FDA expanded use of omalizumab to patients aged 6 years and older with moderate-to-severe persistent asthma.

Chronic Spontaneous Urticaria

The US FDA approved omalizumab on 21st March, 2014 for use in CSU.[2]

The recommended dose is 300 mg by subcutaneous injection every 4 weeks. Some patients may achieve control of their symptoms with a dose of 150 mg every 4 weeks.

In other cases, dose needs to be increased to 300 mg every 2 weeks.

The dose is not based on body weight or serum IgE level. The appropriate duration of omalizumab therapy for CSU has not been evaluated. Periodic reassessment of the need for continued medication is recommended.[4,5]

There are three landmark studies on the use of omalizumab in CSU, namely ASTERIA 1 study, ASTERIA 2 study and GLACIAL study. In the above three studies, a total of 733 patients having CSU received omalizumab and it was found to be effective and safe in the dose of 300 mg 4-weekly subcutaneous injections.

There was 62–71% reduction in itch from baseline at 12 weeks, 34–44% of patients were itch- and hive-free at 12 weeks and 73–78% had improvement in Dermatology Life Quality Index scores at 12 weeks, respectively. Common side effects observed were injection site reactions, headache, joint pain and upper respiratory infections.[6-8]

Omalizumab is a safe and effective alternative to corticosteroids for refractory urticaria patients. It is equally effective and safe for long-term use up to 4 years.[9]

Off-label Use of Omalizumab in Other Diseases

Atopic Dermatitis

It is believed that omalizumab may be useful in the treatment of AD because it is associated with elevated serum IgE levels.[10]

There have been mixed reports about the efficacy of omalizumab in treatment of AD with Lane et al.[11] reporting significant improvement in three patients, Vigo et al.[12] showed improvement in five out of seven patients, while Krathen and Hsu[13] described three cases of severe AD in adults who did not respond to omalizumab. Hotze et al. conducted a pilot study and found omalizumab to be effective in subset of patient with AD, who had absent filaggrin mutation and higher serum level of phosphatidylcholine.[14] Thus, based on these reports, it is currently difficult to make recommendations about use of omalizumab in cases of AD and more studies are needed to validate the effectiveness of omalizumab for AD.

Bullous Pemphigoid

The standard therapy for bullous pemphigoid is systemic steroids plus a potentially steroid-sparing agent. Compared to the standard therapy, omalizumab has a relatively selective effect. Omalizumab may be an effective and relatively safe therapeutic option for patients with bullous pemphigoid who do not respond to or have contraindications to standard treatment. The onset of action is rapid and a dose of 300 mg/month may be sufficient to suppress the blistering.[15]

Systemic Mastocytosis

Omalizumab has been reported to be safe and effective in preventing recurrent anaphylaxis in patients with systemic mastocytosis.[16]

Hyperimmunoglobulin E Syndrome

It is a heterogenous group of immune disorders characterized by very high levels of serum IgE, dermatitis, and recurrent skin and lung infections. Studies report clinical improvement in patients with high serum IgE levels and presenting with severe atopic eczema.[17,18]

ADMINISTRATION

- Available as lyophilized powder and a solvent water for injection.
- One vial of omalizumab 150 mg powder and solvent for solution for injection delivers 150 mg of omalizumab.
- Reconstituted solution contains 125 mg/mL of omalizumab (150 mg in 1.2 mL).
- For omalizumab 150 mg vial, 1.4 mL of water for injection is transferred into the vial.
- The vial is swirled in an upright position (do not shake) for 5–10 seconds every 5 minutes to dissolve the products.
- The lyophilized product takes 15–20 minutes to dissolve completely forming a clear viscous solution.
- The solution may have few small bubbles along the edge of the vial.
- Using a syringe equipped with an 18-gauge needle, the solution is withdrawn from the inverted vial.
- The 18-gauge needle is replaced by a 25-gauge needle for subcutaneous injection.
- The excess solution is expelled to obtain the required 1.2 mL dose.
- As the solution is viscous, the injection takes 5–10 seconds to administer.[19]

Tests to be Done Prior to Administration

Complete blood count, random blood sugar, urine routine and microscopy should be done before starting omalizumab. There is no need to screen for tuberculosis as is done for other biologicals.

- Body weight measurement and baseline serum IgE levels are not required before the administration of omalizumab for CSU.

MONITORING DURING THERAPY

Omalizumab does not necessitate hospital admission for administration.

It should only be administered by a health care professional or a physician, who is trained in the recognition and treatment of anaphylaxis, in a setting where the appropriate equipment is available to respond to an episode of anaphylaxis.[19]

The patient should be observed for a period of 2 hours for the first three injections and for 30 minutes for subsequent injections as an incidence of 0.2% of anaphylaxis has been reported.[20]

There are rare reports of thrombocytopenia hence, monitoring of platelet counts at baseline and during therapy may be advisable.

All reports of thrombocytopenia have been transient and reversible. Currently, there are no guidelines available for monitoring of platelet counts.[14]

ADVERSE EFFECTS

The safety profile of omalizumab is favorable with injection site reaction being the most common reported adverse event.[21]

Anaphylaxis

In the post marketing spontaneous reports, the frequency of anaphylaxis was estimated to be 0.2%.

In the phase 3 study by Maurer et al., the reported adverse events were influenza viral infection, headache, neck pain and discomfort, upper respiratory tract infection, musculoskeletal and connective tissue pain and discomfort, asthenic conditions, mononeuropathies, and urticaria.[1]

Thrombocytopenia is a known side effect.

CONTRAINDICATIONS

Absolute

Known hypersensitivity to omalizumab

Special Situations

- *Renal or hepatic impairment*: As omalizumab is primarily degraded in the reticular endothelial system, no dose adjustment is recommended in renal or hepatic impairment.
- *Pregnancy*: There are no adequate studies of omalizumab in pregnant women, but it is a pregnancy category B drug. It should be administered only if benefit outweighs the risks.[22,23]
- *Lactation*: The presence of omalizumab in human milk and its potential harm to the infant has not been studied, it should be administered with caution to nursing mothers.[18]
- *Geriatric patients*: No dose adjustment required in the elderly patients.
- *Pediatric patients*: Safety and efficacy in this group has not been established. It is approved for use in children aged 12 years and older.

REFERENCES

1. Belliveau PP. Omalizumab: a monoclonal anti-IgE antibody. Med Gen Med. 2005;7:27.
2. Godse K, Mehta A, Patil S, et al. Omalizumab—a review. Indian J Dermatol. 2015;60:381-4.
3. Graves JE, Nunley K, Heffernan MP. Off-label uses of biologics in dermatology: rituximab, omalizumab, infliximab, etanercept, adalimumab, efalizumab and alefacept. J Am Acad Dermatol. 2007;56:55-79.

4. Navines-Ferrer A, Serrano-Candelas E, Molina-Molina G, et al. IgE-related chronic diseases and anti-IgE-based treatments. J Immunol Res. 2016;2016:8163803.
5. U.S. Food and Drug Administration (2016). Xolair (Omalizumab) for injection, for subcutaneous use. Highlights of Prescribing Information. [online] Available from http://www.accessdata.fda.gov/drugsatfda_docs/label/2014/103976s5211lbl.pdf [Accessed December 2017].
6. Maurer M, Rosen K, Hsieh HJ, et al. Omalizumab for the treatment of chronic idiopathic or spontaneous urticaria. N Engl J Med. 2013;368:924-35.
7. Saini S, Rosen KE, Hsieh HJ, et al. A randomized, placebo-controlled, dose-ranging study of single-dose omalizumab in patients with H1-antihistamine-refractory chronic idiopathic urticaria. J Allergy Clin Immunol. 2011;128:567-73.
8. Rottem M, Segal R, Kivity S, et al. Omalizumab therapy for chronic spontaneous urticaria: the Israeli experience. Isr Med Assoc J. 2014;16:487-90.
9. Godse K, Rajagopalan M, Girdhar M, et al. Position statement for the use of Omalizumab in the management of chronic spontaneous urticaria in Indian patients. Indian Dermatol Online J. 2016;7:6-11.
10. Johansson SG, Haahtela T, O'Byrne PM. Omalizumab and the immune system: an overview of preclinical and clinical data. Ann Allergy Asthma Immunol. 2002;89:132-8.
11. Lane Je, Cheyney JM, Lane TN, et al. Treatment of recalcitrant atopic dermatitis with Omalizumab. J Am Acad Dermatol. 2006;54:68-72.
12. Vigo PG, Girgis KR, Pfuetze BL, et al. Efficacy of anti-IgE therapy in patients with atopic dermatitis. J Am Acad Dermatol. 2006;55:168-70.
13. Krathen RA, Hsu S. Failure of omalizumab for treatment of severe adult atopic dermatitis. J Am Acad Dermatol. 2005;53:338-40.
14. Hotze M, Baurecht H, Rodríguez E, et al. Increased efficacy of omalizumab in atopic dermatitis patients with wild-type filaggrin status and higher serum levels of phosphatidylcholines. Allergy. 2014;69(1):132-5.
15. Gonul M, Keseroglu HO, Ergin C, et al. Bullous pemphigoid successfully treated with omalizumab. Indian J Dermatol Venereol Leprol. 2016;82:577-9.
16. Douglass J, Caroll K, Voskamp A, et al. Omalizumab is effective in treating systemic mastocytosis in a nonatopic patient. Allergy. 2010;65(7):926-7.
17. Belloni B, Ziai M, Lim A, et al. Low dose anti-IgE therapy in patients with atopic eczema with high serum IgE levels. J Allergy Clin Immunol. 2007;120(5):1223-5.
18. Chulanrojanamontri L, Wimoolchart S, Tuuchinda P, et al. Role of omalizumab in a patient with hyper-IgE syndrome and review dermatologic manifestations. Asian Pac J Allergy Immunol. 2009;27(4):233-6.
19. Novartis Healthcare Private Limited India. Full prescribing information of Xolair (omalizumab). 2015.
20. Kim HL, Leigh R, Becker A. Omalizumab: practical considerations regarding the risk of anaphylaxis. Allergy Asthma Clin Immunol. 2010;6:32.
21. Cox L, Platts-Mills TA, Finegold I, et al. American Academy of Allergy, Asthma and Immunology/American College of Allergy, Asthma and Immunology Joint Taskforce Report on omalizumab-associated anaphylaxis. J Allergy Clin Immunol. 2007;120:1373-7.
22. Godse K. Omalizumab in severe chronic urticaria. Indian J Dermatol Venereol Leprol. 2008;74:157-8.
23. Godse K, Vasani R. Viva voce on omalizumab. Indian J Drugs Dermatol. 2016;2:121-3.

Chapter

13

Intravenous Immunoglobulins

Rajesh Verma, Vijendran P, Aneesh KP

INTRODUCTION

Intravenous immunoglobulin (IVIg) was originally used for antibody replacement therapies in primary immune deficiencies. A multitude of dermatologic disorders have shown potential for treatment with this unique treatment modality. The dermatoses successfully treated with IVIg include autoimmune bullous diseases, connective tissue diseases, vasculitis, Stevens-Johnson syndrome (SJS), toxic epidermal necrolysis (TEN) and infectious disorders such as streptococcal toxic shock syndrome.[1,2] Lack of randomized controlled trials (RCTs) is a hindrance to the regular use of IVIg. Nevertheless, there is a significant body of evidence demonstrating the efficacy of IVIg in patients with skin diseases that are resistant to treatment with standard agents. IVIg is used as a disease-modifying agent or an adjuvant to conventional therapy.

STRUCTURE OF IMMUNOGLOBULIN

Immunoglobulins are produced by plasma cells in response to an immunogen and are glycoprotein molecules that function as antibodies. They all are built from the same basic units. The structure and the components of an immunoglobulin are depicted in Figures 13.1A and B.

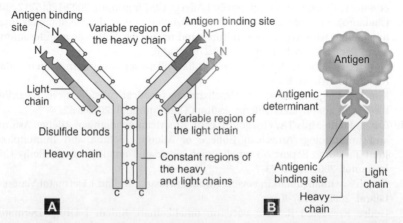

Figs. 13.1A and B: Structure of immunoglobulin.[3] (A) Structure; (B) Antigen binding site.

METHODS OF PREPARATION OF IVIg

Intravenous immunoglobulin contains supraphysiologic levels of IgG and is derived from fractionated human plasma. Immunoglobulin preparations are obtained from purified human plasma of 3,000 to approximately 10,000 individual donors per batch. Pooling is performed to provide repertoire representing all antibodies and also natural autoantibodies.[4] The donors are free from any infections and chronic diseases. They should be screened for hepatitis B surface antigens, anti-HCV antibodies, HIV-1 and HIV-2 antibodies. There is a "look back" screening period of 60 days for donors. Any seroconversion of a donor during this period would result in quarantine and destruction of the plasma obtained.[5,6]

COMPOSITION OF IVIg

Intravenous immunoglobulin is a highly purified IgG preparation which typically contains more than 95% of unmodified IgG with functionally intact Fc-dependent effector functions and only trace amounts of IgA, IgE and IgM.[2] Subclass distribution may vary between preparations, with some products having less than physiological levels of IgG_3 and/or IgG_4.[5] It may also contain small amounts of albumin, sugars, salts, solvents, detergents, and buffers.[5] Variability of the manufacturing processes may lead to differences in the marketed IVIg products. Factors affecting the biological activity and integrity of the IgG molecule, tolerability, and yield depends on production steps like stabilization and purification.

PHARMACOKINETICS

Peak serum concentrations occur immediately after intravenous (IV) injection and are dose related. Up to 30% of the dose may be removed by catabolism and distribution within 24 hours. IVIg distributes in the intravascular (60%) and extravascular (40%) compartments and can cross placenta and is excreted in milk. The serum half-life is 3–5 weeks.[7,8] Higher the concentration of the IVIg product, the less volume required for infusion. For example, a 70 kg individual receiving 1 g/kg would require either 700 mL of a 10% solution or 1400 mL of a 5% solution. In high-risk patients, such as those with cardiac or renal failure, these factors must be taken into consideration. In selecting the most appropriate IVIg for the patient, convenience, efficacy, safety, and tolerability of the different products must be considered.

MECHANISM OF ACTION

The mechanism by which high-dose intravenous immunoglobulin mediates anti-inflammatory activity is not well-understood. The effects are mediated via the Fc portion of IgG or the antigen-binding site and the variable regions of the antibody molecule.[2] The proposed mechanism of action of high-dose IVIg is discussed in Table 13.1.

The complex interplay of these effects is diagrammatically represented in Figure 13.2.

Table 13.1: Mechanism of action of high-dose intravenous immunoglobulin (IVIg).[5,9]

Mechanism	Remarks	Example
Reduced antibody production	By IgG binding via its Fc fragment (crystallizable) to corresponding cellular surface receptors on B lymphocytes	Autoantibodies directed against factor VIII, DNA, intrinsic factor, thyroglobulin and antineutrophil cytoplasmic antibodies (ANCA)
	Downregulation of pathogenic autoantibody production	
Increased catabolism of antibodies	Reduced half-life of circulating immunoglobulins, probably by saturating the protective neonatal Fc receptor (FcRn)	
Effect on complement system	Bind to complement components C3b and C4b	Dermatomyositis
	Block complement activation at an early stage	
	Interfere with the formation of the terminal membrane attack complex (MAC)	
Functional blockade of Fc receptors	Fc receptors are saturated by "anti-idiotypic" antibodies in IVIg	Idiopathic thrombo-cytopenic purpura
	Decreased cellular destruction as a consequence of Fc-mediated phagocytosis of antibody-coated cells in auto-antibody mediated diseases.	
Effect on T-Cell activation	IVIg preparations contain amounts of soluble CD4, CD8, MHC-I and -II molecules which may have the ability to inhibit autoreactive T lymphocytes	--
	Modulates the production of IL-1, -2, -3, -4, -5, -10, TNF-α, GM-CSF and IL-1 receptor antagonist by monocytes, macrophages, and lymphocytes	
	Restoration of a Th1/Th2 cytokine balance by supplying neutralizing antibodies	
Activation or functional blockade of the death receptor Fas (CD95)	IVIg can either inhibit or activate cell death by binding to the death receptor Fas	SJS/TEN
	Mediated by agonistic anti-Fas IgG and antagonistic anti-Fas IgG	
	Inhibitory Fc receptor, FcγRIIB, is shown to be required for protection	

Contd...

Contd...

Mechanism	Remarks	Example
Synergistic effect with corticosteroids	Adjunctive use of IVIg has led to reduced dose requirements for systemic corticosteroids	–
	Because of increased glucocorticoid receptor sensitivity	
	IVIg and corticosteroids can synergistically suppress the lymphocyte activation.	

(IVIg: Intravenous immunoglobulin; CD: Cluster of differentiation; MHC: Major histocompatibility complex; IL: Interleukin; TNF-α: Tumor necrosis factor-α; GM-CSF: Granulocyte-macrophage colony-stimulating factor; SJS: Stevens-Johnson syndrome; TEN: Toxic epidermal necrolysis; FcγRIIB: Fcγ receptor IIB).

INDICATIONS IN DERMATOLOGY

The only Food and Drug Administration (FDA) approved indication for use of IVIg from a dermatology point of view is Kawasaki disease. The other indications and contraindications for use of IVIg in dermatology are listed in Boxes 13.1 and 13.2.

Indications for high-dose IVIg in autoimmune bullous diseases are given in Box 13.3.

DOSAGE REGIMEN

The most commonly used dosage regimen in dermatology to produce desired or expected results is 2 g/kg/cycle, divided into 3 equal doses, given on each of 3 consecutive days. Some studies have advocated the use of 400 mg/kg daily given over a course of 5 days to constitute a cycle. The infusion is given slowly over 4–4.5 hours and vital signs are monitored frequently.[9]

As the half-life of IVIg ranges from 3 to 5 weeks, the infusions are generally spaced at monthly intervals. But in very aggressive diseases it may be shortened up to once in every 2 weeks. A maintenance schedule which has been proposed is to increase the interval between two infusions in the increment of 2 weeks keeping the dose of the infusion the same, till a maximum interval of 16 weeks is achieved.[9,12]

A review of major clinical trials, case series of IVIg in dermatology, European Academy of Dermatology and Venereology (EADV) guidelines, summary of evidence and recommended dosing schedule is summarized in Table 13.2.

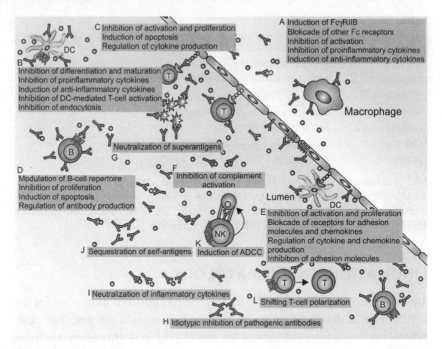

Fig. 13.2: The complex interplay of various effects of high-dose intravenous immunoglobulin (IVIg).[10]

The mechanisms that underlie the beneficial effects of IVIg involve its direct interaction with various cellular and soluble components of the immune system. IVIg stimulates the expression of FcγRIIB on a subset of macrophages while blocking the expression of FcγRIIA (A). IVIg also modulates cytokine secretion, blocks the expression of Fc receptors and inhibits the activation of macrophages (A) and dendritic cells (B). In addition to inhibition of the activation and production of pro-inflammatory cytokines by T cells (C), IVIg downregulates DC-mediated T-cell proliferation. At the B-cell level (D), IVIg modulates antibody synthesis and the B-cell repertoire, inhibits B-cell proliferation and induces B-cell apoptosis. In endothelial cells (E) IVIg blocks the expression of pro-inflammatory cytokines, chemokines, and adhesion molecules. Several other mechanisms of action of IVIg exist: interference with complement activation (F); neutralization of superantigens (G), pathogenic autoantibodies (H) and cytokines (I); sequestration of self antigens (J); induction of ADCC (K) and shifting the balance between T-helper cell subsets (L). The area encompassed by endothelial cells represents the vascular lumen. Adhesion molecules on endothelial cells are depicted. IVIg is depicted in the form of antibody structures with different colors to highlight the fact that it is a polyclonal IgG obtained from pooled plasma from a large number of healthy blood donors. Soluble factors such as complement proteins and cytokines are indicated by colored circles.

(IVIg: Intravenous immunoglobulin; ADCC: Antibody-dependent cell-mediated cytotoxicity; B: B cell; DC: Dendritic cell; EC: Endothelial cell; Fc: Crystallizable fragment; FcγR: Fcγ receptors; NK: Natural killer cell; T: T cell).

Box 13.1: Indications for use of high-dose intravenous immunoglobulin (IVIg).[13-17]

Indications
FDA approved indication
Kawasaki disease
Off-label indications
Autoimmune connective tissue disorders
Systemic lupus erythematosus
Scleroderma
Dermatomyositis/polymyositis
Autoimmune bullous dermatoses
Pemphigus vulgaris and foliaceous
Bullous pemphigoid
Pemphigoid gestationis
Cicatricial pemphigoid
Linear IgA bullous dermatoses
Epidermolysis bullosa acquisita
Steven Johnsons syndrome/Toxic epidermal necrolysis
Other inflammatory dermatoses
Chronic autoimmune urticaria
Atopic dermatitis
Psoriasis
Pyoderma gangrenosum
Graft-Versus-Host disease
Other dermatoses
Scleromyxoedema
Pretibial myxedema
Livedoid vasculopathy
Necrobiotic xanthogranuloma

Box 13.2: Contraindications for use of high-dose intravenous immunoglobulin (IVIg).[9]

Contraindications	
Absolute	*Relative*
Anaphylaxis secondary to previous infections	Renal Failure (risk of fluid overload)
	IgA Deficiency (risk of anaphylaxis)
	Congestive cardiac failure
	Rheumatoid arthritis (risk of renal failure)
	Cryoglobulinemia (risk of renal failure)

Pregnancy Category C

Clinical experience does not suggest harmful effect on pregnancy or fetus. Should be used if benefit outweighs the risk.

(IVIg: Intravenous immunoglobulin).

Box 13.3: Indications for high-dose IVIg in autoimmune bullous diseases.[11]

1. Disease is progressive in spite of administering appropriate maximum yet safe conventional systemic therapy
2. Significant adverse effects of conventional therapy
3. Conventional therapy has failed
4. Absolute and relative contraindications to the use of high-dose long-term systemic steroids or immunosuppressive agents

(IVIg: Intravenous immunoglobulin).

Table 13.2: Summary of evidence and recommended dosing schedule of high-dose intravenous immunoglobulin (IVIg) in various dermatological indications.[4,18-28]

Indications	Summary of evidence	Dosing	Response time	Remarks
Dermatomyositis[4]	Level of evidence I-b, grade of recommendation grade A	2 g/kg (over 2 days). Initially given every month for 6 cycles	1–2 months to response; maximal response at 3 months	Resistant or intolerant to prednisone or immunosuppressives
Kawasaki's disease[4,21]	Level of evidence I a, recommendation grade A	2 g/kg (over 6–12 hours) for a period of 3–6 months	Clinical response in 4.5 months	In addition, acetylsalicylic acid with an initial dose of 50 mg/kg body weight per day is administered
Toxic epidermal necrolysis[18,26-28]	Case series, evidence level II a, recommendation grade B	2–3 gm/kg over 3–5 days	Mean time to response: 2.3 days. Mean time for skin healing: 15 days. Objective response rate: 90% Survival rate: 88%	Administered at the earliest on confirmation of the diagnosis. The onset of reepithelialization is the best clinical parameter for evaluating treatment efficacy.
Pemphigus variants[22,23]	Case series, anecdotal evidence	2 g/kg (over 2–3 days) Initially given every month, maintenance schedule individualized	Clinical response in 4.5 months	Adjunctive or second-line therapy

Contd...

Contd...

Indications	Summary of evidence	Dosing	Response time	Remarks
Bullous pemphigoid[24]	Case series, anecdotal evidence	2 g/kg (over 2–3 days) Initially given every month, maintenance schedule individualized	Mean effective clinical response: 2.9 months	Adjunctive or second-line therapy
Mucous membrane pemphigoid[25]	Case series, anecdotal evidence	2–3 g/kg (over 3 days) Initially given every 2–6 weeks, maintenance schedule individualized	Maximum response between 4 cycles and 12 cycles	Adjunctive or second-line therapy
Epidermolysis bullosa acquisita	Case series, anecdotal evidence	2 g/kg (over 2–3 days) Initially given every month, maintenance schedule individualized	-	Adjunctive or second-line therapy
Wegener's granulomatosis and microscopic polyangiitis[4]	Level of evidence I a, recommendation grade B	2 g/kg (over 2–3 days). Initially given every month, for a period of 3–6 months, maintenance schedule individualized	-	IVIg prevents massive tissue destruction and thus reduce the extent of defects in Wegener's granulomatosis.

(IVIg: Intravenous immunoglobulin).

ADVERSE EFFECTS

High-dose IVIg infusion is a complex therapy and can lead to various adverse effects. Fortunately, most IVIg infusion reactions are back or abdominal aching or pain, nausea, rhinitis, asthma, chills, low grade fever, myalgia, and/or headache. Mild reactions can be reversed by slowing or stopping the infusion for 15–30 minutes.[9] Recalcitrant reactions can be managed by

Table 13.3: Common adverse reactions and precautions to high-dose IVIg.[9]

Adverse reaction	Remarks
Infusion-related general effects	Generally mild, 30–60 min after initiation of infusion
	Easily managed by slowing down the infusion rate or temporarily discontinuing the infusion.
Anaphylaxis and other hypersensitivity reactions	Increased risk in patients with IgA deficiency with anti-IgA antibodies and those with previous infections
	Erythema multiforme, purpura and alopecia have also been reported
Risk of fluid overload	Acute renal failure due to "osmotic nephrosis"
Hematological side effects	Neutropenia and hemolysis in patients with autoantibodies against blood group antigens of the ABO and Rhesus (Rh) system
Neurologic side effects	Aseptic meningitis (11% of neurological patients)
Thromboembolic events	Because of high osmolality and viscosity of the preparation, cerebral and myocardial infarctions reported
	Risk may be reduced by slowing down the rate of infusion.

50–100 mg of injection hydrocortisone and oral NSAIDs. Adverse reactions are particularly likely in patients who have not received IVIg previously and who have or recently have had a bacterial infection. Irrespective of an individual patient's personal experience with IVIg, vigilance needs to be maintained for detecting and managing reactions. The common adverse reactions and precautions to use high-dose IVIg is listed in Table 13.3.

MONITORING GUIDELINES

The monitoring guidelines have been illustrated in Table 13.4.

CONCLUSION

As more and more studies are collated, the understanding of the role of IVIg is increasing. Our knowledge of the properties, clinical management and potential benefits of IVIg has increased greatly over the past several years. Newer processing techniques have improved the quality of the IVIg. Although evidence-based data supporting the use of high dose IVIg is lacking in many indications, one has to bear in mind the fact that its use is beneficial in many dermatological conditions if risk-benefit ratio is considered. Careful matching of the most appropriate IVIg preparation with

Table 13.4: Monitoring guidelines for use of high-dose intravenous immunoglobulin (IVIg).[9]

Baseline
History and physical examination
Complete history and physical with emphasis on cardiopulmonary and renal status
Weigh patient prior to treatment for comparison if at risk of fluid overload
Laboratory
Complete blood count (CBC)
Assess liver function and renal function—LFT and RFT
Immunoglobulin levels—particularly IgA (if defective, anti-IgA titers of the IVIg preparation need to be assessed)
Screen for rheumatoid factor (RA factor) and cryoglobulins
Screening for Hepatitis B, C and HIV
Follow-up
During infusion
Monitor blood pressure and heart rate frequently
Assess for fluid overload: weight of the patient, auscultate lungs and heart
Laboratory
No specific follow-up laboratory testing required

(LFT: Liver function tests; RFT: Renal function tests; HIV: Human immunodeficiency virus).

each patient and his or her risk factors and consideration of the actual cost-benefit ratio of treatment with IVIg compared with alternative therapeutic options are a must before undertaking treatment.

REFERENCES

1. Orange JS, Hossny EM, Weiler CR, et al. Use of intravenous immunoglobulin in human disease: a review of evidence by members of the Primary Immunodeficiency Committee of the American Academy of Allergy, Asthma and Immunology. J Allergy Clin Immunol. 2006;117(4 Suppl):S525-53.
2. Sandipan Dhar. IVIG in dermatology. Indian J Dermatol. 2009;54(1):77-9.
3. RJ Poljak, LM Amzel, HP Avey, et al. Three-dimensional structure of the Fab' fragment of a human immunoglobulin at 2.8-Å resolution. Proc Natl Acad Sci U S A. 1973;70(12):3305-10.
4. Alexander Enk. Guideline on the use of high-dose intravenous immunoglobulin in dermatology: developed by the Guideline Subcommittee of the European Dermatology Forum. Eur J Dermatol. 2009;19(1):90-8.
5. Prins C, Gelfand EW, French LE. French. Intravenous Immunoglobulin: properties, mode of action and practical use in dermatology. Acta Derm Venereol. 2007;87:206-18.
6. Martin TD. IVIG: contents, properties and methods of industrial production—evolving closer to a more physiologic product. Int Immunopharmacol. 2006;6:517-22.

7. Morell A, Schurch B, Ryser D et al. In vivo behaviour of gamma globulin preparations. Vox Sang. 1980;38:272-83.
8. Morell A, Riesen W, Nydegger UE et al. Structure, Function and Catabolism of Immunoglobulins in Immunotherapy. London: Academic Press; 1981.
9. Wolverton SE. Intravenous immunoglobulin therapy, Comprehensive Dermatologic Drug Therapy, Third Edition. Elsevier; 2012. p. 390.
10. Bayry J, Lacroix-Desmazes S, Kazatchkine MD, et al. Monoclonal antibody and intravenous immunoglobulin therapy for rheumatic diseases: rationale and mechanisms of action. Nat Clin Pract Rheumatology. 2007;3:262-72.
11. Ahmed AR, Dahl MV. Consensus statement in the use of intravenous immunoglobulin therapy in the treatment of autoimmune mucocutaneous blistering disease. Arch Dermatol. 2003;139:1051-9.
12. Goodfield M, Davison K, Bowden K. Intravenous immunoglobulin (IVIg) for therapy-resistant cutaneous lupus erythematosus (LE). J Dermatolog Treat. 2004;15: 46-50.
13. Mydlarski PR, Mittmann N, Shear NH. Intravenous immunoglobulin: use in Dermatology. Skin therapy letter. 2004;9(5).
14. Jolles S, Hughes J, Whittaker S. Dermatological uses of high-dose intravenous immunoglobulin. Arch Dermatol. 1998;134:80-6.
15. Rutter A, Luger TA. Intravenous immunoglobulin: an emerging treatment for immune-mediated skin diseases. Curr Opin Investig Drugs. 2002;3:713-9.
16. Bussel JB, Eldor A, Kelton JG, et al. IGIV-C, a novel intravenous immunoglobulin: evaluation of safety, efficacy, mechanisms of action, and impact on quality of life. Thromb Haemost. 2004;91(4):771-8.
17. Ibanez C, Montoro-Ronsano JB. Intravenous immunoglobulin preparations and autoimmune disorders: mechanisms of action. Curr Pharm Biotechnol. 2003;4:239-47.
18. Viard I, Wehrli P, Bullani R, et al. Inhibition of toxic epidermal necrolysis by blockade of CD95 with human intravenous immunoglobulin. Science. 1998;282(5388):490-3.
19. Winston DJ, Antin JH, Wolff SN, et al. A multicenter, randomized, double-blind comparison of different doses of intravenous immunoglobulin for prevention of graft-versushost disease and infection after allogeneic bone marrow transplantation. Bone Marrow Transplant. 2001;28:187-96.
20. Oates-Whitehead R, Baumer J, Haines L, et al. Intravenous immunoglobulin for the treatment of Kawasaki disease in children. Cochrane Database Syst Rev. 2003;4:CD004000.
21. Dalakas MC, Illa I, Dambrosia JM, et al. A controlled trial of high-dose intravenous immune globulin infusions as treatmentfor dermatomyositis. N Engl J Med. 1993;329:1993-2000.
22. Ahmed AR. Intravenous immunoglobulin therapy in the treatment of patients with pemphigus vulgaris unresponsive to conventional immunosuppressive treatment. J Am Acad Dermatol. 2001;45:679-90.
23. Ahmed AR, Sami N. Intravenous immunoglobulin therapy for patients with pemphigus foliaceus unresponsive to conventional therapy. J Am Acad Dermatol. 2002;46:42-9.
24. Ahmed AR. Intravenous immunoglobulin therapy for patients with bullous pemphigoid unresponsive to conventional immunosuppressive treatment. J Am Acad Dermatol. 2001;45:825-35.

25. Foster CS, Ahmed AR. Intravenous immunoglobulin therapy for ocular cicatricial pemphigoid: a preliminary study. Ophthalmology. 1999;106:2136-43.
26. Trent JT, Kirsner RS, Romanelli P, et al. Analysis of intravenous immunoglobulin for the treatment of toxic epidermal necrolysis using SCORTEN: The University of Miami Experience. Arch Dermatol. 2003;139:39-43.
27. Prins C, Kerdel FA, Padilla RS, et al. Treatment of toxic epidermal necrolysis with high-dose intravenous immunoglobulins: multicenter retrospective analysis of 48 consecutive cases. Arch Dermatol. 2003;139:26-32.
28. Bachot N, Revuz J, Roujeau JC. Intravenous immunoglobulin treatment for Stevens-Johnson syndrome and toxic epidermal necrolysis: a prospective noncomparative study showing no benefit on mortality or progression. Arch Dermatol. 2003;139:33-6.

Chapter 14

Miscellaneous Uses of Biologics

Dipali Rathod, Manas Chatterjee

▌ INTRODUCTION

The biologic agents are the latest addition to the dermatologist's treatment armamentarium, owing to the advent of latest technology and better understanding of the disease pathophysiology. Biologic agents, produced by recombinant DNA technology target specific proteins involved in various immune-mediated diseases without affecting the rest of the pathogenic pathway; hence, are presumed to have fewer side-effects in comparison to the conventional systemic immunosuppressive agents. With the continued evolution of biologics, in a quest to offer more targeted treatment, newer biologics continue to be introduced with a ray of new hope in the battle against these chronic conditions.

The Food and Drug Administration (FDA)-approved indications of different biologics have been covered in detail in respective chapters and therefore, in this chapter we shall discuss only the miscellaneous or uncommon uses of biologics currently available in India [Infliximab, adalimumab, etanercept, secukinumab, itolizumab, rituximab, omalizumab and intravenous immunoglobulin (IVIg)].

The various biologic agents with their FDA-approved and off-label indications have been summarized in Table 14.1. The sections beneath outline brief descriptions of the various biologic agents, and the available evidences for their off-label dermatological uses have been summarized in Table 14.2.

Table 14.1: Biologic agents with their Food and Drug Administration (FDA)-approved and off-label indications.

Sr No	Biologic agents	FDA-approved indications	Off-label indications
1.	Infliximab[1,2]	• Psoriasis vulgaris • Pustular psoriasis • Psoriatic arthropathy	• Erythrodermic psoriasis, nail psoriasis, generalized pustular psoriasis • Hidradenitis suppurativa • Pyoderma gangrenosum • Sweet's syndrome • Subcorneal pustular dermatosis
			• Immunobullous disorders

Contd...

Contd...

Sr No	Biologic agents	FDA-approved indications	Off-label indications
			• Behçet's disease • Cutaneous sarcoidosis • Generalized granuloma annulare[3,4] • Dermatomyositis • Systemic sclerosis • Generalized morphea[5] • Pityriasis rubra pilaris • Cutaneous vasculitis[6] • Wegener's granulomatosis • Granulomatous cheilitis • Necrobiosis lipoidica[9] • Atopic dermatitis • Graft versus host disease (GvHD)[7] • Toxic epidermal necrolysis (TEN) • SAPHO syndrome (synovitis, acne, pustulosis, hyperostosis and osteitis)
2.	*Adalimumab*[1,8]	• Moderate to severe chronic plaque psoriasis • Psoriatic arthritis • Hidradenitis suppurativa	• Cutaneous sarcoidosis • Systemic vasculitis • Neutrophilic dermatoses • Generalized granuloma annulare[9] – Immunobullous disorders[13] • Multicentric reticulohistiocytosis[10] • Aphthous stomatitis[11] • Dermatomyositis • Systemic sclerosis • Necrobiosis lipoidica[12] • GvHD • Pityriasis rubra pilaris
3.	*Etanercept*[1]	• Moderate to severe chronic plaque psoriasis • Psoriatic arthritis	• Hidradenitis suppurativa • Pyoderma gangrenosum • Dermatomyositis • Scleroderma • Aphthous stomatitis • Behçet's disease • Immunobullous disorders[17,18] • Granuloma annulare[13] • Cutaneous sarcoidosis • Necrobiosis lipoidica

Contd...

Contd...

Sr No	Biologic agents	FDA-approved indications	Off-label indications
			• GvHD • Pityriasis rubra pilaris[14] • Multicentric reticulo-histiocytosis[15]
4.	*Secukinumab*	• Moderate to severe plaque psoriasis • Psoriatic arthritis	• Palmoplantar psoriasis[16] • Pustular psoriasis and erythrodermic psoriasis • Nail psoriasis
5.	*Itolizumab[17]*	• Moderate to severe chronic plaque psoriasis	• Palmoplantar psoriasis • Psoriatic arthritis • Sjögren's syndrome[18]
6.	*Omalizumab[1]*	• Moderate to severe persistent asthma • Chronic urticaria[19]	• Atopic dermatitis[20] • Subacute cutaneous lupus erythematosus • Urticarial vasculitis • Cold urticaria[21] • Systemic mastocytosis[22] • Hyperimmunoglobulin E syndrome (HIES) • Bullous pemphigoid[23]
7.	*Rituximab[1,2]*	• Microscopic polyangiitis • Granulomatosis with polyangiitis	• Primary cutaneous B cell lymphoma • Autoimmune bullous disorders (pemphigus vulgaris, paraneoplastic pemphigus, epidermolysis bullosa acquisita, bullous pemphigoid) • Acute and chronic GvHD • Urticarial vasculitis • Vasculitic syndromes (Wegener granulomatosis, Churg-Strauss syndrome and microscopic poly-angiitis) • Systemic lupus erythematosus • Systemic sclerosis • Dermatomyositis • Atopic eczema
8.	*Intravenous immunoglo-bulin (IVIg)[25,26]*	• Primary immuno-deficiencies • Idiopathic thrombo-cytopenic purpura • Kawasaki disease	• Autoimmune bullous disorders • Connective tissue diseases (dermatomyositis)

Contd...

Contd...

Sr No	Biologic agents	FDA-approved indications	Off-label indications
			• Stevens-Johnson syndrome (SJS) or TEN spectrum • Vasculitic syndromes • Urticaria • Atopic dermatitis • Pyoderma gangrenosum

Table 14.2: Biologic agents with their off-label indications and the available evidence.

Biologic agent	Off-label indications	Dosage	Evidence available	Remarks
Infliximab	Pemphigus vulgaris	3 doses (5 mg/kg) intravenous (IV) infusion at weeks 0, 2 and 6, 8 weeks thereafter	Case reports have shown it to be effective[27-29]	Anti-tumor necrosis factor (TNF)-α inhibitors are not very effective for the management of immunobullous disorders and with availability of rituximab, not used in the present scenario.[30] However, it should be used with caution as induction of paradoxical pemphigus foliaceus and linear immunoglobulin A (IgA) bullous dermatosis has been observed.[31,32]
	Recalcitrant subcorneal pustular dermatosis	5 mg/kg IV infusion	Case reports[33-35]	Although the patients were successfully treated, the response was transient.
	Hidradenitis suppurativa (HS)	5 mg/kg/dose IV infusion at 0, 2 and 6 weeks and 8 weekly thereafter	Randomized controlled trial (RCT) of 38 patients and other studies reported significant improvement[36-40]	Effective alternative to adalimumab for management of HS

Contd...

Contd...

Biologic agent	Off-label indications	Dosage	Evidence available	Remarks
	Pyoderma gangrenosum	5 mg/kg IV infusion	RCT with 30 subjects and other case series[41-44]	Effective alternative in patients not responding to first-line therapy
	Sweet's syndrome	3–5 mg/kg IV infusion	Case reports[45,46]	Although effective in these patients, it must be borne in mind that it may aggravate infections
	Behçet's disease (ocular and oral or genital involvement)	5 mg/kg IV infusion	Case reports[47,48]	Significant improvement was observed in the vision and extraocular manifestations with reduction in the frequency of uveitis.[49] Also found effective in the treatment of progressive Neuro-Behçet's disease.[50]
	Sarcoidosis	3–10 mg/kg/dose IV infusion at 0, 2, 6 and every 8–19 week subsequently	Case series showed improvement[51]	Care should be taken to rule out tuberculosis objectively as it can be difficult to rule out tuberculosis and infliximab can result in potential problem in this scenario[52,53]
	Generalized morphea	5 mg/kg IV infusion every month × 4 months	Case report with promising result[5]	Mixed results observed; however, it resulted in clinical stabilization
	Dermatomyositis	5 mg/kg IV infusion at 0, 2, 6, 10 week and every 8 weeks thereafter	Case reports with successful outcome[54]	Rituximab is the first-line biologic therapy
	Pityriasis rubra pilaris (PRP)	5 mg/kg IV infusion	Case series with successful outcome[55,56]	Effective in patients not responding to first-line therapy

Contd...

Contd...

Biologic agent	Off-label indications	Dosage	Evidence available	Remarks
	Atopic dermatitis	5 mg/kg IV infusion at weeks 0, 2, 6, 14, 22, 30 and 38	A pilot study of 9 patients demonstrated significant clinical improvement with induction therapy; however, the response was not maintained[57]	Not used routinely and has no place in day-to-day care of the disease
Adalimu-mab	Pemphigus vulgaris	40 mg subcuta-neous(SC) every other week	Case report achieved a very good clinical response[58]	Same as other TNF-α inhibitors, not very effective. Should be used with caution[31]
	IgA pemphigus of the subcorneal pustular dermatosis subtype	40 mg SC biweekly with 1 g mycophe-nolate mofetil daily	Case report showed successful outcome in an aggressive case[59]	
	Pyoderma gangre-nosum	80 mg SC week 0, followed by 40 mg week 1, then 40 mg every other week	Case reports[60-64]	Showed variations of successes and failures; may be useful after other systemic therapies and TNF-α inhibitors are ineffective
	Behçet's disease	40 mg SC, 2 weekly	Case series[65-66]	As effective as infliximab in maintaining disease remission and preventing relapse
	Sweet's syndrome	40 mg SC weekly	Case report with longstanding improvement in a patient with lung involvement[67]	

Contd...

Contd...

Biologic agent	Off-label indications	Dosage	Evidence available	Remarks
	Sarcoidosis	40 mg SC every 2 weekly	Case reports and a double-blind RCT showed effective outcome[68-71]	Not as effective as infliximab; however, proved effective in a patient with multiorgan sarcoidosis[68]
Etanercept	Pemphigus vulgaris (PV), pemphigus vegetans and foliaceous	25–50 mg SC twice weekly	Case reports[72-74]	
	Sneddon-Wilkinson disease	50 mg SC twice weekly	Case report showed successful outcome[75]	Proved effective in patients refractory to numerous treatments
	Bullous pemphigoid	50 mg SC weekly-twice weekly	Case report with effective control[76]	
	Cicatricial pemphigoid	25 mg SC twice weekly	Case reports[77,78]	Alternative treatment option in recalcitrant patients or those who require aggressive systemic therapy
	Pyoderma gangrenosum	25–50 mg SC twice weekly	Case reports[79]	Alternative therapeutic option
	Hidradenitis suppurativa	50 mg SC once weekly × 12 weeks	2 small open-label studies[80,81] and case reports have shown clinical improvement	Adalimumab and infliximab is much more effective as compared to etanercept for management of HS and it is not preferred for its management
	Sweet's syndrome	50 mg SC weekly	Case reports[82,83]	Alternative therapeutic option for patients with recurrent Sweet's syndrome

Contd...

Contd...

Biologic agent	Off-label indications	Dosage	Evidence available	Remarks
	Erythema nodosum leprosum	50 mg SC weekly	Case reports	It can be used for management of erythema nodosum leprosum not responding to steroids and thalidomide
Secukinu-mab	Nail psoriasis	150–300 mg SC weekly for 0–4 weeks and 4 weekly, with primary endpoint evaluated at week 16	A double-blind, randomized, placebo-controlled, parallel-group, phase 3b study reported effective response[84]	Efficacy was measured by Nail Psoriasis Severity Index (NAPSI) percent change
	Generalized pustular psoriasis	150–300 mg SC weekly, with primary endpoint evaluated at week 16	An open label phase 3 study of 12 patients reported effective treatment[85]	
	Extensive alopecia areata	300 mg SC at weeks 0, 1, 2, 3, 4 and every 4 weeks thereafter up to and including week 20	Being tested in a double-blind, randomized, placebo-controlled clinical trial[86]	Ongoing and future clinical trials shall be able to better elucidate its role
Itolizu-mab	Sjögren's syndrome		A study in 6 patients support the rational for anti-CD6 treatment[18]	Its role needs further validation
	B-cell chronic lymphocytic leukemia and cutaneous T-cell lymphoma	0.8 mg/kg/IV weekly × 12 weeks	A preliminary study showed promising results[87]	

Contd...

Contd...

Biologic agent	Off-label indications	Dosage	Evidence available	Remarks
Omalizu-mab	Moderate to severe persistent allergic asthma and atopic dermatitis (AD)	150 or 300 mg SC every 2 weeks based on pretreatment serum IgE levels and body weight in kg 300 mg SC every 2 weekly	A pilot study of 21 patients showed effective response[88] Several case reports have shown mixed response[89-91]	Effective in treating patients with severe AD unresponsive to other therapeutic measures and improved the quality of life; however, RCT studies with large population are required to validate its efficacy
	Cold urticaria	375 mg SC every 2 weeks	Case report showed efficacy[92]	Needs further research to validate its efficacy
	Bullous pemphigoid	300 mg SC per month	Effective in suppressing the blistering and is a relatively safe therapeutic option[23]	Useful in patients who have contraindications or do not respond to the standard treatment
	Systemic mastocytosis	150 mg SC fortnightly for the first month and then monthly	Safe and effective in preventing recurrent anaphylaxis[22]	Useful in nonatopic individuals as well
	Hyperimmu-noglobulin E syndrome (HIES)	300 mg SC every 2 weeks	Report showed clinical improve-ment[93]	
Rituximab	Dermato-myositis	Rheumatoid arthritis (RA) regimen—1000 mg every 2 weeks × 2 doses Lymphoma regimen–375 mg/m² per week × 4 doses	Clinical trials showed efficacy[94,95]	Discussed in chapter on connective tissue diseases

Contd...

Contd...

Biologic agent	Off-label indications	Dosage	Evidence available	Remarks
	Systemic lupus erythema-tosus	Both RA and lymphoma regimen	Clinical trials and case reports[96]	Discussed in separate chapter
	Bullous systemic lupus erythema-tosus	Along with prednisone maintenance therapy	Case report showed complete clinical response[97]	
	Melanoma	375 mg/m^2 IV infusion once a week × 4 weeks followed by a maintenance therapy every 8 weeks	A pilot trial reported clinical improve-ment[98]	Well-tolerated and proves to be a potential therapeutic option
	Atopic eczema (AE)	Two IV infusions each 1000 mg, 2 weeks apart	Case series[99]	Appears to be promising in severe AE cases recalcitrant to other therapies. Further clinical studies are recommended
	Graft-versus-host disease (GvHD)	Lymphoma protocol	Few studies demonstrated reduction in the rate of chronic GvHD[100]	Effective for patients with corticosteroid-refractory chronic GvHD that is not advanced
Intra-venous immuno-globulin (IVIg)	Pemphigus vulgaris	2 g/kg/cycle over 3–5 consecutive days	Combined with rituximab for recalcitrant disease[101]	No observable side effects were noted and both the agents resulted in sustained and complete remission
	Pemphigus variants	2 g/kg/cycle over 3–5 consecutive days	Case series[102,103]	Discussed in chapter on IVIg, can be used as short-term measure to control the disease
	Bullous pemphigoid	2 g/kg/cycle over 3–5 con-secutive days	Case series[104]	

Contd...

Contd...

Biologic agent	Off-label indications	Dosage	Evidence available	Remarks
	Mucous membrane pemphigoid[105]	2–3 g/kg/cycle, divided over 3 days and repeated every 2–6 weeks	Proved be a safe and effective therapy	
	Dermatomyositis (DM)	2 g/kg/cycle per month × 3 months	Double-blind, placebo-controlled trial showed efficacy[106]	A safe and effective treatment for refractory DM
	Toxic epidermal necrolysis[107,108]	2 g/kg in a single day or in divided doses × 5 days	Differing reports exist on efficacy of IVIg.	Limited literature, lack of treatment regimen uniformity, lack of adequate control data and size of studies conducted
	Pyoderma gangrenosum	2 g/kg/cycle over 3–5 consecutive days	Case series in combination with steroids and other immunosuppressants[109]	Useful therapeutic option in refractory pyoderma gangrenosum
	Wegener's granulomatosis and microscopic polyangiitis	2 g/kg (over 2–3 days) every month × 3–6 months, later maintenance schedule may be individualized	Prevents massive tissue destruction and minimizes the extent of defects[110]	
	Atopic dermatitis resistant to treatment	2 g/kg/month for 6 cycles, with a 3-month follow-up period	Case series[111,112]	Double-blind placebo-controlled trials are required to validate these findings

CONCLUSION

Biologics are becoming increasingly useful for the treatment of many dermatological diseases, particularly as an alternative for patients who have failed to tolerate or respond to the conventional systemic therapies.

Drug interactions for biologics are minimal, a fact which is important while choosing them for patients with multiple comorbidities.

With so many new and effective existing treatments and many more in the pipeline, there is a promising future for the dermatologist who treats these conditions with the options available in biologic agents and offers hope for the patient's flawless skin. The use of biologic agents in dermatology is evolving; however, the clinical trials so far have not showed consistent results. So, further research on a larger scale in this field is needed to evaluate the efficacy, safety and cost-effectiveness of the biological therapies currently available, so as to elucidate the risk-benefit ratio of these agents in various dermatological conditions and support the development of new treatments options. Although these agents have revolutionized the therapy of many recalcitrant dermatological diseases, the cost factor should be borne in mind before considering them over other conventional management options. However, considering the efficacy of these agents, their cost may be spurned by the fact that it increases patient satisfaction and reduce the hospital stay as well as use of other systemic therapies.[113]

▌ REFERENCES

1. Graves JE, Nunley K, Heffernan MP. Off-label uses of biologics in dermatology: rituximab, omalizumab, infliximab, etanercept, adalimumab, efalizumab, and alefacept (part 2 of 2). J Am Acad Dermatol. 2007;56:e55-79.
2. de Ridder L, Benninga MA, Taminiau JA, et al. Infliximab use in children and adolescents with inflammatory bowel disease. J Pediatr Gastroenterol Nutr. 2007;45:3-14.
3. Murdaca G, Colombo BM, Barabino G, et al. Anti-tumor necrosis factor-α treatment with infliximab for disseminated granuloma annulare. Am J Clin Dermatol. 2010;11:437-9.
4. Hertl MS, Haendle I, Schuler G, et al. Rapid improvement of recalcitrant disseminated granuloma annulare upon treatment with the tumour necrosis factor-α inhibitor, infliximab. Br J Dermatol. 2005;152:552-5.
5. Diab M, Coloe JR, Magro C, et al. Treatment of recalcitrant generalized morphea with infliximab. Arch Dermatol. 2010;146:601-4.
6. Josselin L, Mahr A, Cohen P, et al. Infliximab efficacy and safety against refractory systemic necrotising vasculitides: long-term follow-up of 15 patients. Ann Rheum Dis. 2008;67:1343-6.
7. Couriel DR, Saliba R, de Lima M, et al. A phase-III study of infliximab and corticosteroids for the initial treatment of acute graft-versus-host disease. Biol Blood Marrow Transplant. 2009;15:1555-62.
8. Richardson S, Getfand J. Immunobiologicals, cytokines and growth factors in dermatology. In: Wolff K, Goldsmith LA, Katz SI, Gilchrest BA, Paller AS, Leffell DJ (Eds). Fitzpatrick's Dermatology in General Medicine, 7th edition. New Delhi: McGraw Hill; 2008. pp. 2223-31.
9. Kozic H, Webster GF. Treatment of widespread granuloma annulare with adalimumab: a case report. J Clin Aesthet Dermatol. 2011;4:42-3.

10. Shannon SE, Schumacher HR, Self S, et al. Multicentric reticulohistiocytosis responding to tumor necrosis factor-alpha inhibition in a renal transplant patient. J Rheumatol. 2005;32:565-7.
11. Vujevich J, Zirwas M. Treatment of severe, recalcitrant major aphthous stomatitis with adalimumab. Cutis. 2005;76:129-32.
12. Zhang KS, Quan LT, Hsu S. Treatment of necrobiosis lipoidica with etanercept and adalimumab. Dermatol Online J. 2009;15:12.
13. Shupack J, Siu K. Resolving granuloma annulare with etanercept. Arch Dermatol. 2006;142:394-5.
14. Vasher M, Smithberger E, Lien MH, et al. Familial pityriasis rubra pilaris: report of a family and therapeutic response to etanercept. J Drugs Dermatol. 2010;9:844-50.
15. Lovelace K, Loyd A, Adelson D, et al. Etanercept and the treatment of multicentric reticulohistiocytosis. Arch Dermatol. 2005;141:1167-8.
16. Gottlieb A, Sullivan J, van Doorn M, et al. Secukinumab shows significant efficacy in palmoplantar psoriasis: results from GESTURE, a randomized controlled trial. J Am Acad Dermatol. 2017;76(1):70-80.
17. Menon R, David BG. Itolizumab—a humanized anti-CD6 monoclonal antibody with a better side effects profile for treatment of psoriasis. Clin Cosmet Investig Dermatol. 2015;8:215-22.
18. Le Dantec C, Alonso R, Fali T, et al. Rationale for treating primary Sjögren's syndrome patients with an anti-CD6 monoclonal antibody (Itolizumab). Immunol Res. 2013;56(2-3):341-7.
19. Godse KV. Omalizumab in severe chronic urticaria. Indian J Dermatol Venereol Leprol. 2008;74:157-8.
20. Schmitt J, Schäkel K. Omalizumab as a therapeutic option in atopic eczema: current evidence and potential benefit. Hautarzt. 2007;58:128,130-2.
21. Boyce JA. Successful treatment of cold-induced urticaria/anaphylaxis with anti-IgE. J Allergy Clin Immunol. 2006;117:1415-8.
22. Douglass J, Caroll K, Voskamp A, et al. Omalizumab is effective in treating systemic mastocytosis in a nonatopic patient. Allergy. 2010;65(7):926-7.
23. Gonul M, Keseroglu HO, Ergin C, et al. Bullous pemphigoid successfully treated with omalizumab. Indian J Dermatol Venereol Leprol. 2016;82:577-9.
24. Carr DR, Heffernan MP. Off-label uses of rituximab in dermatology. Dermatol Ther. 2007;20(4):277-87.
25. Fernandez AP, Kerdel FA. The use of IV IG therapy in dermatology. Dermatol Ther. 2007;20:288-305.
26. Smith DI, Swamy PM, Heffernan MP. Off-label uses of biologics in dermatology: interferon and intravenous immunoglobulin (part 1 of 2). J Am Acad Dermatol. 2007;56:e1-54.
27. Jacobi A, Shuler G, Hertl M. Rapid control of therapy-refractory pemphigus vulgaris by treatment with the tumour necrosis factor-alpha inhibitor infliximab. Br J Dermatol. 2005;153:448-9.
28. Pardo J, Mercader P, Mahiques L, et al. Infliximab in the management of severe pemphigus vulgaris. Br J Dermatol. 2005;153:222-3.
29. García-Rabasco A, Alsina-Gibert M, Pau-Charles I, et al. Infliximab therapy failure in two patients with pemphigus vulgaris. J Am Acad Dermatol. 2012;67:e196-7.
30. Hall RP, Fairley J, Woodley D, et al. A multicentre randomized trial of the treatment of patients with pemphigus vulgaris with infliximab and prednisone compared with prednisone alone. Br J Dermatol. 2015;172(3):760-8.

31. Boussemart L, Jacobelli S, Batteux F, et al. Autoimmune bullous skin diseases occurring under anti-tumor necrosis factor therapy: two case reports. Dermatology. 2010;221:201-5.

32. Hoffmann J, Hadaschik E, Enk A, et al. Linear IgA bullous dermatosis secondary to infliximab therapy in a patient with ulcerative colitis. Dermatology. 2015;231:112-5.

33. Voigtländer C, Lüftl M, Schuler G, et al. Infliximab (anti-tumor necrosis factor alpha antibody): A novel, highly effective treatment of recalcitrant subcorneal pustular dermatosis (Sneddon-Wilkinson disease). Arch Dermatol. 2001;137:1571-4.

34. Naretto C, Baldovino S, Rossi E, et al. The case of SLE associated Sneddon-Wilkinson pustular disease successfully and safely treated with infliximab. Lupus. 2009;18:856-7.

35. Bonifati C, Trento E, Cordiali Fei P, et al. Early but not lasting improvement of recalcitrant subcorneal pustular dermatosis (Sneddon-Wilkinson disease) after infliximab therapy: relationships with variations in cytokine levels in suction blister fluids. Clin Exp Dermatol. 2005;30:662-5.

36. Grant A, Gonzalez T, Montgomery MO, et al. Infliximab therapy for patients with moderate to severe hidradenitis suppurativa: a randomized, double-blind, placebocontrolled crossover trial. J Am Acad Dermatol. 2010;62(2):205-17.

37. Sullivan TP, Welsh E, Kerdel FA, et al. Infliximab for hidradenitis suppurativa. Br J Dermatol. 2003;149:1046-9.

38. Hassan I, Aleem S, Sheikh G, et al. Biologics in dermatology: a brief review. BJMP. 2013;6(4):a629.

39. Lebwohl B, Sapadin AN. Infliximab for the treatment of hidradenitis suppurativa. J Am Acad Dermatol. 2003;49:S275-6.

40. Adams DR, Gordon KB, Devenyi AG, et al. Severe hidradenitis suppurativa treated with infliximab infusion. Arch Dermatol. 2003;139:1540-2.

41. Brooklyn TN, Dunnill MG, Shetty A, et al. Infliximab for the treatment of pyoderma gangrenosum: a randomised, double-blind, placebo-controlled trial. Gut. 2006;55:505-9.

42. Mooij JE, van Rappard DC, Mekkes JR. Six patients with pyoderma gangrenosum successfully treated with infliximab. Int J Dermatol. 2013;52(11):1418-20.

43. Hayashi H, Kuwabara C, Tarumi K, et al. Successful treatment with infliximab for refractory pyoderma gangrenosum associated with inflammatory bowel disease. J Dermatol. 2012;39:576-8.

44. Carrasco Cubero C, Ruiz Tudela MM, Salaberri Maestrojuan JJ, et al. Pyoderma gangrenosum associated with inflammatory bowel disease. A report of two cases with good response to infliximab. Reumatol Clin. 2012;8:90-2.

45. Matzkies FG, Manger B, Schmitt-Haendle M, et al. Severe septicaemia in a patient with polychondritis and Sweet's syndrome after initiation of treatment with infliximab. Ann Rheum Dis. 2003;62:81-2.

46. Foster EN, Nguyen KK, Sheikh RA, et al. Crohn's disease associated with Sweet's syndrome and Sjogren's syndrome treated with infliximab. Clin Dev Immunol. 2005;12:145-9.

47. Haugeberg G, Velken M, Johnsen V. Successful treatment of genital ulcers with infliximab in Behçet's disease. Ann Rheum Dis. 2004;63:744-5.

48. Goossens PH, Verburg RJ, Breedveld FC. Remission of Behçet's syndrome with tumour necrosis factor alpha blocking therapy. Ann Rheum Dis. 2001;60:637.

49. Accorinti M, Pirraglia MP, Paroli MP, et al. Infliximab treatment for ocular and extraocular manifestations of Behcet's disease. Jpn J Ophthalmol. 2007;51:191-6.

50. Yamada Y, Sugita S, Tanaka H, et al. Comparison of infliximab versus ciclosporin during the initial 6-month treatment period in Behcet disease. Br J Ophthalmol. 2010;94:284-8.
51. Doty JD, Mazur JE, Judson MA. Treatment of sarcoidosis with infliximab. Chest. 2005;127(3):1064-71.
52. Clementine RR, Lyman J, Zakem J, et al. Tumor necrosis factor-alpha antagonist-induced sarcoidosis. J Clin Rheumatol. 2010;16:274-9.
53. Santos G, Sousa LE, João AM. Exacerbation of recalcitrant cutaneous sarcoidosis with adalimumab—a paradoxical effect: a case report. An Bras Dermatol. 2013;88:26-8.
54. Hengstman GJ, van den Hoogen FH, Barrera P, et al. Successful treatment of dermatomyositis and polymyositis with anti-tumor-necrosis-factor-alpha: preliminary observations. Eur Neurol. 2003;50:10-5.
55. Müller H, Gattringer C, Zelger B, et al. Infliximab monotherapy as first-line treatment for adult-onset pityriasis rubra pilaris: case report and review of the literature on biologic therapy. J Am Acad Dermatol. 2008;59(Suppl. 5):S65-70.
56. Garcovich S1, Di Giampetruzzi AR, Antonelli G, et al. Treatment of refractory adult-onset pityriasis rubra pilaris with TNF-alpha antagonists: a case series. J Eur Acad Dermatol Venereol. 2010;24:881-4.
57. Jacobi A1, Antoni C, Manger B, et al. Infliximab in the treatment of moderate to severe atopic dermatitis. J Am Acad Dermatol. 2005;52:522-6.
58. Vojáèková N, Fialová J, Vaòusová D, et al. Pemphigus vulgaris treated with adalimumab: case study. Dermatol Ther. 2012;25:95-7.
59. Howell SM, Bessinger GT, Altman CE, et al. Rapid response of IgA pemphigus of the subcorneal pustular dermatosis subtype to treatment with adalimumab and mycophenolate mofetil. J Am Acad Dermatol. 2005;53:541-3.
60. Hinterberger L, Muller CS, Vogt T, et al. Adalimumab: a treatment option for pyoderma gangrenosum after failure of systemic standard therapies. Dermatol Ther. 2012;2(1):6.
61. Heffernan MP, Anadkat MJ, Smith DJ. Adalimumab treatment for pyoderma gangrenosum. Arch Dermatol. 2007;143:306-8.
62. Pomerantz RG, Husni ME, Mody E, et al. Adalimumab for treatment of pyoderma gangrenosum. Br J Dermatol. 2007;157:1267-304.
63. Hubbard VG, Friedman AC, Goldsmith P. Systemic pyoderma responding to infliximab and adalimumab. Br J Dermatol. 2005;152:1059-61.
64. Margaret AF, Cummins DL, Ehst BD. Adalimumab therapy for recalcitrant pyoderma gangrenosum. J Burns Wounds. 2006;5:e8.
65. Mushtaq B, Saeed T, Situnayake RD, et al. Adalimumab for sight-threatening uveitis in Behçet disease. Eye. 2007;21:824-5.
66. van Laar JA, Missoten T, van Daele PL. Adalimumab: a new modality of Behçet disease? Ann Rheum Dis. 2007;66:565-6.
67. Karamlou K, Gorn AH. Refractory Sweets syndrome with autoimmune organizing pneumonia treated with monoclonal antibodies to tumor necrosis factor. J Clin Reumatol. 2004;10:331-5.
68. Callejas-Rubio JL, Ortego-Centeno N, Lopez-Perez L, et al. Treatment of therapy-resistant sarcoidosis with adalimumab. Clin Rheumatol. 2006;25:596-7.
69. Heffernan MP, Smith DJ. Adalimumab for treatment of cutaneous sarcoidosis. Arch Dermatol. 2006;142:17-9.
70. Philips MA, Lynch J, Azmi FH. Ulcerative cutaneous sarcoidosis responding to adalimumab. J Am Acad Dermatol. 2005;53:917.

71. Pariser RJ, Paul J, Hirano S, et al. A double-blind, randomized, placebo controlled trial of adalimumab in the treatment of cutaneous sarcoidosis. J Am Acad Dermatol. 2013;68(5):765-73.
72. Shetty A, Marcum CB, Glass LF, et al. Successful treatment of pemphigus vulgaris with etanercept in four patients. J Drugs Dermatol. 2009;8:940-3.
73. Lin MH, Hsu CK, Lee JY. Successful treatment of recalcitrant pemphigus vulgaris and pemphigus vegetans with etanercept and carbon dioxide laser. Arch Dermatol. 2005;141:680-2.
74. Gubinelli E, Bergamo F, Didona B, et al. Pemphigus foliaceus treated with etanercept. J Am Acad Dermatol. 2006;55:1107-8.
75. Berk DR, Hurt MA, Mann C, et al. Sneddon-Wilkinson disease treated with etanercept: Report of two cases. Clin Exp Dermatol. 2009;34:347-51.
76. Yamauchi PS, Lowe NJ, Gindi V. Treatment of coexisting bullous pemphigoid and psoriasis with the tumor necrosis factor antagonist etanercept. J Am Acad Dermatol. 2006;54(3 Suppl 2):S121-2.
77. Sacher C, Rubbert A, König C, et al. Treatment of recalcitrant cicatricial pemphigoid with the tumor necrosis factor alpha antagonist etanercept. J Am Acad Dermatol. 2002;46:113-5.
78. Canizares MJ, Smith DI, Conners MS, et al. Successful treatment of mucous membrane pemphigoid with etanercept in 3 patients. Arch Dermatol. 2006;142:1457-61.
79. Patel F, Fitzmaurice S, Duong C, et al. Effective strategies for the management of pyoderma gangrenosum: a comprehensive review. Acta Dermato Venereologica. 2015;95(5):525-31.
80. Pelekanou A, Kanni T, Savva A, et al. Long-term efficacy of etanercept in hidradenitis suppurativa: results from an open-label phase-II prospective trial. Exp Dermatol. 2010;19:538-40.
81. Giamarellos-Bourboulis EJ, Pelekanou E, Antonopoulou A, et al. An open-label phase-II study of the safety and efficacy of etanercept for the therapy of hidradenitis suppurativa. Br J Dermatol. 2008;158:567-72.
82. Ambrose NL, Tobin AM, Howard D. Etanercept treatment in Sweet's syndrome with inflammatory arthritis. J Rheumatol. 2009;36:1348-9.
83. Yamauchi PS, Turner L, Lowe NJ, et al. Treatment of recurrent Sweet's syndrome with coexisting rheumatoid arthritis with the tumor necrosis factor antagonist etanercept. J Am Acad Dermatol. 2006;54(Suppl 2):S122-6.
84. Reich K, Sullivan J, Arenberger P, et al. Secukinumab is effective in subjects with moderate to severe plaque psoriasis with significant nail involvement: 16-week results from the TRANSFIGURE study. Presented at 23rd World Congress of Dermatology. Vancouver, Canada: International League of Dermatological Societies; 2015.
85. Armstrong AW, Vender R, Kircik L. Secukinumab in the treatment of palmoplantar, nail, scalp, and pustular psoriasis. J Clin Aesthet Dermatol. 2016; 9(6 Suppl 1):S12-6.
86. Yuval R, Yassky G. A novel therapeutic paradigm for patients with extensive alopecia areata. Expert Opin Biol Ther. 2016;16(8):1005-14.
87. Izquierdo CLM, Espinosa EEE, Hernández PC, et al. Itolizumab humanized monoclonal antibody (anti-cd6) in patients with cd6 + lymphoproliferative disorders. Preliminary experience. Rev Cubana Hematol Inmunol Hemoter. 2014;30(3):257-64.

88. Sheinkopf LE, Rafi AW, Do LT, et al. Efficacy of omalizumab in the treatment of atopic dermatitis: a pilot study. Allergy Asthma Proc. 2008;29:530-7.
89. Lane JE, Cheyney JM, Lane TN, et al. Treatment of recalcitrant atopic dermatitis with omalizumab. J Am Acad Dermatol. 2006;54:68-72.
90. Vigo PG, Girgis KR, Pfuetze BL, et al. Efficacy of anti-IgE therapy in patients with atopic dermatitis. J Am Acad Dermatol. 2006;55:168-70.
91. Forman SB, Garrett AB. Success of omalizumab as monotherapy in adult atopic dermatitis: case report and discussion of the high-affinity immunoglobulin E receptor, Fcepsilon RI. Cutis. 2007;80:38-40.
92. Boyce JA. Successful treatment of cold-induced urticaria/anaphylaxis with anti-IgE. J Allergy Clin Immunol. 2006;117:1415-8.
93. Chulanrojanamontri L, Wimoolchart S, Tuuchinda P, et al. Role of omalizumab in a patient with hyper-IgE syndrome and review dermatologic manifestations. Asian Pac J Allergy Immunol. 2009;27(4):233-6.
94. Oddis CV, Reed AM, Aggarwal R, et al. Rituximab in the treatment of refractory adult and juvenile dermatomyositis and adult polymyositis: a randomized, placebo-phase trial. Arthritis Rheum. 2013;65(2):314-24.
95. Chung L, Genovese MC, Fiorentino DF. A pilot trial of rituximab in the treatment of patients with dermatomyositis. Arch Dermatol. 2007;143:763-7.
96. Ramos-Casals M, Soto MJ, Cuadrado MJ, et al. Rituximab in systemic lupus erythematosus: a systematic review of off-label use in 188 cases. Lupus. 2009;18:767-76.
97. Alsanafi S, Kovarik C, Mermelstein AL, et al. Rituximab in the treatment of bullous systemic lupus erythematosus. J Clin Rheumatol. 2011;17:142-4.
98. Pinc A, Somasundaram R, Wagner C, et al. Targeting CD20 in melanoma patients at high risk of disease recurrence. Mol Ther. 2012;20:1056-62.
99. Simon D, Hösli S, Kostylina G, et al. Anti-CD20 (rituximab) treatment improves atopic eczema. J Allergy Clin Immunol. 2008;121:122-8.
100. Teshima T, Nagafuji K, Henzan H, et al. Rituximab for the treatment of corticosteroid-refractory chronic graft-versus-host disease. Int J Hematol. 2009;90:253-60.
101. Ahmed AR, Spigelman Z, Cavacini LA, et al. Treatment of pemphigus vulgaris with rituximab and intravenous immune globulin. N Engl J Med. 2006;355(17):1772-9.
102. Ahmed AR. Intravenous immunoglobulin therapy in the treatment of patients with pemphigus vulgaris unresponsive to conventional immunosuppressive treatment. J Am Acad Dermatol. 2001;45:679-90.
103. Ahmed AR, Sami N. Intravenous immunoglobulin therapy for patients with pemphigus foliaceus unresponsive to conventional therapy. J Am Acad Dermatol. 2002;46:42-9.
104. Ahmed AR. Intravenous immunoglobulin therapy for patients with bullous pemphigoid unresponsive to conventional immunosuppressive treatment. J Am Acad Dermatol. 2001;45:825-35.
105. Foster CS, Ahmed AR. Intravenous immunoglobulin therapy for ocular cicatricial pemphigoid: a preliminary study. Ophthalmology. 1999;106:2136-43.
106. Dalakas MC, Illa I, Dambrosia JM, et al. A controlled trial of high-dose intravenous immune globulin infusions as treatment for dermatomyositis. N Engl J Med. 1993;329(27):1993-2000.

107. Prins C, Kerdel FA, Padilla RS, et al. Treatment of toxic epidermal necrolysis with high-dose intravenous immunoglobulins: multicenter retrospective analysis of 48 consecutive cases. Arch Dermatol. 2003;139(1):26-32.

108. Bachot N, Revuz J, Roujeau JC. Intravenous immunoglobulin treatment for Stevens-Johnson syndrome and toxic epidermal necrolysis: a prospective noncomparative study showing no benefit on mortality or progression. Arch Dermatol. 2003;139(1):33-6.

109. Kreuter A, Reich-Schupke S, Stucker M, et al. Intravenous immunoglobulin for pyoderma gangrenosum. Br J Dermatol. 2008;158(4):856-7.

110. Alexander Enk. Guideline on the use of high-dose intravenous immunoglobulin in dermatology developed by the Guideline Subcommittee of the European Dermatology Forum. Eur J Dermatol. 2009;19(1):90-8.

111. Jolles S, Hughes J, Rustin M. The treatment of atopic dermatitis with adjunctive high-dose intravenous immunoglobulin: a report of three patients and review of the literature. Br J Dermatol. 2000;142(3):551-4.

112. Jolles S, Sewell C, Webster D, et al. Adjunctive high-dose intravenous immunoglobulin treatment for resistant atopic dermatitis: efficacy and effects on intracellular cytokine levels and CD4 counts. Acta Derm Venereol. 2003;83: 433-7.

113. Cheng J, Feldman SR. The cost of biologics for psoriasis is increasing. Drugs Context. 2014;3:212266.

Chapter

15

Biologic Approach to Management of Psoriasis

Muralidhar Rajagopalan, Shekhar Neema, Manish Khandare, Manas Chatterjee

▌ INTRODUCTION

Psoriasis is a common disease affecting approximately 1% of general population. Approximately, 30–40% of affected individuals have severe psoriasis requiring systemic therapy. Choice of systemic therapy depends on factors like availability, affordability, comorbidities, ease of administration, tolerability, rapidity of response desired, adverse effect profile, and previous treatment administered and comfort level of the physician with available treatment. The advent of biological therapy in psoriasis has increased our armamentarium in management of psoriasis. Biologics have been a game changer in management of psoriasis as they yield a more targeted therapy, result in rapid improvement and are associated with less adverse effects in comparison to the conventional systemic therapy. This chapter will deal with the practical aspects of choosing a biologic in a psoriasis patient reporting to the OPD. Also, an algorithm on what all investigations are required before initiating a patient on biologics will be briefly discussed here.

There are three scenarios in which one needs to initiate biologics:

Scenario 1: These are the most common presentations where a physician thinks about initiating biologics

1. Failure, intolerance or toxicity of conventional systemic therapy
2. Comorbidities precluding use of conventional therapy
3. Comorbidities like psoriatic arthritis
4. When rapid control is desired because of social or economic pressure—this is especially when psoriasis affects high impact areas. This could include the face, palms, soles, and genitals.

Scenario 2: As a first-line therapy, especially when rapid control and complete clearance is desirable and there are no financial constraints. This could depend on the patients choice too as some patients do want a faster clearance. Studies have shown that most patients who are treated for psoriasis are not very happy with the treatment approach when complete clearance is not achieved. It is not practical to expect a patient to be philosophical about his disease, especially when he himself suffers and the disease, through comorbidities, could affect his lifespan and mental and social health.

Scenario 3: When patient has failed the conventional systemic therapy. This happens when patients are kept indefinitely on conventional therapy and considering the relapsing and remitting course of the disease the patient starts failing conventional therapy. One must the same time be compassionate and not lead a patient to believe that being on a biological leads to cure of the disease. This has not been demonstrated with any therapy for psoriasis so far.

▍SYSTEMIC THERAPY IN PSORIASIS[1]

Systemic therapy in psoriasis should be initiated when topical therapy and phototherapy has failed. Indication to start systemic therapy are:
• Psoriasis Area and Severity Index (PASI) >10, Dermatology Life Quality Index (DLQI) >10 and body surface area >10%
• Involvement of high impact sites like palm, soles, nails, and genitalia
• Associated psoriatic arthritis
• Significant cosmetic or psychosocial impact.
    This supposes that we are treating severe psoriasis. However, the definition of moderate psoriasis is in flux today with a lot of discussion going on about what is moderate disease and how do we really classify moderate disease. A linking of disease extent to the quality of life score seems to be a better method to decide on when to escalate therapy for a psoriasis patient.

▍WHEN TO START BIOLOGICALS?

To answer the first question, when to start biologic therapy in a patient who presents to us with severe psoriasis, most of the current literature complies with the fact that biologicals should be used when conventional therapy fails. However, biologics may be offered as first-line therapy, if the clinical situation demands. Some examples have been stated above. People who fulfill the disease severity criteria, have disease at high impact site, failure of conventional therapy or toxicity resulting from conventional systemic therapy should be offered biologic therapy. Patient with large impact on social functioning should be offered biologic therapy if their disease is not well controlled with conventional therapy.[2]

Scenario 1: We will be discussing chronic plaque psoriasis in general. Other variants of psoriasis shall be dealt with separately.

    Methotrexate is most commonly used systemic agent for management of psoriasis and often is first line for its management. It is started in the dose of 5–10 mg per week and dose can be escalated to maximum of 25 mg per week. Limitations of methotrexate are hepatotoxicity in long-term use, ineffectiveness in many cases and gastrointestinal intolerance. We should also understand that many methotrexate naïve patients of psoriasis already have NAFLD, which would preclude the use of methotrexate in these patients. When on methotrexate, we do not have dependable algorithms to predict hepatic damage as normal enzyme levels do not always correlate with no structural damage to the liver. Cyclosporine is another systemic option for management of psoriasis especially when rapid control of disease is desired. Cyclosporine is initiated in the dose of 2.5–3 mg/kg and increased up to 5 mg/kg in case of poor response after 4 weeks. Cyclosporine cannot be continued for more than a year at a time. Acitretin can also be used for management of plaque psoriasis. It is not very effective as monotherapy in 25 mg daily dose and associated with unacceptable mucocutaneous adverse effects with 50 mg daily dose. This drug takes time to act and the action is unpredictable. The patient who is prone for the metabolic syndrome due to psoriasis, may well have his dyslipidemia unmasked once acitretin is started. There is a shortage of good studies to document what happens to the dyslipidemia once the acitretin is stopped.

In case, where patient has not been able to tolerate conventional systemic therapy, developed unacceptable adverse effect like hepatotoxicity with methotrexate or did not respond to conventional systemic therapy; which biologic should be offered? The available biologics for management of psoriasis as of now in India are etanercept, infliximab, adalimumab, itolizumab and secukinumab. Etanercept and infliximab are available both as originator and biosimilar molecule while adalimumab only as biosimilar is available. However, none of these molecules have been recognized by the US FDA as a true biosimilar. Etanercept and infliximab are only intended biosimilar and it is incorrect to term their Indian versions as true biosimilars. Immunogenicity studies for these molecules are also lacking. Mechanism of action of various biologics and prebiologic investigations has been dealt in detail in separate chapters and we will only deal with the concept of administering biologic in this chapter.

Once patient is ready for biologic, the choice of biologic depends on many factors. The most important factor in our setting is economic as majority of our patients are self-financed and finally choice of biologic depends much more on economics than science. Notwithstanding these factors, we will try to understand why we choose one biologic over another in a particular scenario for benefit of the patient. Does it really make a difference or is it just a matter of familiarity with the particular drug? We have tried to deal with the matter of cost effectiveness of various biologics in detail in a separate chapter and will not discuss that part here.

▎STEPS WHILE STARTING THE PATIENT ON A BIOLOGIC AGENT

1. Counseling patient about the need for biologic, economic impact and understanding that despite being expensive therapy, it is not a cure for your disease.

2. Pretreatment history and investigations
   a. History suggestive of multiple sclerosis, congestive cardiac failure, inflammatory bowel disease or tuberculosis
   b. Complete blood count, urine examination, blood urea, serum creatinine, blood sugar fasting and post-prandial
   c. Liver function test, hepatitis B surface antigen, anti-hepatitis C virus, immunoglobulin M (IgM), hepatitis B core total antibody.
   d. Chest X-ray, interferon-gamma release assays (IGRA) for latent tuberculosis (details in separate chapter).
3. Planning vaccination (details in separate chapter)
4. Choosing biologic
   a. Rapidity of response desired
   b. Comorbidities
   c. Facilities available
5. Administering biologic
6. Follow-up.

Choosing Biologic in Chronic Plaque Psoriasis

With the availability of multiple biologics and majority of the dermatology practice being an outpatient practice, use of infliximab for management of chronic plaque psoriasis is limited to institutions and in crisis situations. Infliximab and itolizumab, both are given by infusion and require hospital visit or admission, which is a big hindrance for their use in daily practice. Infliximab is reserved for patients who require rapid control of disease or have failed other biologics and will be discussed somewhere else. So, the choice is between etanercept, adalimumab (intended biosimilar), secukinumab and itolizumab (Table 15.1).

These results are from trial data and includes originator molecule. We should remember that clinical trial data will never mimic real life experience. Hence, the need for a proper registry of patients on biologics. The similar studies from biosimilars, biomimics and intended copies are lacking and these issues have been discussed in detail in separate chapter. Real world experience differs from trial data in various ways because in real world majority of patients are not treatment naive and expect faster improvement because of cost involved in treatment as compared to trials where treatment is generally offered free of cost.

• If rapid and complete clearance is desired, secukinumab appears to be the best option for treatment. Real world experience also suggests that even in therapy experienced patients, use of 300 mg dose results in achievement of PASI-75 as early as 6 weeks after starting therapy.

Table 15.1: Psoriasis area and severity index (PASI) response of available biologics.

S. No.	Drug	Dose	PASI-75	PASI-90	PASI-100	Remarks
1.	Etanercept[3,4]	50 mg twice a week	49%	20.7%	4.3%	After 12 weeks
		25 mg twice a week	34%			
		25 mg once a week	14%			
2.	Adalimumab[5]	80 mg day 0, 40 mg week 1 and every other week	71%	45%	20%	After 16 weeks (Trial data for 12 weeks not available)
		40 mg every week	80%	–		After 12 weeks (PASI-90 and PASI-100 data not available in this study)
3.	Secukinumab[3]	300 mg	77%	54%	24%	After 12 weeks
		150 mg	67%	42%	14%	
4.	Itolizumab[6]	1.6 mg/kg body weight, once every 2 weeks for 12 weeks, followed by monthly for next 12 weeks	45%	21%	–	After 28 weeks (Trial data after 12 weeks is not available)

- Adalimumab biosimilar is a cost-effective option for management of psoriasis. In case where patient can wait, it is an excellent choice because of its cost effectiveness. It achieves clearance in reasonable number of patients.
- Etanercept in a standard dose of 50 mg twice a week appears to be more expensive than adalimumab, which is also administered subcutaneously. Adalimumab is more effective as compared to etanercept. Only benefit of using etanercept is its best safety profile, as it is the safest among all biologics and can be used in children and has been used in pregnant women and HIV patients. Etanercept can also be used as an add-on

therapy when patient is not responding adequately to methotrexate. The risk of infections and tuberculosis is highest with infliximab and adalimumab.

• Itolizumab does not offer any advantage over other biologics in terms of rapidity and clearance as it has poor response rate and needs to be given as an infusion.

Comorbidities

Psoriasis is a chronic disease and many of the patients with psoriasis have other comorbidities. The presence of comorbidities can alter the choice of biologic in a particular patient. Absolute and relative contraindications of various biologics have been discussed in detail in various chapters, here we shall discuss about how to approach patients with psoriasis using biologic in presence of these comorbidities (Table 15.2).

Presence of other concomitant diseases like pyoderma gangrenosum, hidradenitis suppurativa, or inflammatory bowel disease which may benefit from treatment with the use of anti-TNF-α therapy and can reduce the threshold for using biologics. Biologic during pregnancy and lactation has been discussed in detail in separate chapter.

Table 15.2: Choice of biologic with comorbidities.		
Infection	*How to screen?*	*What to do?*
Tuberculosis[7] a. Active tuberculosis	History, clinical examination, investigations like chest X-ray and sputum for AFB	Initiate biologic after completion of therapy in consultation with the pulmonologist
b. Latent tuberculosis	Screening with tuberculin skin test or IGRA (IGRA preferred) Annual screening in patients on biologics	• Treat with INH monotherapy for 9 months or INH and rifampicin for 3 months—current recommendation is to avoid monotherapy and uses combination of INH and rifampicin for 2 months • Initiate or resume biologic after 1 month of therapy • Secukinumab and etanercept have lowest risk of reactivation of latent tuberculosis infection and are preferred biologic. Available literature on secukinumab is scarce, it can be used being a nonTNF-α biologic

Contd...

Contd...

Infection	How to screen?	What to do?
Hepatitis B[8,9]	HbsAg	• Secukinumab is the first choice as per expert opinion • Use of TNF-α inhibitor can lead to viral reactivation • Anti-TNF-α therapy can be used in combination with oral antivirals • Oral antivirals should be started 2–4 weeks before starting biologics • Frequent monitoring of LFT and viral load in consultation with the hepatologist • Data with secukinumab and itolizumab is not available
Hepatitis C[10]	Anti-hepatitis C virus, immunoglobulin M	• Etanercept used as a second-line therapy • Frequent monitoring of LFT and viral load in consultation with the hepatologist
HIV infection	HIV serology	• Etanercept preferred • In combination with anti-retroviral, monitor CD4 count and viral load.

Comorbidities	Screening	What to do?
Psoriatic arthropathy	History, examination, X-ray joints, MRI-spine	• Adalimumab as first-line biologic therapy when psoriatic arthritis is predominant • Secukinumab as first-line biologic therapy when psoriasis is more extensive • Secukinumab when patient does not respond to TNF-α inhibitors
Multiple sclerosis	History, examination, neurologist consultation	• Secukinumab preferred • Anti-TNF-α inhibitors contraindicated
Congestive heart failure	History, examination, 2D echocardiography, cardiologist consultation	• Secukinumab preferred • New York Heart Association (NYHA) class I/II—antiTNF-α therapy (with caution) recommended • NYHA class III/IV—secukinumab recommended

Contd...

Contd...

Comorbidities	Screening	What to do?
Coronary artery disease	History and examination	• Anti-TNF-α therapy preferred
Inflammatory bowel disease	History and examination	• Anti-TNF-α therapy—Adalimumab and infliximab preferred • Secukinumab—contraindicated
Autoimmune diseases[11]	ANA and ANA profile	• Antinuclear antibodies may develop while patient is on infliximab • Anti-ds DNA and drug-induced lupus may develop rarely, but the severity of symptoms is not bad • Development of ANA is associated with treatment failure • Prospective studies are available in which ANA was determined before starting antiTNF-α therapy and patients were followed up on treatment • Though development of drug-induced lupus in patient treated with anti-TNF-α therapy is rare, it is prudent to consider biologic therapy in this scenario with caution
Chronic liver disease of noninfectious etiology	Liver function test	• Pharmacokinetic data of biologics in presence of liver disease is not available • Various case reports of successful use of TNF-α inhibitors in presence of chronic liver disease exist • Etanercept or adalimumab preferred • Secukinumab may also be used in compensated liver disease, while this can be done, it is important to remember that some degree of TNF alpha blockade does occur with secukinumab • Most TNF alpha blockers can induce changes in liver enzymes and even worsening of liver disease • However, literature is scant

Contd...

Contd...

Comorbidities	Screening	What to do?
Chronic renal failure	Renal function test	• Metabolized by proteolysis • Etanercept preferred • Caution: risk of infection
Cancer[12]		• Data is scant • Possible increase risk of recurrence of solid organ malignancy • Should be used with caution, avoid, if possible
Obesity[13]		• Secukinumab preferred • TNF-α inhibitors can be used, associated with mean weight gain of 1–4 kg • Use biologic with lifestyle modification • Weight reduction is associated with better efficacy of biologic therapy

(IGRA: Interferon-gamma release assays; AFB: Acid-fast bacillus; INH: Isoniazid; HBsAg: Hepatitis B virus surface antigen; LFT: Liver function test; HIV: Human immunodeficiency virus; MRI: Magnetic resonance imaging; ANA: Antinuclear antibody).

Choosing A Biologic: Based on the Facilities Available and Preferred Route of Administration

While it is a reasonable assumption that patient will prefer subcutaneous injections over infusions as patients need to come to hospital or daycare center to take infusion, there are studies which suggest that lot of patients prefer intravenous therapy over subcutaneous therapy because of reasons like interactions with staff during injection, dislike for self-injection and less frequent injections.[14]

Most of the physicians prefer the use of subcutaneous route as these can be injected in a clinic-based setting and subsequent injections can be administered by the carer or patient himself. Schedule of treatment can also determine the choice of biologic. Ustekinumab requires injection once in 12 weeks for maintenance and has become first-line biologic therapy for management of plaque psoriasis in western world. Infliximab has dosing schedule of 0, 2, 6 weeks and 8 weekly thereafter; however, it is given as infusion and most of the physicians do not prefer to use it for this indication. Etanercept has initial dosing of 50 mg twice a week or once a week for 12 weeks and patient or caregiver should be ready to learn to self-inject.

Adalimumab has once in fortnightly maintenance dosing and secukinumab has once-in-a-month maintenance dosing; however, secukinumab requires weekly injections for initial 5 weeks as induction therapy.

Thus, choosing a biologic not only depends on science of pathogenesis and targeted therapy of psoriasis but it also depends on numerous other factors, which requires consideration by physicians before prescribing biologic else best of the science can fail because of the circumstances.

Combination with Biologics

Biologics can be either used as monotherapy or can be combined with other form of systemic therapy. Combination therapy can enhance efficacy of treatment, decrease the side effects by allowing dose reductions and increase the onset of remission. Combination therapy can be used in following settings:

- Synergistic mechanism of action:
  - *Rescue therapy*: Use of additional conventional systemic agent at the initiation of biologic therapy for <120 days
  - *Bridging therapy*: Initiation of conventional systemic therapy before starting biologic therapy and used concomitantly with biologics for <120 days
  - *Concomitant therapy*: Systemic therapy used for >120 days along with biologics.
- *Rotational therapy*: Faster action of biologic and continued action of second drug can reduce cost of therapy.
- *To reduce adverse effect of biologics*: Use of methotrexate for prevention of development of human antichimeric antibody while using infliximab.

It is not possible to combine all forms of systemic therapy with biologics as it may lead to unacceptable immunosuppression in some cases. There are no approved indications for combining biologic with conventional systemic agents in psoriasis; however, in real world adding conventional systemic agents offers multiple advantages like better efficacy, improved pharmacoeconomics and improved long-term disease management. We shall discuss briefly regarding the systemic therapies that can be combined safely with biologics in the scenarios given in Table 15.3.

Combining Biologics with Biologics

We have come to a point where multiple biologics of different class with different mechanism of actions are available. Since, biomarker for efficacy of particular biologic in a subset of patients is not available, we have some percentage of patients who do not respond to a biologic in a desired manner. When a patient does not achieve desirable response with one biologic, there is a scope for using combination biologic. However, there is a fear

Table 15.3: Systemic therapies combined with biologics.

Biologic therapy	Systemic therapy	Baseline (biologic)		Combination		Literature
		PASI-75	PASI-90	PASI-75	PASI-90	
Etaner-cept	Photo-therapy (NBUVB)	55%	23%	85%	58%	Kircik et al.[15]

- Etanercept is used in dose of 50 mg twice weekly and NBUVB given thrice weekly
- 26% patients also achieved PASI-100
- Caution should be exercised as there is higher risk of development of cutaneous malignancy and combination should be limited to shortest period of time
- Phototherapy has been used with standard dosing of etanercept for faster clearance, reduced dosing of etanercept (50 mg weekly) or as rescue therapy in patients not responding adequately after 12 weeks of etanercept

	Metho-trexate	55%	23%	70.2%	34%	Gottlieb AB[16]

- Methotrexate was used in the dose of 7.5–15 mg per week
- Patients who can tolerate and do not have any contraindications to the use of methotrexate should be given a combination of low dose methotrexate with etanercept
- There are no safety issues in this combination and faster clearance can be achieved

	Acitretin	55%	23%	57.9%		Lee JH[17]

- In this randomized controlled trial, acitretin 10 mg twice a day and etanercept 25 mg twice weekly was compared with etanercept 50 mg twice weekly
- Similar PASI score could be achieved even at half the etanercept dose

	Cyclo-sporine	55%	23%	-	-	Cohen Barak E[18]

- No guidelines for combination, risk of infection and malignancy prevents combined use of these drugs. It has been used safely in many difficult cases. It has role in the following scenarios
  - o Patient already on anti-TNF alpha therapy and has exacerbation and needs a rescue therapy
  - o Patient on cyclosporine for long and requires transition from cyclosporine, should be slowly tapered to prevent rebound
  - o May be used as a combination therapy rarely in severe recalcitrant psoriasis

Adali-mumab	Photo-therapy	71%	45%	95%	75%	Bagel J[19]

- Adalimumab was given in approved dose and NBUVB was given three times a week, 55% patients also achieved PASI-100 in combination group as compared to 20% with monotherapy
- Erythema is the only adverse effect encountered. Can be used as rescue therapy, bridge therapy, concomitant or maintenance therapy. Caution as already been discussed

Contd...

Contd...

Biologic therapy	Systemic therapy	Efficacy					
		Baseline (biologic)		Combination		
		PASI-75	PASI-90	PASI-75	PASI-90	Literature
	Metho-trexate	71%	45%	-	-	-

- There are no studies in clinical efficacy of combination of adalimumab and methotrexate in psoriasis
- Studies in rheumatoid arthritis found combination to be safe and effective

| | Acitretin | 71% | 45% | - | - | - |

- There are no studies showing clinical efficacy of combination of adalimumab and acitretin
- Case reports of safe and efficacious combination exists. Combination can be used safely as bridging therapy or as maintenance therapy in case one wants to reduce the maintenance dose of biologics

| | Cyclo-sporine | 71% | 45% | - | - | Cohen Barak E[18] |

- No guidelines for combinations; issues are same as has been discussed with etanercept and cyclosporine combination

| Inflixi-mab | Photo-therapy | 80% | 57% | - | - | - |

- No guidelines for combination, combination can be used as rescue therapy when biologic is losing its efficacy or as maintenance therapy

| | Metho-trexate | 80% | 57% | - | - | Spertino J[20] |

- Minor increase in efficacy on combining low dose methotrexate to infliximab; however, it improves drug survival (duration for which infliximab is effective), decreases infusion reactions and development of anti-drug antibodies. Thus, low dose methotrexate should always be combined with infliximab

| | Acitretin | 80% | 57% | - | - | - |

- No studies in plaque psoriasis. Has been combined in erythrodermic psoriasis as maintenance therapy and found to be safe and effective. Can be used as a rescue therapy or maintenance therapy

| | Cyclo-sporine | 80% | 57% | - | - | - |

- No guidelines for combination. Avoid combination as risk of infection is high

| Itolizu-mab | Cyclo-sporine | 45% | 21% | - | - | Gupta et al.[21] |

- In this case report, treatment was initiated with cyclosporine 100 mg twice a day for 2 weeks followed by standard dosing of itolizumab, this resulted in PASI-90 response in 12 weeks
- Studies of combination therapy of itolizumab with other systemic therapy like methotrexate, acitretin and phototherapy is lacking

Contd...

Contd...

Biologic therapy	Systemic therapy	Efficacy				Literature
		Baseline (biologic)		Combination		
		PASI-75	PASI-90	PASI-75	PASI-90	
Secuki-numab	-	81%	60%	-	-	-

- Reports of combination therapy with secukinumab with other systemic therapy are not available, possibly because it achieves clearance of disease in majority of patients when used as monotherapy and it is a relatively new drug
- It is reasonable to assume that it can be combined with acitretin and phototherapy safely if required.

that blocking multiple immune pathways by using multiple biologics can lead to severe immune suppression and can be counter-productive. There are reports of use of combination of IL-12/23 monoclonal antibody with anti-TNF-α therapy for management of recalcitrant psoriasis.[22] Combining different classes of biologics should be avoided unless there is a strong clinical need and patient should be closely followed-up for the risk of infection.

Scenario 2: As a first-line therapy, especially when rapid control and complete clearance is desirable and there are no financial constraints.

- Patient who wants rapid control and complete clearance of disease because of social reasons often comes to dermatologist in distress. What can be done in this scenario? Secukinumab is the only biologic which is Food and Drug Administration-approved as first line for management of chronic plaque psoriasis and provide rapid clearance in this scenario. Infliximab is another option to gain rapid control of disease; however, safety should not be compromised and all investigations should be conducted prior to the initiation of biologics.

Scenario 3: When patient has failed conventional systemic therapy and at least one biologic therapy.

When patient does not respond to one biologic therapy, how to use another biologic therapy?

SWITCHING BIOLOGICS

Patient may be required to switch from one biologic to another because of various reasons like primary failure, secondary failure, adverse effects like infusion reactions or other factors like patients request and cost of therapy.

When switching is performed for safety reasons, a wash out period should be allowed to normalize the safety parameter. However, when a switch is performed for inadequate response, wash out period is not necessary. A switch should be considered when patient does not achieve PASI-50 at the end of induction phase (in real world, if patient does not achieve PASI-75, switch should be considered as PASI-75 is considered as the meaningful response).

Switching for Inefficacy

If switching is done for inefficacy, switching can be done between same classes of biologic or a new class of biologic can be introduced. Inefficacy in biologics is not a class action unlike adverse effects and they can be interchanged within the same class. For example, patient not responding to etanercept can be given adalimumab or infliximab, similarly patient not responding to infliximab can be given a trial of adalimumab or etanercept. There is no pecking order or hierarchy in anti-TNF-α inhibitor, a patient who shows poor response to drugs with superior efficacy (infliximab) can be switched to adalimumab or etanercept. In general, response in biologic-experienced patient is not as good as biologic-naive patient.[23]

Switching from etanercept—switch to adalimumab, infliximab, secukinumab or itolizumab, start 1 week after last dose (when next dose is due).

Switching from adalimumab—switch to etanercept, adalimumab, infliximab, secukinumab or itolizumab, start 2 weeks after last dose (when next dose is due).

Switching from infliximab—switch to adalimumab, etanercept, secukinumab or itolizumab, start 2–4 weeks after last dose.

Switching from itolizumab—switch to any of the anti-TNF-α inhibitors or secukinumab, exact timing to start new biologic not available but can be started at 2 weeks.

Switching from secukinumab—switch to any of the anti-TNF-α inhibitors, start between 2 and 4 weeks.

Switching for Adverse Effects

If a patient develops adverse effects while on biologic, one needs to switch biologic. This switch depends on whether adverse effect is due to the class effect or it is due to the specific adverse effect of the biologic.

- Anti-drug antibodies (ADA) to TNF-α inhibitors do not cross react. Patient who develop ADA and develops loss of response can be started on another anti-TNF-α inhibitor.
- Patients who develop infectious complications like reactivation of latent tuberculosis or hepatitis B infection require stoppage of drug and institution of appropriate therapy. Since, this reactivation is a class action of anti-TNF-α inhibitor, it should be restarted only after clinical

evaluation. Ideally, a different class of biologic like secukinumab should be used.

- Patients who develop other class action adverse effects of anti-TNF-α inhibitors like worsening of congestive heart failure or precipitation of multiple sclerosis in a rare event, these drugs should be avoided for future use.
- Patients who develop worsening or new onset inflammatory bowel disease while on secukinumab should not be restarted on secukinumab, while patients who develop vulvovaginal candidiasis can be possibly treated for candidiasis and treatment can be continued.

Switching of biologic in this scenario can be better understood by knowing the use of biologic in presence of comorbidities and contraindications of various biologics discussed in previous sections and earlier chapters.

▋ BIOLOGICS FOR LESS COMMON FORMS OF PSORIASIS

Nail Psoriasis

Nail involvement occurs in up to 50% of patients with psoriasis. Nail psoriasis is associated with more severe disease, duration of skin lesions and arthropathy. Involvement of nail even without arthritis has negative impact on functioning and quality of life. Patient can have constant pain, which can result in restriction of day-to-day activities. Nail involvement is objectively measured using Nail Psoriasis Severity Index (NAPSI). Topical and systemic therapies are not very effective for management of nail psoriasis. Data using biologic for management of nail psoriasis is not robust.

TNF-α inhibitors like etanercept, adalimumab and infliximab has been used for the management of nail psoriasis (Table 15.4).

Since many available biologics work on nail psoriasis, choice of biologic should depend on other factors which have been discussed before.

Table 15.4: Biologics used for the management of nail psoriasis.

Biologic	Schedule	Outcome	Literature
Infliximab	5 mg/kg 0, 2, 6 and 8 weekly	Nail Psoriasis Severity Index (NAPSI)-75 in 65% patients at 22 weeks and 82% at 38 weeks	Fabroni C[24]
Adalimumab	40 mg every other week	NAPSI 75 in 46% patients at 26 weeks	Elewski BE[25]
Secukinumab	300 mg 0, 1, 2, 3, 4 and every 4 weeks	NAPSI reduction by 45% at 16 weeks	Kristian Reich[26]

Palmoplantar Psoriasis, Scalp Psoriasis, and Other Variants of Psoriasis

Psoriasis involving palms and soles and other difficult-to-treat areas like genital and scalp can be quite disabling and can severely impair the quality of life despite involving less body surface area. Biologics can be used for these areas when conventional systemic therapy does not work adequately; however, biologics have not been studied rigorously for these forms of psoriasis. Use of TNF-α inhibitors for treatment of other diseases resulted in development of paradoxical development of psoriasis rarely, commonest of which was palmoplantar variant. That may be the reason that there were no trials for management of palmoplantar psoriasis using TNF-α inhibitors. There are many case reports of successful management of palmoplantar psoriasis using TNF-α inhibitors and same can be tried in recalcitrant cases.[27,28]

Secukinumab has been studied in double-blind, randomized, placebo-controlled trial for management of palmoplantar psoriasis and found to be very effective in 300 mg dose. At week 16, Palmoplantar Psoriasis Area and Severity Index (ppPASI) reduced by 54% and almost 33% patients achieved clear palms.[29]

Erythrodermic Psoriasis

Psoriatic erythroderma can occur de novo or it can occur as an extension of chronic plaque psoriasis. Erythrodermic flare of psoriasis is associated with chills, edema, weight loss and altered temperature regulation. Untreated disease is associated with serious morbidity and even mortality in some cases.[30] As erythrodermic psoriasis is an uncommon disease, high quality scientific data is lacking and treatment is based on the experience and expert opinions.

Erythroderma causes severe physiological disturbance, drugs, which act faster, should be used so that physiology can be restored at the earliest. National Psoriasis Foundation guidelines for management of erythrodermic psoriasis recommended cyclosporine and infliximab as first-line agent. Etanercept can also be used as second-line agent along with methotrexate.[31]

Secukinumab has also been successfully used recently by various authors for the management of erythrodermic psoriasis; however, it is relatively a new drug and data regarding its use in erythrodermic psoriasis is scant.[32]

Infliximab and secukinumab are good options for treating erythrodermic psoriasis with biologics as they result in rapid response.

Generalized Pustular Psoriasis

Generalized pustular psoriasis (GPP) is a rare form of life-threatening psoriasis, characterized by development of sterile pustules with widespread erythema. GPP variants includes childhood GPP, von Zumbush type and impetigo herpetiformis (GPP in pregnant women). Extensive GPP can be life-threatening and needs faster control of the disease. Robust evidence-based data for treatment of this variant is lacking and guidelines are based on limited data and expert recommendations.

National Psoriasis Foundation recommends acitretin, methotrexate, cyclosporine, and infliximab as the first-line therapy. However, many experts believe that in extensive disease, infliximab should be used as first-line option because of its rapid onset of action. Adalimumab, etanercept and combination therapy is a second-line therapy for management of GPP.

Etanercept can be used as first-line therapy for childhood GPP as etanercept is approved for pediatric use. Adalimumab and infliximab can be used as second-line therapy apart from conventional systemic therapy for management of childhood GPP.

Generalized pustular psoriasis in pregnancy is difficult to manage as it can be life threatening for both mother and child. Cyclosporine and oral steroids are traditionally considered first-line therapy for management of GPP in pregnancy. Infliximab has been used safely for management of GPP in pregnancy, care should be taken about vaccination of neonate post-delivery (details have been discussed in the Chapter on Biologics in Special Situations).[33]

Recently, a phase 3 open label, multicenter study has been conducted in Japan for use of secukinumab in management of GPP. This study concluded that 83% patients improved with secukinumab at week 16.[34]

Infliximab appears to be the first-line biologic option for management of GPP. Evidence for the use of secukinumab in GPP is rapidly accumulating and is being safer and easier to administer the drug. Therefore, it can definitely be tried in the clinical scenario if indicated.

▌ HOW LONG TO USE BIOLOGICS?

Physician who counsel patients to start biologic is always faced with this question by patients and sometimes by himself. How long can we use them continuously? Should we use them continuously once we start using them to maintain remission or we can use them as on required basis, thus reducing the cost of therapy? There are multiple studies, which have been done which have looked at efficacy of various biologics in continuous or intermittent manner.

Study involving intermittent and continuous therapy of infliximab had to be terminated because of higher adverse effects in intermittent group and most of the experts agree that infliximab should be used in continuous manner.[35] Long-term safety and efficacy in real world practice for infliximab has been studied for up to 98 weeks.[36]

Etanercept has been studied as continuous and intermittent therapy. Patient with interrupted therapy had longer survival of biologic. Another study found that retreatment requires almost 4 weeks more than initial treatment to achieve remission.[37]

Adalimumab results in PASI-75 response in 80% patients. Study done by Papp et al. found that patient in whom treatment was withdrawn after remission was achieved and reinitiated on relapse, 69% patient achieved PASI-75. There were no safety issues in intermittent and continuous therapy groups. In real world, patient stops therapy in between and it is reassuring that majority of these patients regain control of the disease without any major safety issues.[38] Adalimumab has been used continuously for 3 years safely and its efficacy has been maintained in a phase 3 trial.[39]

Secukinumab has also been studied in as needed versus fixed interval maintenance regime in a randomized, double-blind trial. Study concluded that fixed interval dosing is much more efficacious as compared to as needed basis; however, safety in both groups were found to be comparable. However, an extension of the ERASURE and FIXTURE trials by Blauvelt et al. showed that intermittent treatment with secukinumab brought down the efficacy of the drug. Long-term safety data from various trials is available for up to 2 years of continuous use in psoriasis and psoriatic arthritis.[40,41]

CONCLUSION

Successful use of biologics for management of psoriasis requires basic understanding of the pathogenesis of disease, availability of conventional systemic therapy, comorbid diseases and financial constraints of patient.

REFERENCES

1. National Institute for Health and Care Excellence. Psoriasis: assessment and management. Clinical Guideline CG153. 2012. [online] Available from: https://www.nice.org.uk/guidance/cg153. [Accessed December 2017].
2. Smith CH, Jabbar-Lopez ZK, Yiu ZZ, et al. British Association of Dermatologists guidelines for biologic therapy for psoriasis 2017. Br J Dermatol. 2017;177(3): 628-36.
3. Langley RG, Elewski BE, Lebwohl M, et al. Secukinumab in plaque psoriasis results of two phase 3 trials. N Engl J Med. 2014;371:326-38.
4. Leonardi CL, Powers JL, Matheson RT, et al. Etanercept as monotherapy in patients with psoriasis. N Engl J Med. 2003;349(21):2014-22.
5. Menter A, Tyring SK, Gordon K, et al. Adalimumab therapy for moderate to severe psoriasis: a randomized, controlled phase III trial. J Am Acad Dermatol. 2008;58(1):106-15.
6. Krupashankar DS, Dogra S, Kura M, et al. Efficacy and safety of itolizumab, a novel anti-CD6 monoclonal antibody, in patients with moderate to severe chronic plaque psoriasis: results of a double-blind, randomized, placebo-controlled, phase-III study. J Am Acad Dermatol. 2014;71(3):484-92.

7. Cantini F, Nannini C, Niccoli L, et al. Guidance for the management of patients with latent tuberculosis infection requiring biologic therapy in rheumatology and dermatology clinical practice. Autoimmun Rev. 2015;14(6):503-9.

8. Vassilopoulos D, Apostolopoulou A, Hadziyannis E, et al. Long-term safety of anti-TNF treatment in patients with rheumatic diseases and chronic or resolved hepatitis B virus infection. Ann Rheum Dis. 2010;69(7):1352-5.

9. Amin M, No DJ, Egeberg A, et al. Choosing first-line biologic treatment for moderate-to-severe psoriasis: what does the evidence say? Am J Clin Dermatol. 2017 Oct 27.

10. Di Nuzzo S, Boccaletti V, Fantini C, et al. Are anti-TNF-α agents safe for treating psoriasis in hepatitis C virus patients with advanced liver disease? Case reports and review of the literature. Dermatology. 2016;232(1):102-6.

11. Silvy F, Bertin D, Bardin N, et al. Antinuclear antibodies in patients with psoriatic arthritis treated or not with biologics. PloS one. 2015;10(7):e0134218.

12. Majewksi S, Kheterpal M, Nardone B, et al. First line biologic agent therapy for moderate-to-severe psoriasis in cancer survivors. J Am Acad Dermatol. 2016;74 (5);(Suppl.1):AB250.

13. Briot K, Garnero P, Le Henanff A, et al. Body weight, body composition, and bone turnover changes in patients with spondyloarthropathy receiving anti-tumour necrosis factor α treatment. Ann Rheum Dis. 2005;64(8):1137-40.

14. Scarpato S, Antivalle M, Favalli EG, et al. Patient preferences in the choice of anti-TNF therapies in rheumatoid arthritis. Results from a questionnaire survey (RIVIERA study). Rheumatology (Oxford). 2010;49:289-94.

15. Kircik L, Bagel J, Korman N, et al. Utilization of narrow-band ultraviolet light b therapy and etanercept for the treatment of psoriasis (UNITE): efficacy, safety, and patient-reported outcomes. J Drugs Dermatol. 2008;7(3):245-53.

16. Gottlieb AB, Langley RG, Strober BE, et al. A randomized, double-blind, placebo-controlled study to evaluate the addition of methotrexate to etanercept in patients with moderate to severe plaque psoriasis. Br J Dermatol. 2012;167(3):649-57.

17. Lee JH, Youn JI, Kim TY, et al. A multicenter, randomized, open-label pilot trial assessing the efficacy and safety of etanercept 50 mg twice weekly followed by etanercept 25 mg twice weekly, the combination of etanercept 25 mg twice weekly and acitretin and acitretin alone in patients with moderate to severe psoriasis. BMC Dermatol. 2016;16(1):11.

18. Cohen Barak E, Kerner M, Rozenman D, et al. Combination therapy of cyclosporine and anti-tumor necrosis factor α in psoriasis: a case series of 10 patients. Dermatol Ther. 2015;28(3):126-30.

19. Bagel J. Adalimumab plus narrowband ultraviolet-B light phototherapy for the treatment of moderate to severe psoriasis. J Drugs Dermatol. 2011;10(4):366-71.

20. Spertino J, López-Ferrer A, Vilarrasa E, et al. Long-term study of infliximab for psoriasis in daily practice: drug survival depends on combined treatment, obesity and infusion reactions. J Eur Acad Dermatol Venereol. 2014;28(11):1514-21.

21. Gupta A, Sharma YK, Deo K, et al. Severe recalcitrant psoriasis treated with itolizumab, a novel anti-CD6 monoclonal antibody. Indian J Dermatol Venereol Leprol. 2016;82(4):459.

22. Gniadecki R, Bang B, Sand C. Combination of anti-tumour necrosis factor-α and anti-interleukin-12/23 antibodies in refractory psoriasis and psoriatic arthritis: a long-term case-series observational study. Br J Dermatol. 2016;174(5):1145-6.

23. Kerdel F, Zaiac M. An evolution in switching therapy for psoriasis patients who fail to meet treatment goals. Dermatol Ther. 2015;28(6):390-403.
24. Fabroni C, Gori A, Troiano M, et al. Infliximab efficacy in nail psoriasis. A retrospective study in 48 patients. J Eur Acad Dermatol Venereol. 2011;25(5): 549-53.
25. Elewski BE, Okun MM, Papp K, et al. Adalimumab for nail psoriasis: efficacy and safety from the first 26 weeks of a phase 3, randomized, placebo-controlled trial. J Am Acad Dermatol. 2017 Oct 6.
26. Reich K, Arenberger P, Mrowietz U, et al. Secukinumab shows high and sustained efficacy in nail psoriasis: week 80 results from the TRANSFIGURE study. J Am Acad Dermatol. 2017;76(6):AB232.
27. Ko JM, Gottlieb AB, Kerbleski JF. Induction and exacerbation of psoriasis with TNF-blockade therapy: a review and analysis of 127 cases. J Dermatolog Treat. 2009;20(2):100-8.
28. Weinberg JM. Successful treatment of recalcitrant palmoplantar psoriasis with etanercept. Cutis. 2003;72(5):396-8.
29. Gottlieb A, Sullivan J, van Doorn M, et al. Secukinumab shows significant efficacy in palmoplantar psoriasis: results from GESTURE, a randomized controlled trial. J Am Acad Dermatol. 2017;76(1):70-80.
30. Boyd AS, Menter A. Erythrodermic psoriasis: precipitating factors, course, and prognosis in 50 patients. J Am Acad Dermatol. 1989;21:985-91.
31. Rosenbach M, Hsu S, Korman NJ, et al. Treatment of erythrodermic psoriasis: from the medical board of the National Psoriasis Foundation. J Am Acad Dermatol. 2010;62(4):655-62.
32. Mugheddu C, Atzori L, Lappi A, et al. Successful secukinumab treatment of generalized pustular psoriasis and erythrodermic psoriasis. J Eur Acad Dermatol Venereol. 2017;31(9):e420-1.
33. Robinson A, Van Voorhees AS, Hsu S, et al. Treatment of pustular psoriasis: from the Medical Board of the National Psoriasis Foundation. J Am Acad Dermatol. 2012;67(2):279-88.
34. Imafuku S, Honma M, Okubo Y, et al. Efficacy and safety of secukinumab in patients with generalized pustular psoriasis: a 52-week analysis from phase III open-label multicenter Japanese study. J Dermatol. 2016;43(9):1011-7.
35. Menter A, Feldman SR, Weinstein GD, et al. A randomized comparison of continuous vs. intermittent infliximab maintenance regimens over 1 year in the treatment of moderate-to-severe plaque psoriasis. J Am Acad Dermatol. 2007;56(1):31.
36. Shear NH, Hartmann M, Toledo-Bahena M, et al. Long-term efficacy and safety of infliximab maintenance therapy in patients with plaque-type psoriasis in real-world practice. Br J Dermatol. 2014;171(3):631-41.
37. Ortonne JP, Taieb A, Ormerod AD, et al. Patients with moderate-to-severe psoriasis recapture clinical response during re-treatment with etanercept. Br J Dermatol. 2009;161(5):1190-5.
38. Papp K, Crowley J, Ortonne JP, et al. Adalimumab for moderate to severe chronic plaque psoriasis: efficacy and safety of retreatment and disease recurrence following withdrawal from therapy. Br J Dermatol. 2011;164(2):434-41.
39. Gordon K, Papp K, Poulin Y, et al. Long-term efficacy and safety of adalimumab in patients with moderate to severe psoriasis treated continuously over 3 years: results from an open-label extension study for patients from REVEAL. J Am Acad Dermatol. 2012;66(2):241-51.

40. Kavanaugh A, Mease PJ, Reimold AM, et al. Secukinumab for long-term treatment of psoriatic arthritis: a two-year follow-up from a phase iii, randomized, double-blind placebo-controlled study. Arthritis Care Res. 2017;69(3):347-55.

41. Mrowietz U, Leonardi CL, Girolomoni G, et al. Secukinumab retreatment-as-needed versus fixed-interval maintenance regimen for moderate to severe plaque psoriasis: a randomized, double-blind, noninferiority trial (SCULPTURE). J Am Acad Dermatol. 2015;73(1):27-36.

Biologic Approach to Management of Immunobullous Diseases

Manish Khandare, Ankan Gupta

INTRODUCTION

Pemphigus is a group of related autoimmune disorders characterized by flaccid vesiculobullous lesions over skin and mucosae. Pemphigus vulgaris and pemphigus foliaceus are the most common types and are fatal if not treated. Management of both the types is similar but pemphigus vulgaris is more difficult to treat. The management of pemphigus vulgaris will be discussed henceforth. Systemic steroids have been the cornerstone of therapy and continue to be the most common drug used to attain clinical remission. The role of steroid sparing agents (SSA) is for maintenance and assisting in decreasing the cumulative dose of systemic steroids. The SSA traditionally employed, in decreasing order of preference, include azathioprine (AZA), mycophenolate mofetil (MMF) and dapsone. Cyclophosphamide (CYC) is a common SSA used in India with steroids orally and as pulse dosing but western literature supports its use in only refractory cases. Rituximab has been a revelation in the last decade for treating autoimmune vesiculobullous disorders. We suggest rituximab to be the first-line SSA in all fresh cases. It is essential for readers to know the definitions of disease process and therapy before proceeding further.[1]

INITIAL MANAGEMENT[2,3]

Systemic steroids at the dose of 1–2 mg/kg are universally accepted as the treatment option of choice to control the disease activity. In refractory cases, intravenous immunoglobulin (IVIg) is the only other option to bring control. Few physicians still prefer starting an SSA in conjunction with steroids but the rationale suggests otherwise. Firstly, the SSA are slow to act and do not help in acute control of the disease and secondly, it increases immunosuppression which makes the patient more susceptible to infections, which in turn is responsible for higher disease activity. For this reason precisely, we suggest rituximab (and other SSA) to not be used in the acute stage of the disease.

We believe that each and every pemphigus patient once diagnosed should be given at least 1 mg/kg of steroids regardless of the pemphigus disease area index (PDAI) score to prevent a smoldering disease process which ultimately leads to a higher cumulative steroid dosing. We also believe rituximab to be offered to each and every patient unless contraindicated, as it does have a higher efficacy, higher safety, and offers a much better quality of life than other SSA. Our experience with cyclophosphamide and pulse dosing is limited and its use will not be discussed further in this chapter.

The role of adequate antibiotic coverage proactively, skin cleansing and oral care, antiseptic baths and compresses, and topical and intralesional steroids cannot be overemphasized. Early recognition of bacterial infection and/or superadded herpetic infection is foremost and helps in decreasing the cumulative steroid dosing and early disease control. The management would also include vitamin D correction, calcium and bisphosphonate therapy, analgesia before dressings, requisite glycemic control, and management of hypertension. Initial management of pemphigus should be done in an inpatient setting.

MAINTENANCE AND STEROID TAPERING

Most clinicians start SSA along with steroids with the rationale of SSA taking over the mantle on disease control as the steroids are tapered. We, however, prefer to increase the steroid dose to "2-step-back" dose during acute flare rather than adding an SSA. If disease continues to be active, we restart at the initial dose and then taper the steroid at a slower rate. The speed of tapering steroids does not have a consensus with decreasing the dose every 15 days by 20 mg till 40 mg, by 10 mg till 20 mg and slower thereafter is an acceptable approach. In patients worsening on tapering of steroids, a slow tapering by 2.5–5 mg every fortnightly also results in a fruitful result. In refractory cases where disease flares up with tapering of steroids at a very high dose of steroids, adding an SSA after going 2 steps back is a reasonable plan.

INTRODUCTION OF SSA

The ultimate aim in management of pemphigus is to have a long remission period completely off therapy.[1] SSA are the drugs to maintain remission and rituximab has proved to be a boon in this regard with several case series suggesting it to be the most effective SSA in management of pemphigus.[4-6] There is no ideal time for introducing the SSA and the therapy is individualized in most cases but logic says adding the SSA when the dose of steroids are low would prevent higher depth of immunosuppression at one point of time and hence a better control of secondary infection, thereby effectively preventing infection related flares. Steroid dose of 20 mg or less constitutes "low-dose immunosuppression" and ideally the SSA should be introduced after achieving that dose but practically SSA often have to be introduced at doses as high as 40 mg. Introducing another immunosuppressive at higher doses is discouraged. Because of longer and much higher immunosuppression with rituximab than other SSA, the first infusion should preferably be started at steroid doses of 20 mg or less. Hence, the decision on SSA can wait during the initial management period and can be made later on depending upon the comorbidities, hepatic and renal profile, and after excluding the contraindications for each SSA.

Rituximab is offered as the first option for all patients, especially if the disease is of recent onset. Financial constraints notwithstanding, the total cost of management of disease over a long period are discussed with the patient and relatives and they are encouraged to opt for rituximab as the SSA. The cost of investigations done prior to clearing the patient for rituximab infusion is itself a financial burden and can be distributed over time to decrease a onetime strain. A negative viral screening including the core antigen of hepatitis B, eliminating the possibility of latent and active tuberculosis, antinuclear antibodies (ANA) negativity, cardiac clearance and normal immunoglobulin levels are fundamental requisites before planning for rituximab. Most of these investigations take a few weeks to show up and can be planned sequentially to allay the cost. Any contradictory result deters the use of rituximab and warrants a discussion with the concerned specialist physician regarding the feasibility of using rituximab or opting for an alternative SSA.

Azathioprine is the second choice for SSA and requires an initial thiopurine methyltransferase (TPMT) enzyme level to decide on its use and dosing. If the TPMT assay is not available, starting with 1 mg/kg of AZA and stringent monitoring on the blood counts and hepatic profile is required. MMF is another option, which is safer than AZA but not as effective as AZA.[4]

DISCONTINUATION OF THERAPY

After rituximab infusion, the steroid dose can be tapered to physiological dose and maintained till immunological remission.

With other SSA, there is a controversy where few physicians taper and discontinue the steroids and start tapering the SSA after 6–8 weeks. We prefer tapering the steroid to the physiological dose and start tapering of SSA within 4–8 weeks depending upon the clinical remission. AZA can be tapered by 50 mg and MMF by 500 mg every 8 weeks and discontinued. Steroids at physiological dose are continued till immunological remission. Occasional flares can be managed in a similar way by "2-step-back" method if required. Additional dose of rituximab after 12–18 months might be needed, decision for which should be strictly clinical rather than immunological.[7]

TIMING FOR VACCINATION

The timing for vaccination with use of rituximab in pemphigus is tricky. For vaccines to be effective maximally, the ideal timing should be such that the disease activity is minimal and iatrogenic immunosuppression should be in "low-dose immunosuppression" range as discussed in chapter on vaccines. The other important aspect is to vaccinate prior to using a biologic. We find a window of 2 weeks period after tapering the steroids to 20 mg and then vaccinate them. It is important to be patient while using rituximab in pemphigus as the risk of acquiring infections can be fatal and outweigh the benefits of its use.

DOSING OF RITUXIMAB

The "rheumatoid arthritis" protocol of infusing 1,000 mg of rituximab 2 weeks apart is the standard regimen used by most dermatologists.[8] The lymphoma protocol is not superior and uses higher amount of total rituximab. The lower dose rituximab protocol employs 500 mg rituximab 2 weeks apart and is proving to be effective but the duration of remission might be lower.[9] We still await a head-to-head trial on dosing of rituximab in pemphigus.[10]

RITUXIMAB FOR PEMPHIGUS IN CHILDREN

Pemphigus is rare in children and data of use of rituximab in children is scarce. Though the long-term effects of rituximab are yet to be seen, it does appear to be a safe SSA for use.[11]

RITUXIMAB FOR PEMPHIGUS IN PREGNANCY

Pemphigus is an uncommon disease in pregnancy and can be mostly managed with steroids alone or steroids and IVIg. Severe pemphigus requiring biologic therapy for management is rare. Rituximab is a pregnancy category C drug. Its prescribing information states that contraception should be advised during and after 12 months of rituximab use in women in reproductive age-group. British Society for Rheumatology (BSR) guidelines recommend rituximab should be stopped 6 months prior to conception, however pregnant patients who were exposed to rituximab have had uneventful pregnancy outcomes.[12,13] Rituximab can cause neonatal cytopenia or B-cell depletion and can increase risk of infections in neonate.[14] The vaccination of neonate needs to be discussed with the neonatologists and avoidance of live vaccines is advised.

ADVERSE EFFECTS WITH USE OF RITUXIMAB

The adverse events with use of rituximab are mostly infusion reactions, which can be minimized with premedications. Rituximab desensitization protocols are also available if rituximab therapy is highly desired.[15] Infections though definitely a risk, remain incalculable because of the concomitant use of steroids. Other rare idiosyncratic side effects include thromboembolic phenomenon, long-term persistent hypogammaglobulinemia, and progressive multifocal leukoencephalopathy.[16,17]

ALTERNATIVE TREATMENT OPTIONS FOR PEMPHIGUS

Rarely, patients do not respond to most standard therapies or may have contraindications to their use. Other drugs in our arsenal with proven efficacy include dapsone, methotrexate,[18] cyclosporine,[19] and tetracyclines.[20] Cyclophosphamide, immunoadsorption, and plasmapheresis are reserved for most refractory cases.

PROPOSED PROTOCOL FOR USE OF RITUXIMAB IN A PATIENT WITH PEMPHIGUS (ADULT WEIGHING 60 KG)

- Step I (Control of disease activity)
  - Establish the diagnosis with biopsy, direct immunofluorescence and ELISA (enzyme-linked immunosorbent assay) for desmogleins.
  - Do a presteroid investigation and discuss with patient the options of SSA with benefits of using rituximab over other SSA.
  - Start the patient on steroid equivalent to 1 mg/kg (up to 2 mg/kg as required).
- Step II (Maintenance)
  - Taper the steroids after new lesions stop appearing and older lesions start epithelializing.
  - Taper steroids every fortnightly thereafter as 60, 40, 30, 20, 15, 10, 7.5, 5, 2.5.
  - A slower tapering may be required as described in the text.
- Step III (Introduction of rituximab)
  - After meticulously ruling out all contraindications for rituximab, plan for the 1st infusion after achieving 20 mg dose of steroids.
  - Complete vaccination 2 weeks prior to infusion of rituximab.
- Step IV (Premedication and infusion)
  - Regular vital and cardiac monitoring has to be done. Make sure that the resuscitation kit is available and accessible.
  - Withhold the steroid dose on the day and the antihypertensives on the day of infusion.

- Premedicate 1 hour prior to the infusion with:
    - Injection methylprednisolone 100 mg as intravenous infusion in 100 mL of normal saline over 30 minutes
    - Tablet paracetamol 1 g
    - Injection avil 25 mg intravenously.
- Monitor vitals every 30 minutes during infusion
- Speed of infusion
    - 25 mL/hour for the 1st 30 minutes
    - 50 mL/hour for the next 30 minutes
    - Increase by 50 mL/hour every 30 minutes thereafter to a maximum 200 mL/hour
    - Rate of infusion can be doubled for subsequent infusions if no infusion reaction occurs in the 1st infusion.
- Step V (Surveillance)
    - Immunological recovery takes at least 6 months and steroids are tapered and maintained at physiological dose till immunological remission.
    - Continue the vaccination protocol for the rest of their lives with annual influenza shots, 5-yearly pneumococcal shots and hepatitis B boosters.

▌REFERENCES

1. Murrell DF, Dick S, Ahmed AR, et al. Consensus statement on definitions of disease, end points, and therapeutic response for pemphigus. J Am Acad Dermatol. 2008;58(6):1043-6.
2. Kasperkiewicz M, Schmidt E, Zillikens D. Current therapy of the pemphigus group. Clin Dermatol. 2012;30(1):84-94.
3. Martin LK, Werth VP, Villanueva EV, et al. A systematic review of randomized controlled trials for pemphigus vulgaris and pemphigus foliaceus. J Am Acad Dermatol. 2011;64(5):903-8.
4. Chams-Davatchi C, Esmaili N, Daneshpazhooh M, et al. Randomized controlled open-label trial of four treatment regimens for pemphigus vulgaris. J Am Acad Dermatol. 2007;57(4):622-8.
5. Joly P, Maho-Vaillant M, Prost-Squarcioni C, et al. French study group on autoimmune bullous skin diseases. First-line rituximab combined with short-term prednisone versus prednisone alone for the treatment of pemphigus (Ritux 3): a prospective, multicentre, parallel-group, open-label randomised trial. Lancet. 2017;389(10083):2031-40.
6. Ingen-Housz-Oro S, Valeyrie-Allanore L, Cosnes A, et al. First-line treatment of pemphigus vulgaris with a combination of rituximab and high-potency topical corticosteroids. JAMA Dermatol. 2015;151(2):200-3.
7. Colliou N, Picard D, Caillot F, et al. Long-term remissions of severe pemphigus after rituximab therapy are associated with prolonged failure of desmoglein B cell response. Sci Transl Med. 2013;5(175):175.

8. Leshem YA, Hodak E, David M, et al. Successful treatment of pemphigus with biweekly 1-g infusions of rituximab: a retrospective study of 47 patients. J Am Acad Dermatol. 2013;68(3):404-11.

9. Horváth B, Huizinga J, Pas HH, et al. Low-dose rituximab is effective in pemphigus. Br J Dermatol. 2012;166(2):405-12.

10. Kanwar AJ, Vinay K, Sawatkar GU, et al. Clinical and immunological outcomes of high- and low-dose rituximab treatments in patients with pemphigus: a randomized, comparative, observer-blinded study. Br J Dermatol. 2014;170(6): 1341-9.

11. Vinay K, Kanwar AJ, Sawatkar GU, et al. Successful use of rituximab in the treatment of childhood and juvenile pemphigus. J Am Acad Dermatol. 2014; 71(4):669-75.

12. De Cock D, Birmingham L, Watson KD, et al. Pregnancy outcomes in women with rheumatoid arthritis ever treated with rituximab. Rheumatology. 2017; 56(4):661-3.

13. Chakravarty EF, Murray ER, Kelman A, et al. Pregnancy outcomes after maternal exposure to rituximab. Blood. 2011;117(5):1499-506.

14. Soh MC, MacKillop L. Biologics in pregnancy–for the obstetrician. The Obstetrician & Gynaecologist. 2016;18(1):25-32.

15. Abadoglu O, Epozturk K, Atayik E, et al. Successful rapid rituximab desensitization for hypersensitivity reactions to monoclonal antibodies in a patient with rheumatoid arthritis: a remarkable option. J Investig Allergol Clin Immunol. 2011;21(4):319-21.

16. Chakraborty S, Tarantolo SR, Treves J, et al. Progressive multifocal leukoencephalopathy in a HIV-Negative patient with small lymphocytic leukemia following treatment with rituximab. Case Rep Oncol. 2011;4(1):136-42.

17. Clifford DB, Ances B, Costello C, et al. Rituximab-associated progressive multifocal leukoencephalopathy in rheumatoid arthritis. Arch Neurol. 2011; 68(9):1156-64.

18. Tran KD, Wolverton JE, Soter NA. Methotrexate in the treatment of pemphigus vulgaris: experience in 23 patients. Br J Dermatol. 2013;169(4):916-21.

19. Vardy DA, Cohen AD. Cyclosporine therapy should be considered for maintenance of remission in patients with pemphigus. Arch Dermatol. 2001; 137(4):505-6.

20. McCarty M, Fivenson D. Two decades of using the combination of tetracycline derivatives and niacinamide as steroid-sparing agents in the management of pemphigus: defining a niche for these low toxicity agents. J Am Acad Dermatol. 2014;71(3):475-9.

Chapter 17

Biologic Approach to Management of Hidradenitis Suppurativa

Rakesh Bharti, Nidhi Sharma

INTRODUCTION

Hidradenitis suppurativa (HS) is a painful, debilitating and chronic inflammatory disease predominantly affecting the apocrine gland bearing skin in axillae, buttocks, groin and the submammary area. Exact pathogenesis of this disease is not known; however, currently it is considered an autoinflammatory disease with involvement of Th17 and Th1 pathway. Follicular hyperkeratosis and subsequent follicular occlusion plays a role in pathogenesis of hidradenitis suppurativa (HS).[1]

It affects 0.5–4% of the global population. It generally starts around puberty and is more common in females. The primary lesions are tender, deep-seated follicular papules and pustules, which may enlarge to become nodules or pus discharging abscesses and ultimately leading to nodular scars and interconnected sinuses. Prevalence of metabolic syndrome in patients with hidradenitis suppurativa was found to be higher as compared to controls in one of the study.[2]

It is associated with significant morbidity and poor quality of life. The etiopathogenesis is multifactorial, with immunological, genetic, hormonal factors, smoking and obesity all playing some role in the causation of the disease (Fig. 17.1).

DISEASE STAGING

Staging of the disease is important to know the extent of disease and plan treatment for the patient. Hurley's and Sartorius staging system are most

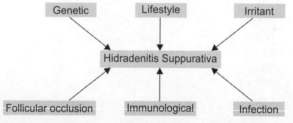

Fig. 17.1: Factors responsible for causing hidradenitis suppurativa.

commonly used for staging of the HS. Hurley's staging system is simpler and hence more commonly used in clinical setting. The Dermatology Life Quality Index (DLQI) can also be done know the impact of disease on quality of life of patient.

Hurley's Staging System[3]

Stage I – Abscess formation without sinus tracts.
Stage II – Recurrent abscess with sinus tract and scar formation.
Stage III – Multiple interconnected tracts and abscess.

Sartorius Staging System[4]

It is a more objective staging system in which numerical scoring is done in following manner.
- Anatomical regions involved—axilla, groin, gluteal (left or right) – 3 points per region.
- Number and scores of lesions—nodules -2, fistula -4, scars 1, others 1
- Distance between two relevant lesions – <5 cm -2; <10 cm, 4; > 10 cm 8.
- Are lesions clearly separated by normal skin? In each region (yes 0/ No 6).

Besides weight reduction and cessation of smoking, HS[5] is commonly managed by:
- Systemic antibiotics
- Retinoids
- Hormonal therapy
- Biologicals
- Surgical interventions.

▍IMMUNOPATHOGENESIS AND BASIS OF TREATMENT WITH BIOLOGICS

The exact immunopathogenesis of HS has not been delineated and is still under investigation. Tumor necrosis factor alpha (TNF-α) level were found to be higher in skin and serum of patients with HS.[6] This finding is consistent with effectiveness of anti-TNF-α drugs in its management. Interleukin (IL-1β) receptors are upregulated in affected and perilesional skin in HS patients.[7] Th17 cells and IL-17, IL-23 were also found to be raised in HS skin, which also implicates Th17 pathway in causation of HS and opens newer targets in management of this chronic, debilitating condition.[8]

Biologicals are the newer agents used for treating HS. They are mainly used for recalcitrant HS either as monotherapy or to supplement surgical excision. Although the US Food and Drug Administration (US FDA) has only approved adalimumab to treat HS, a few more biological agents have been explored to treat it in recent years.

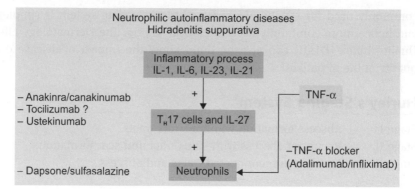

Fig. 17.2: Mechanism and site of action of various biologic agents used in managing hidradenitis suppurativa (HS).

Biologicals, which have been used are:
- Monoclonal antibodies
  - Anti-TNF-α
    - Infliximab
    - Adalimumab
  - Anti-IL-12 and anti-IL-23
    - Ustekinumab
  - Anti-IL- 1β
    - Canakinumab
- Fusion antibody proteins
  - Etanercept
- Recombinant human cytokines and growth factors
  - Interleukin-1 receptor antagonist (IL1Ra)
    - Anakinra
  - Interleukin-6 receptor antagonist (IL-6Ra)
    - Tocilizumab

Figure 17.2 explains the mechanism and site of action of various biologic agents being used in managing hidradenitis suppurativa (HS).

We will discuss biologicals available and used in India for management of HS in detail. Detailed descriptions of individual biologics have been given elsewhere in this book. Our aim is to discuss biologics usage specifically in HS.

Infliximab

Infliximab has the longest tradition of being used as an off-label biologic in the management of HS not responding to topical and systemic antibiotics. The potential of TNF-α inhibition was serendipitously observed in a patient of HS undergoing infliximab treatment for Crohn's disease in 2001 (Table 17.1).[9]

Table 17.1: Dosage of infliximab.

Dose	Schedule	Outcome	Reference
5 mg/kg	Treatment phase: 0,2,6 weeks and 8 weekly till week 22 Observation phase: Week 22–week 52	Week 8: 50% improvement in hidradenitis suppurativa (HSSI) and mean dermatology life quality index (DLQI) change was 10.	Grant A[10]
5 mg/kg	0, 2, 6 weeks and follow-up every 8 weeks	Follow-up duration: 112 weeks 3 months: Pain reduction 96.2%, Discharge reduction: 69.5% 24 months: Pain reduction: 34.8%, discharge reduction: 30.5%. (There is reduction in efficacy of infliximab with continuous treatment)	Brunasso AM[11]
Comparison of adalimumab and infliximab	Infliximab 5 mg/kg – 0, 2, 6 (3 infusions) Adalimumab – 40 mg every other week	Follow-up period: One year Reduction in 54% of baseline for infliximab group and 66% of baseline in adalimumab group Significant reduction in DQLI in infliximab group	Van Rappard DC[12]
	• Adalimumab was used in dose less than FDA approved dosing, which might have resulted in poor result in adalimumab group.		

Adalimumab

Adalimumab is supported by the highest levels of evidence (including data from randomized Pioneer I and Pioneer II clinical trials) and has been approved by US Food and Drug Administration in September 2015 for the management of Hurley's stage II and III HS. FDA approved dose for treatment of HS is 160 mg on day 0, 80 mg on day 15 and 40 mg on day 29, followed by every week (Table 17.2).

Response Rate

Adalimumab is more convenient to administer and more tolerable than infliximab.

Ustekinumab

Ustekinumab is a human p40 monoclonal antibody against p40 subunit of IL-12/IL-23. Th1 and Th17 response is mediated by IL-12 and 23. It is used to treat patients with moderate to severe recalcitrant plaque psoriasis and

Table 17.2: Dosage of adalimumab.

Dose	Schedule	Outcome	Reference
40 mg every other week.	Increased to 40 mg every week in patients with poorly controlled disease and every three weeks in patient in remission.	Follow-up: 21.5 months Decrease in nodules, fistula at one month and one year Significant improvement in DLQI	Blanco et al.[13]
	6 patients with refractory HS (patient who did not respond to oral antibiotics, contraceptive, isotretinoin, surgery) were included in this study.		

Dose	Schedule	Outcome	Reference
80 mg baseline followed by 40 mg sec every other week	Placebo controlled trial (n-21), 15 adalimumab and 6 placebo Treatment for 12 weeks and follow-up for 12 weeks.	Significant reduction in Sartorius score at end of 6 weeks and 24 weeks. No significant change after 12 weeks during follow-up period.	Miller et al.[14]
Week 0 – 160 mg Week 2 – 80 mg Week 4 onwards – 40 mg weekly	Placebo controlled trial Period 1 – till week 12 Period 2 – Re-randomization and continue for 24 weeks Assessment based on hidradenitis suppurative clinical response (HSCR)	Week 12 – PIONEER I – 41.8% vs 26 % (placebo) PIONEER II -58.9% vs 27.6 % (placebo)	PIONEER I and II[15]

psoriatic arthritis. IL-23 were also found to be raised in HS skin, which also implicates Th17 pathway in causation of HS. This involvement of Th 17 pathway might explain the observed therapeutic effect of ustekinumab in HS.[16,17] It is not available in India as of now.

Dosage and Duration of Treatment

Route

Subcutaneous injections are available as prefilled syringe or vial of 45 mg/ 0.5 mL and 90 mg/mL. 45 or 90 mg {(if the weight is > 100 kg) subcutaneous injections are administered at weeks 0, 4, 16 and 28 weeks (children 0.75 mg/kg).

Response rate

In a recent open-label prospective study, 17 patients of HS were treated with 4 doses of ustekinumab. Moderate-to-marked improvement of the modified Sartorius score was achieved in 82% of patients at week 40 and the Hidradenitis Suppurativa Clinical Response 50 were achieved in 47%.[18]

Etanercept

Etanercept is a recombinant fully human dimeric fusion protein comprising of the human TNF-α p75 receptor and the Fc portion of human IgG1 molecule that can bind to two TNF molecules, thereby effectively removing them from circulation. It functions as a TNF-α inhibitor, thereby preventing interaction with its cell surface receptors on target cells and blocking its pro-inflammatory effects (Table 17.3).

Response Rate

The response rate of etanercept is discussed in detail in Table 17.3.

Table 17.3: Dosage of etanercept.			
Dose	*Schedule*	*Outcome*	*Reference*
25 mg twice a week.	Started with 25 mg twice a week, Increased to 50 mg twice a week in cases with poor response (2 out of 6 cases)	Maximum follow-up period: 40 weeks. Initial response: 16 days (9–20 days) 24 weeks: DLQI reduced by 61%	Cusack C et al.[19]
	• Objective measure of clinical severity was not used in the study. • Previous treatment included high dose antibiotics, dapsone, isotretinoin, oral contraceptives and surgery. • Two out of six patients relapsed within 2–3 weeks and one who was restarted on etanercept improved in 3 weeks.		
50 mg once a week	For 24 weeks in 10 patients	Sartorius score: >50% improvement in score in 6 patients at week 12 and 7 patients at week 24. 30% improvement in all patients at week 12.	Giamarellos-Bourboulis EJ et al.[20,21]
	• Long-term follow-up of these patients were published in different paper. • Follow-up period of 144 weeks. Three patients did not report any recurrence. • Seven patients required a second course of therapy. Improvement was seen in five patients, while two patients failed treatment.[21]		

Contd...

Contd...

Dose	Schedule	Outcome	Reference
50 mg twice a week	Placebo controlled trial Etanercept or placebo for 12 weeks. 12–24 weeks all patients received etanercept.	Follow-up: 24 weeks No difference between placebo and treatment group in patient global assessment (PGA) or DLQI either at 12 or 24 weeks	Adams DR et al.[22]

▍ INTERLEUKIN-1 RECEPTOR ANTAGONIST/SECOND-LINE BIOLOGIC THERAPIES

Interleukin-1 is a pro-inflammatory cytokine that plays an important role in the regulation of inflammation and immune response. IL-1Ra is a naturally occurring antagonist that competes with IL-1α and IL-1β for the IL-1 receptor. The relative amounts of IL-1α, IL-1β and IL-1Ra influence the severity of inflammation.

Anakinra

It is a recombinant non-glycosylated form of the human IL-1Ra competitively inhibiting the biologic activity of IL-1α and IL-1β. The US Food and Drug Administration and the European Medical Agency have approved the use of anakinra for the treatment of moderate to severe rheumatoid arthritis. It is not available in India and is prohibitively expensive.

Dosage and Duration of Treatment

Route

Subcutaneous Injection
- Administered as a daily subcutaneous dose of 100 mg (children: 1–2 mg/kg) initially; may increase by 0.5–1 mg/kg increments to control active inflammation, not to exceed 8 mg/kg.
- The daily dosing schedule of anakinra is a major disadvantage over other biologics.

Response rate

In a double-blind, randomized, placebo-controlled clinical trial, anakinra was administered subcutaneously once daily for 12 weeks in the treatment phase and after 12-week follow-up phase. Hidradenitis suppurativa clinical response was achieved in 30% (3 of 10) of the placebo and in 78% (7 of 9) of the patients receiving anakinra (P = 0.04).[23] There have been case series reporting failure of anakinra therapy in treating HS.[24]

COCHRANE REVIEW FOR TREATMENT OF HIDRADENITIS SUPPURATIVA

A Cochrane review was published in May 2016 on interventions used for management of HS. The review concluded that high quality data is not available for management of HS. Adalimumab 40 mg every week improves quality of life, while available evidence suggests that adalimumab 40 mg every other week and etanercept 50 mg twice weekly are ineffective for management of HS. Infliximab is an effective option for management of hidradenitis suppurativa, however data is not robust due to small number of patients included in randomized controlled trial (RCT).[25]

SUMMARY

Trials demonstrating the efficacy of biologic therapy for moderate to severe hidradenitis suppurativa have inspired new multidisciplinary treatment strategies especially combined biologic and surgical therapy for recalcitrant HS. Lower rates of recurrence and disease progression, as well as a longer disease-free interval may be achieved with the use of adjuvant biologic therapy including infliximab (n = 8) and ustekinumab (n = 3) which were initiated 2 to 3 weeks after closure and were continued for an average of 10.5 months after radical resection for recalcitrant HS.[26]

Hidradenitis suppurativa (HS) is a rare paradoxical adverse effect of biologics exposure observed in 25 patients treated with these 5 biologics (adalimumab, infliximab, etanercept, rituximab, tocilizumab). Median duration of biologics exposure before HS onset was 12 (range 1–120) months. There was a trend towards better outcome when the biologics were discontinued or switched. Reintroducing the same biologics resulted in HS relapse in three patients.[27,28]

To conclude, the short-term side effects of biologics are usually minimal with regard to the risk/benefit ratio. The long-term effects ultimately determine the utility of each biologic therapy and the most appropriate disease–therapeutic pairing. Higher response rate could be associated with higher doses and several authors have suggested use of biological drugs with higher doses in HS than those used in psoriasis. Not all biologics are equally effective, but finding the optimal biological to achieve optimal control is goal in biologic treatment of HS.

For the ease of readers, Box 17.1 and Table 17.4 for clinical trials and algorithm for biologics used in treatment of hidradenitis suppurativa.

Box 17.1: Algorithm for incorporating biologics into treatment of hidradenitis suppurativa.

When to use

Moderate to severe Hidradenitis Suppurativa (Hurley stage II and III)

Stage I – one or more abscesses with no sinus tract or scar formation

Stage II – one or more widely separated recurrent abscesses, with sinus tract and scar formation

Stage III – multiple interconnected tracts and abscesses throughout an affected region

Which all to choose

- Infliximab
- Adalimumab
- Etanercept

How to choose

Step 1

Check the suitability for an individual: know the safety profile of each biologic.

SAFETY PROFILE OF EACH BIOLOGIC

TNF-α antagonists

- Serious infection
- Malignancy
- Demyelinating disease
- Congestive heart failure
- Hepatitis B
- Hematologic
- Lupus like syndrome
- Live vaccines

Step 2

Evaluate for comorbidities

- Inflammatory bowel diseases especially Crohn's disease—favor TNF-α antagonists
- Pyoderma gangrenosum—favor canakinumab
- Behcet's disease, Psoriasis—favor ustekinumab
- Metabolic syndrome
  - Obesity—disfavor etanercept
  - Cardiovascular disease (CVD)
- Coronary artery disease—favor TNF-α antagonists
  - Arthropathies spondyloarthropathy (joint disease),
- Favor- TNF-α antagonists > IL- 12/23 antagonists
  - Squamous cell carcinoma- disfavor TNF-α antagonists

Contd...

Contd...

Step 3	
Consider concomitant medical issues	
Serious infections	**Multiple sclerosis**
Caution: All biologicals	Caution: TNF-α antagonists
Tuberculosis	
Caution: All biologicals	**Prior malignancy**
Hepatitis	Caution: All biological
Hepatitis B: Caution- TNF-α antagonists	Cutaneous SCC
Hepatitis C:	Caution: TNF-α antagonists
Favor- TNF-α antagonists - etanercept	Solid tumors
Deep fungal infections	Depends upon type, severity and
Cation - TNF-α antagonists	duration, risk-benefit ratio
Congestive heart failure (mod to severe)	
Caution TNF-α antagonists	
Step 4	
Choose best method of administration and frequency of administration.	
Self-administration/Subcutaneous	In-office administration/Infusion
Adalimumab: every other week or every weeks	Infliximab: 0, 2, 6 and every 8 weeks
Etanercept: every week or twice a week	

Table 17.4: Summary of clinical trials of biologics used in the treatment of hidradenitis suppurativa.

Biologics	Author and trial design	N	Dose/Frequency	Follow-up from treatment initiation	Results
Adalimu-mab	Miller et al. (2011), double-blind randomized controlled trial	15	Adalimumab 80 mg SC at baseline followed by 40 mg SC every other week.	12 weeks	Reduction in Sartorius score of 10.7 points at 6 weeks and 11.3 points at 12 weeks was seen in the treatment group compared to 7.5 points and 5.8 points in the placebo group, respectively.

Contd...

Contd...

Biologics	Author and trial design	N	Dose/Frequency	Follow-up from treatment initiation	Results
	Kimball et al. (2012), phase 2, randomized, placebo controlled parallel trial consisting of a blinded 16-week period (period 1) and an open-label 36-week period (period 2)	154	Adalimumab 40 mg/week; adalimumab, 40 mg every other week or placebo. All patients received adalimumab 40 mg every other week at the beginning of period 2 but switched to weekly dosing if the response was suboptimal at weeks 28 or 31.	16 weeks	At week 16, 3.9% of patients receiving placebo (2 of 51), 9.6% of patients receiving adalimumab every other week (5 of 52), and 17.6% of patients treated weekly (9 of 51) achieved minimal or mild HS-PGA score by week 16.
Infliximab	Paradela et al. (2012), prospective trial	10	Infliximab 5 mg/kg every 8 weeks after initial standard loading dose	37 weeks	2 patients (20%) had no response to treatment after 5 doses; five (50%) patients experienced disease recurrence.
	Grant et al. (2010), randomized double-blind placebo-controlled crossover trial	38	Infliximab 5 mg/kg infusions at 0, 2 and 6	8 weeks	60% of patients in the infliximab group compared to 5.6% of patients in the placebo group achieved 25–50% decrease in their severity scores.

Contd...

Contd...

Biologics	Author and trial design	N	Dose/Frequency	Follow-up from treatment initiation	Results
	Moriarty et al. (2014), prospective cohort trial	11	Infliximab 5 mg/kg infusion every 4 weeks after initial standard loading dose.	60.3 months	Nine patients had measurable improvement after undergoing treatment; 2 had treatment failure at 12 and 19 months
Usteki-numab	Gulliver (2012), prospective cohort trial	3	45 mg SC injections at 0, 1 and 4 months	6 months	1 patient had remission of disease, the second patient improved and the third had no response
	Blok (2016)	17	45 or 90 mg (if the weight is >100 kg) SC injections administered at weeks 0, 4, 16 and 28 weeks	40 weeks	Moderate-to-marked improvement of the modified Sartorius score was achieved in 82% of patients at week 40 and the Hidradenitis Suppurativa Clinical Response 50 in 47%.
Etanercept	Adams et al. (2010), double-blind, placebo-controlled study	20	Etanercept 50 mg SC was administered twice weekly for 3 months, followed by open-label etanercept 50 mg SC, twice weekly for an additional 3 months	6 months	No statistically significant difference among PGA, patient global assessment and DLQI at 12 or 24 weeks between treatment and placebo groups

Contd...

Contd...

Biologics	Author and trial design	N	Dose/Frequency	Follow-up from treatment initiation	Results
Anakinra	Leslie (2014), prospective cohort	N	Anakinra 100 mg SC daily	8 weeks	Mean decrease in modified Sartorius score of 34.8 points
	Tzanetakou V (2016) Double-blind, randomized, placebo-controlled clinical trial	15	Anakinra 100 mg SC daily	12 weeks	Clinical response at 12 weeks was achieved in 78% of the anakinra than in 30% of the placebo (P = 0.04)

(N: Number of patients; SC: Subcutaneous; DLQI: Dermatologic quality of life Index; PGA: Physician global assessment; EOW: Every other week).

REFERENCES

1. Attanoos RL, Appleton MA, Douglas-Jones AG. The pathogenesis of hidradenitis suppurativa: a closer look at apocrine and apoeccrine glands. Br J Dermatol. 1995;133(2):254-8.
2. Shalom G, Freud T, Harman-Boehm I, et al. Hidradenitis suppurativa and metabolic syndrome: a comparative cross-sectional study of 3207 patients. Br J Dermatol. 2015;173(2):464-70.
3. Hurley H. Dermatologic surgery, principles and practice. In: Rocnigk RK, Rocnigk HH (Eds). New York: Marcel Dekker; 1989. pp. 729-39.
4. Sartorius K, Lapins J, Emtestam L, et al. Suggestions for uniform outcome variables when reporting treatment effects in hidradenitis suppurativa. Br J Dermatol. 2003;149(1):211-3.
5. Martinez F, Nos P, Benlloch S, et al. Hidradenitis suppurativa and Crohn's disease: response to treatment with infliximab. Inflamm Bowel Dis. 2001;7(4):323-6.
6. Mozeika E, Pilmane M, Nurnberg BM, et al. Tumor necrosis factor-alpha and matrix metalloproteinase-2 are expressed strongly in hidradenitis suppurativa. Acta Derm Venereol. 2013;93(3):301-4.
7. Van der Zee HH, de Ruiter L, van den Broecke DG, et al. Elevated levels of tumour necrosis factor (TNF)-alpha, interleukin (IL)-1beta and IL-10 in hidradenitis suppurativa skin: a rationale for targeting TNF-alpha and IL-1beta. Br J Dermatol. 2011;164(6):1292-8.
8. Schlapbach C, Hanni T, Yawalkar N, et al. Expression of the IL-23/Th17 pathway in lesions of hidradenitis suppurativa. J Am Acad Dermatol. 2011;65(4):790-8.
9. Mekkes JR, Bos JD. Long-term efficacy of a single course of infliximab in hidradenitis suppurativa. Br J Dermatol. 2008;158(2):370-4.

10. Grant A, Gonzalez T, Montgomery MO, et al. Infliximab therapy for patients with moderate to severe hidradenitis suppurativa: a randomized, double-blind, placebo-controlled crossover trial. J Am Acad Dermatol. 2010;62(2):205-17.

11. Brunasso AM, Delfino C, Massone C. Hidradenitis suppurativa: are tumour necrosis factor-α blockers the ultimate alternative? British Journal of Dermatology. 2008;159(3):761-3.

12. Van Rappard DC, Leenarts MF, Meijerink-van't Oost L, et al. Comparing treatment outcome of infliximab and adalimumab in patients with severe hidradenitis suppurativa. J Dermatolog Treat. 2012;23(4):284-9.

13. Blanco R, Martinez-Taboada VM, Villa I, et al. Long-term successful adalimumab therapy in severe hidradenitis suppurativa. Arch Dermatol. 2009;145(5):580-4.

14. Miller I, Lynggaard CD, Lophaven S, et al. A double-blind placebo-controlled randomized trial of adalimumab in the treatment of hidradenitis suppurativa. Br J Dermatol. 2011;165(2):391-8.

15. Kimball AB, Okun MM, Williams DA, et al. Two phase 3 trials of adalimumab for hidradenitis suppurativa. N Engl J Med. 2016;375(5):422-34.

16. Sharon VR, Garcia MS, Bagheri S, et al. Management of recalcitrant hidradenitis suppurativa with ustekinumab. Acta Derm Venereol. 2012;92(3):320-1.

17. Baerveldt EM, Kappen JH, Thio HB, et al. Successful long-term triple disease control by ustekinumab in a patient with Behçet's disease, psoriasis and hidradenitis suppurativa. Ann Rheum Dis. 2012.

18. Blok JL, Li K, Brodmerkel C, et al. Ustekinumab in hidradenitis suppurativa: clinical results and a search for potential biomarkers in serum. Br J Dermatol. 2016;174(4):839-46.

19. Cusack C, Buckley C. Etanercept: effective in the management of hidradenitis suppurativa. Br J Dermatol. 2006;154(4):726-9.

20. Giamarellos-Bourboulis EJ, Pelekanou E, Antonopoulou A, et al. An open-label phase II study of the safety and efficacy of etanercept for the therapy of hidradenitis suppurativa. Br J Dermatol. 2008;158(3):567-72.

21. Pelekanou A, Kanni T, Savva A, et al. Long-term efficacy of etanercept in hidradenitis suppurativa: results from an open-label phase II prospective trial. Exp Dermatol. 2010;19(6):538-40.

22. Adams DR, Yankura JA, Fogelberg AC, et al. Treatment of hidradenitis suppurativa with etanercept injection. Arch Dermatol. 2010;146(5):501-4.

23. Tzanetakou V, Kanni T, Giatrakou S, et al. Safety and efficacy of anakinra in severe hidradenitis suppurativa: a randomized clinical trial. JAMA Dermatol. 2016;152(1):52-9.

24. Van der Zee HH, Prens EP. Failure of anti-interleukin-1 therapy in severe hidradenitis suppurativa: a case report. Dermatology. 2013;226(2):97-100.

25. Ingram JR, Woo PN, Chua SL, et al. Interventions for hidradenitis suppurativa: a Cochrane systematic review incorporating GRADE assessment of evidence quality. Br J Dermatol. 2016;174(5):970-8.

26. DeFazio M, Economides JM, King KS, et al. Outcomes after combined radical resection and targeted biologic therapy for the management of recalcitrant hidradenitis suppurativa. Ann Plast Surg. 2016;77(2):217-22.

27. Harvin G, Kasarala G. Two cases of paradoxical hidradenitis suppurativa while on adalimumab. Case Rep Gastroenterol. 2016;10(1):88-94.

28. Faivre C, Villani AP, Aubin F, et al. Hidradenitis suppurativa (HS): an unrecognized paradoxical effect of biologic agents (BA) used in chronic inflammatory diseases. J Am Acad Dermatol. 2016;74(6):1153-9.

Chapter 18

Biologic Approach to Management of Connective Tissue Diseases

Abhishek Kumar

INTRODUCTION

Connective tissue disorders (CTDs) are characterized by heterogeneity in immunopathogenesis, clinical and laboratory features, and prognosis. A number of immunological pathways across the adaptive and innate immune systems interact and result in various specific and nonspecific clinical features seen in CTDs. Cutaneous involvement in CTDs have varied manifestations and responses to available immunosuppressants are also different. It is a challenge for the physician to balance between the desired response to treatment and undesired adverse effects of immunosuppression. The availability of biological disease-modifying antirheumatic drugs (bDMARDs) has heralded novel possibilities in the field of therapeutics in autoimmune disorders.

The available literature on clinical efficacy of bDMARDs on cutaneous manifestations of CTDs is limited due to many reasons. The biologics have been introduced in clinical practice in the recent past. The cost of treatment has been a major hurdle for its use across the patients of different socioeconomic status. In majority of the clinical trials on efficacy of biologics in CTDs, composite disease activity scoring and response criteria have been used rather than skin specific measures. Aim of this chapter is to analyze the available data and interprets them to make clinical decisions on pharmacotherapy of cutaneous manifestation of CTDs.

CUTANEOUS LUPUS ERYTHEMATOSUS

Gillian classification describes cutaneous manifestations of systemic lupus erythematosus (SLE) as SLE specific and nonspecific manifestations. SLE-specific manifestations are further classified as acute cutaneous lupus erythematosus (ACLE), subacute cutaneous lupus erythematosus (SCLE), and chronic cutaneous lupus erythematosus (CCLE).[1] In this chapter, these terms have been used as defined by the Gillian classification and an attempt has been made to study the effects of biologic treatment on various subtypes of cutaneous lupus erythematosus (CLE).

The scoring systems are required to evaluate the disease activity and to know the effectiveness of the drug in clinical trials. The most commonly used scoring system for SLE are Systemic Lupus Erythematosus Disease Activity Index (SLEDAI) and British Isles Lupus Activity Group (BILAG). While SLEDAI measures SLE disease activity in general, BILAG is an organ-specific study instrument and can be modified depending on the intent of the treating physician. Clinical manifestations and laboratory investigations are combined into a single score for the organ. The score can be from A to E.

- A—very active disease
- B—moderate disease
- C—mild stable disease
- D—resolved activity
- E—organ was never involved.

Evidence on use of biologics in SLE in general are available as part of nonrenal lupus trials. There is no large study, which has been conducted exclusively on use of bDMARDs in CLE. The only group of biologic, which has been found to be effective in CLE, is B-cell depletion (BCD) agents. The different BCD agents will be discussed here.

Rituximab

Rituximab has been evaluated in several clinical trials in SLE. Review of most of these trials show inconsistency in the efficacy of rituximab in CLE.

In a brief report by Vital EM et al., 26 patients of CLE were treated with rituximab.[2] Mucocutaneous disease burden was assessed using BILAG score. Rituximab was given at a dose of 1,000 mg on day 1 and 15. Patients were followed-up for 6 months at least. Concomitant immunosuppression therapy or antimalarial was allowed to continue. Clinical assessment was performed at baseline and 6 months using BILAG 2004.[3]

Among different subtypes of CLE exposed to rituximab, ACLE (malar rash or photosensitive maculopapular rash) was the most common involvement with 14 patients and other subtypes consisted of SCLE (two patients, papulosquamous), CCLE (eight patients), and nonspecific lupus lesions (two patients). Clinical response was achieved in six (42.9%) of ACLE patients, one (50%) of SCLE, and two patients (100%) of nonspecific lupus lesions. None of the eight patients with CCLE [cutaneous or mucosal discoid lupus erythematosus (DLE) or chilblains] could achieve clinical response. Clinical response was associated with anti-dsDNA positivity (nine of 15 ACLE patients, P = 0.075) while anti-SSA Ro positivity (six of eight CCLE patients, P = 0.031) was associated with no response. None of the seven anti-RNP positive patients (four out of 14 of ACLE and two of the CCLE) could achieve clinical response (P = 0.024). Concomitant immunosuppressants or antimalarials were not associated with clinical response.

Explorer study was a randomized phase II/III double-blinded study on efficacy and safety of rituximab in moderately to severely active nonrenal SLE patients.[4] The disease activity was assessed using BILAG score in individual domains. Most of the patients in this study had mucocutaneous involvement at baseline. However, the details on subtypes of CLE are not available. The placebo group had 88 patients and rituximab group included 169 patients of SLE. For mucocutaneous domain 58% and 13.6% patients had BILAG B and BILAG A scores, respectively. In rituximab group 56.2% and 16% patients had BILAG B and BILAG A scores, respectively. Patients were followed-up for 52 weeks. At week 52 there was no difference in major or partial clinical response in the placebo and rituximab groups.

In a systemic review of literature, rituximab has shown inconsistent results with mucocutaneous manifestations in SLE patients, with partial or complete response rates ranging from 33% to 71% and significant disease relapse rates.[5]

Notably, these studies are limited by the lack of CLE-specific assessments.

Belimumab

Belimumab is a human monoclonal antibody against the cytokine B-lymphocyte stimulator (BLyS).[6] Overexpression of BLyS has been found to have a major role in the pathogenesis of SLE.[7] Belimumab has an immunomodulatory effect exerted by suppressing the B-cell survival and differentiation mediated by BLyS.[8] It has been approved for use in SLE in the USA, Canada, and Europe. However, it is not indicated for lupus nephritis and neuropsychiatric SLE.

BLISS-76 study was a phase III randomized controlled trial (RCT) on use of belimumab in SLE patients. Patients with active disease (SELENA-SLEDAI score ≥6 were randomized in 1:1:1 ratio to receive placebo, belimumab 1 mg/kg or belimumab 10 mg/kg on days 0, 14, and 28 days followed by every 28 days for 76 weeks. Mucocutaneous involvement (BILAG A or B) was present in 178 (64.7%), 159 (58.7%), and 141 (51.6%) patients, respectively in placebo, belimumab 1 mg/kg and belimumab 10 mg/kg groups, respectively.[9]

BLISS-52 was a similar study in which 172 (60%), 167 (58%), and 174 (60%) patients had BILAG A or B scores in mucocutaneous domain at baseline. At 52 and 72 weeks significantly more number of patients improved in both belimumab 1 mg//kg and belimumab 10 mg/kg groups. The standard of care treatment was allowed to continue during belimumab treatment, which consisted of corticosteroids, immunosuppressants, and antimalarials. In mucocutaneous domain improvement was noticed in alopecia, mucosal ulcers, and rash.[10] The proportion of patients with improvement from baseline consisted of 48%, 51.1%, and 54.5% (P < 0.01) in placebo, belimumab 1 mg/kg and belimumab 10 mg/kg groups.

Anti-interferon Approaches: Novel Therapies on the Block in Systemic Lupus Erythematosus

Lately, immune dysregulation emanating from activation of type I interferon (IFN) system has been found to be central to the pathogenesis of SLE.[11] Several phase I and II trials have been conducted with agents blocking the type I IFN system.[12] Sifalimumab, anifrolumab, and rontalizumab are the monoclonal antibodies developed targeting the IFN receptors. Rontalizumab failed to meet the primary and secondary endpoints in a phase II study in SLE patients.[13] Sifalimumab had shown only modest clinical efficacy, but did meet the primary and few secondary endpoints.[14]

Positive aspects of these trials have been specific scoring method. Cutaneous Lupus Erythematosus Disease Area and Severity Index (CLASI) was used to measure the response to therapy.[15,16] Both sifalimumab and anifrolumab was found to benefit patients with moderate to severe baseline mucocutaneous disease with 50% decrease in CLASI activity.[17,18] A phase III study is being conducted with anifrolumab.[19]

Other Biological Disease-modifying Antirheumatic Drugs

CTLA4-Ig fusion protein abatacept failed to show clinical efficacy in phase II trial involving nonrenal lupus patients.[20]

Preliminary efficacy of tocilizumab in SLE has been studied in phase I study.[21] Cutaneous involvement has not been reported in this study.

In a case report JAK, 1/2 inhibitor ruxolitinib has been reported to improve a case of chilblain lupus.[22]

▌DERMATOMYOSITIS

Cutaneous manifestations of dermatomyositis (DM) vary from the pathognomonic Gottron's papules and heliotrope rash to nonspecific lesion like calcinosis, panniculitis, photosensitivity, and others. Cutaneous manifestations specially calcinosis and vasculopathic can be a source of considerable morbidity and may pose a difficult challenge in management. Cutaneous lesions may heal with improvement in myositis, however, in significant proportion of patients these lesions remain active and are difficult to manage.[23]

Antitumor Necrosis Factor-α Therapy

Evidence on use of antitumor necrosis factor-α (anti-TNF-α) in DM is scarce and there is no conclusive evidence in favor of or against use of these agents in DM. In a case report, one patient was reported to benefit in skin rash with infliximab.[24] In another case report by Robert Norman, etanercept was found to be beneficial in cutaneous manifestations of DM.[25]

However, in pilot trial published in 2011, which compared etanercept to placebo in DM, five out of 11 patients treated with etanercept developed a worsening rash.[26] These evidences are complicated by several reports of de novo DM appearance or DM-like rashes with use of anti-TNF-α agent for other indications.[27,28]

Rituximab

In a pilot study by Loringa Chung et al., rituximab was found to have limited effect on skin lesions in eight patients subjected to this treatment. In this study, cutaneous disease severity was quantified by the Dermatomyositis Skin Severity Index (DSSI), (Carroll CL, Jorizzo JL, unpublished data, 2002-2004). A score of less than 2 is classified as mild disease while severe disease is score greater than 6. All patients had more than 7 DSSI score at baseline. During rituximab treatment it was observed that mean percentage of change in DSSI was 9.5% (95% confidence interval, −35.8% to 16.7%; P = 0.42). Periungual telangiectasias remained unchanged in all patients while poikiloderma improved in 50% and worsened in rest 50% patients. Only one out of eight patients had improvement in heliotrope rash while in six others there was no change. At baseline, three patients had Gottron's papules which did not improve at 24 weeks.[29] In another pilot study involving seven patients, Levine TD reported improvement in skin rash and regrowth of hair in two patients suffering from alopecia.[30] Improvement in vasculitic ulcer was reported by Joshi N et al.[31] There is no RCT for efficacy of rituximab in cutaneous DM.

Others

Efalizumab, a monoclonal antibody against CD11a, was reported in a single case of resistant DM with improvement in erythematous skin rash; however, drug has been withdrawn due to increased risk of progressive multifocal leukoencephalopathy.[32]

SYSTEMIC SCLEROSIS

Rituximab

Scleroderma or thickening of skin is the hallmark of systemic sclerosis (SSc). Several observational studies have shown benefit of rituximab on skin thickening as measured by modified Rodnan skin score (mRSS). The largest study published as by the European Scleroderma Trial and Research (EUSTAR) group included 63 patients out of which data on cutaneous manifestations was available for 46 patients.[33] Mean disease duration of the patient was 5 (3–10) years. Out of 46 patients, 35 had diffuse and remaining

11 had limited cutaneous disease. Patients were followed-up for 7–9 months and mRSS decreased significantly from 18.1 ± 1.6 to 14.4 ± 1.5 (P = 0.0002) and the percentage change achieved in mRSS was –15.0 ± 5.3% (P = 0.008). In 35 patients with diffuse cutaneous disease mean mRSS, decreased from 22.1 ± 1.6 to 17.7 ± 1.6 (P = 0.0005) after 6 (3–9) months follow-up with percentage change of mRSS versus baseline –16.7 ± 5.5% (P = 0.005). These results favor use of rituximab for severe refractory cutaneous involvement in SSc, however, further studies are required to confirm long-term efficacy and safety of rituximab in SSc. An ongoing trial on comparison of rituximab and cyclophosphamide in SSc may further provide evidences to formulate recommendations for use of rituximab.[34]

Tocilizumab

Lately there has been interest in use of anti-interleukin (IL)-6 receptor antibody therapy for skin and other organ fibrosis in SSc due to high IL-6 expression with disease severity and outcome and possible role of neutrophil-dependent IL-6 trans-signaling in scleroderma microvasculopathy.[35,36] In observational study by EUSTAR group, 15 patients received tocilizumab and no effect on skin fibrosis was noted at the end of 7 months.[37] There have been case reports and a phase II randomized trial suggesting that blocking IL-6 activity may benefit skin and other outcomes in SSc and other studies have suggested that higher circulating levels of IL-6 are associated with worse survival or more progressive lung fibrosis.[38,39]

In the phase II randomized trial, 43 patients treated with tocilizumab were compared with placebo group of 44 patients. The changes in two groups were not statistically significant; however, authors recommended further studies to conclude upon the potential of IL-6 based therapy in SSc as the results met the definitions for minimal clinically important differences.[39] A larger, phase III trial to further evaluate IL-6 receptor antagonism in SSc is ongoing.[40]

In EUSTAR study group observational study abatacept was also shown to suggest some benefit in systemic sclerosis and one phase II clinical trial is ongoing.[41]

Calcinosis cutis associated with SSc pose a serious challenge to physicians for treatment. However, few case reports have found rituximab and infliximab to be of some benefit in these cases.[42,43]

PRIMARY SJÖGREN'S SYNDROME

Primary Sjögren's syndrome (PSS) is characterized by fewer skin manifestations as compared to other CTDs and includes annular erythema and cutaneous vasculitis. Annular erythema responds well to topical therapy and conventional immunosuppressants. Cutaneous vasculitis, which is refractory to conventional immunosuppressants or medium-sized vessel involved in biopsy sample is recommended to be treated by rituximab.[44]

RHEUMATOID ARTHRITIS

Rheumatoid arthritis (RA) may be complicated by cutaneous vasculitis, which many manifest as skin fold infarcts or single or multiple skin ulcers. Ulcers resistant to treatment with topical measures or those associated with systemic vasculitis require systemic immunosuppression and rituximab has shown to benefit rheumatoid vasculitis (RV).[45]

Anti-TNF therapies have shown to have limited role in RV.[46] Moreover, anti-TNF therapy and abatacept have been shown to be associated with development of RV.[47]

CONCLUSION

Use of biologic DMARDs in cutaneous manifestations of connective tissue disorders is in evolutionary stage. The literature in the use of these diseases is scant and at present benefit is not very impressive possibly because they are used in refractory diseases. With improved safety profile of these drugs, better understanding of pathogenesis of diseases and development of precise targets, there is a potential possibility of treating these morbid diseases in a better manner.

REFERENCES

1. Gilliam JN, Sontheimer RD. Distinctive cutaneous subsets in the spectrum of lupus erythematosus. J Am Acad Dermatol. 1981;4(4):471-5.
2. Vital EM, Wittmann M, Edward S, et al. Brief report: responses to rituximab suggest B cell-independent inflammation in cutaneous systemic lupus erythematosus. Arthritis Rheumatol. 2015;67(6):1586-91.
3. Isenberg DA, Rahman A, Allen E, et al. BILAG 2004. Development and initial validation of an updated version of the British Isles Lupus Assessment Group's disease activity index for patients with systemic lupus erythematosus. Rheumatology (Oxford). 2005;44(7):902-6.
4. Merrill JT, Neuwelt CM, Wallace DJ, et al. Efficacy and safety of rituximab in moderately-to-severely active systemic lupus erythematosus: the randomized, double-blind, phase II/III systemic lupus erythematosus evaluation of rituximab trial. Arthritis Rheum. 2010;62(1):222-33.
5. Cobo-Ibanez T, Loza-Santamaria E, Pego-Reigosa JM, et al. Efficacy and safety of rituximab in the treatment of non-renal systemic lupus erythematosus: a systematic review. Semin Arthritis Rheum. 2014;44(2):175-85.
6. Baker KP, Edwards BM, Main SH, et al. Generation and characterization of LymphoStat-B, a human monoclonal antibody that antagonizes the bioactivities of B lymphocyte stimulator. Arthritis Rheum. 2003;48(11):3253-65.

7. Vincent FB, Morand EF, Schneider P, et al. The BAFF/APRIL system in SLE pathogenesis. Nat Rev Rheumatol. 2014;10(6):365-73.
8. Halpern WG, Lappin P, Zanardi T, et al. Chronic administration of belimumab, a BLyS antagonist, decreases tissue and peripheral blood B-lymphocyte populations in cynomolgus monkeys: pharmacokinetic, pharmacodynamic, and toxicologic effects. Toxicol Sci. 2006;91(2):586-99.
9. Furie R, Petri M, Zamani O, et al. A phase III, randomized, placebo-controlled study of belimumab, a monoclonal antibody that inhibits B lymphocyte stimulator, in patients with systemic lupus erythematosus. Arthritis Rheum. 2011;63(12):3918-30.
10. Manzi S, Sánchez-Guerrero J, Merrill JT, et al. Effects of belimumab, a B lymphocyte stimulator-specific inhibitor, on disease activity across multiple organ domains in patients with systemic lupus erythematosus: combined results from two phase III trials. Ann Rheum Dis. 2012;71(11):1833-8.
11. Crow MK. Type I interferon in the pathogenesis of lupus. J Immunol. 2014;192(12):5459-68.
12. Lichtman EI, Helfgott SM, Kriegel MA. Emerging therapies for systemic lupus erythematosus—focus on targeting interferon-alpha. Clin Immunol. 2012;143(3):210-21.
13. Kalunian KC, Merrill JT, Maciuca R, et al. A Phase II study of the efficacy and safety of rontalizumab (rhuMAb interferon-α) in patients with systemic lupus erythematosus (ROSE). Ann Rheum Dis. 2016;75(1):196-202.
14. Khamashta M, Merrill JT, Werth VP, et al. Sifalimumab, an anti-interferon-α monoclonal antibody, in moderate to severe systemic lupus erythematosus: a randomised, double-blind, placebo-controlled study. Ann Rheum Dis. 2016;75(11):1909-16.
15. Albrecht J, Taylor L, Berlin JA, et al. The CLASI (Cutaneous Lupus Erythematosus Disease Area and Severity Index): an outcome instrument for cutaneous lupus erythematosus. J Invest Dermatol. 2005;125(5):889-94.
16. Klein R, Moghadam-Kia S, LoMonico J, et al. Development of the CLASI as a tool to measure disease severity and responsiveness to therapy in cutaneous lupus erythematosus. Arch Dermatol. 2011;147(2):203-8.
17. Merrill JT, Werth VP, Furie R, et al. Safety and efficacy of sifalimumab, an anti IFN-alpha monoclonal antibody, in a phase 2b study of moderate to severe systemic lupus erythematosus (SLE). Arthritis Rheum. 2014;66:3530-1.
18. Furie R, Khamashta M, Merrill JT, et al. Anifrolumab, an anti-interferon-α receptor monoclonal antibody, in moderate-to-severe systemic lupus erythematosus. Arthritis Rheumatol. 2017;69(2):376-86.
19. National Institutes of Health (NIH). Efficacy and safety of anifrolumab compared to placebo in adult subjects with active systemic lupus erythematosus. [online] 2015. Available from: www.clinicaltrials.gov/ct2/show/NCT02446899. [Accessed December, 2017].
20. Merrill JT, Burgos-Vargas R, Westhovens R, et al. The efficacy and safety of abatacept in patients with non-life-threatening manifestations of systemic lupus erythematosus: results of a twelve-month, multicenter, exploratory, phase IIb, randomized, double-blind, placebo-controlled trial. Arthritis Rheum. 2010;62(10):3077-87.
21. Illei GG, Shirota Y, Yarboro CH, et al. Tocilizumab in systemic lupus erythematosus: data on safety, preliminary efficacy, and impact on circulating

plasma cells from an open-label phase I dosage-escalation study. Arthritis Rheum. 2010;62(2):542-52.

22. Wenzel J, van Holt N, Maier J, et al. JAK1/2 inhibitor ruxolitinib controls a case of chilblain lupus erythematosus. J Invest Dermatol. 2016;136(6):1281-3.

23. Sontheimer RD. The management of dermatomyositis: current treatment options. Exp Opin Pharmacother. 2004;57(6):937-43.

24. Dold S, Justiniano ME, Marquez J, et al. Treatment of early and refractory dermatomyositis with infliximab: a report of two cases. Clin Rheumatol. 2007;26(7):1186-8.

25. Norman R, Greenberg RG, Jackson JM. Case reports of etanercept in inflammatory dermatoses. J Am Acad Dermatol. 2006;54(3 Suppl 2):S139-42.

26. The Muscle Study Group. A randomized, pilot trial of etanercept in dermatomyositis. Ann Neurol. 2011;70(3):427-36.

27. Flendrie M, Vissers WH, Creemers MC, et al. Dermatological conditions during TNF-alpha-blocking therapy in patients with rheumatoid arthritis: a prospective study. Arthritis Res Ther. 2005;7(3):R666-76.

28. Hall HA, Zimmermann B. Evolution of dermatomyositis during therapy with a tumor necrosis factor-alpha inhibitor. Arthritis Rheum. 2006;55(6):982-4.

29. Chung L, Genovese MC, Fiorentino DF. A pilot trial of rituximab in the treatment of patients with dermatomyositis. Arch Dermatol. 2007;143(6):763-7.

30. Levine TD. Rituximab in the treatment of dermatomyositis: an open-label pilot study. Arthritis Rheum. 2005;52(2):601-7.

31. Joshi N, Nautiyal A, Davies PG. Successful use of rituximab in recalcitrant skin predominant dermatomyositis. J Clin Rheumatol. 2011;17(2):111-2.

32. Vleugels RA, Callen JP. Dermatomyositis: current and future treatments. Exp Rev Dermatol. 2009;4(6):581-94.

33. Jordan S, Distler JH, Maurer B, et al. Effects and safety of rituximab in systemic sclerosis: an analysis from the European Scleroderma Trial and Research (EUSTAR) group. Ann Rheum Dis. 2015;74(6):1188-94.

34. National Institutes of Health (NIH). Rituximab versus cyclophosphamide in connective tissue disease-ILD (RECITAL) 2013. [online] Available from: www.clinicaltrials.gov/ct2/show/NCT01862926. [Accessed December, 2017].

35. Khan K, Xu S, Nihtyanova S, et al. Clinical and pathological significance of interleukin-6 overexpression in systemic sclerosis. Ann Rheum Dis. 2012;71(7):1235-42.

36. Barnes TC, Spiller DG, Anderson ME, et al. Endothelial activation and apoptosis mediated by neutrophil-dependent interleukin-6 trans-signalling: a novel target for systemic sclerosis? Ann Rheum Dis. 2011;70(2):366-72.

37. Elhai M, Meunier M, Matucci-Cerinic M, et al. Outcomes of patients with systemic sclerosis-associated polyarthritis and myopathy treated with tocilizumab or abatacept: a EUSTAR observational study. Ann Rheum Dis. 2013;72(7):1217-20.

38. Shima Y, Kuwahara Y, Murota H, et al. The skin of patients with systemic sclerosis softened during the treatment with anti-IL-6 receptor antibody tocilizumab. Rheumatology (Oxford). 2010;49(12): 2408-12.

39. Khanna D, Denton CP, Jahreis A, et al. Safety and efficacy of subcutaneous tocilizumab in adults with systemic sclerosis (faSScinate): a phase 2, randomised, controlled trial. Lancet. 2016;387(10038):2630-40.

40. National Institutes of Health (NIH). A study of the efficacy and safety of tocilizumab in participants with systemic sclerosis (SSc) (focuSSced) 2015.

[online] Available from: www.clinicaltrials.gov/ct2/show/NCT02453256. [Accessed December, 2017].

41. National Institutes of Health (NIH). A study of subcutaneous abatacept to treat diffuse cutaneous systemic sclerosis (ASSET) 2014. [online] Available from: www.clinicaltrials.gov/ct2/show/NCT02161406. [Accessed December, 2017].

42. Tosounidou S, MacDonald H, Situnayake D. Successful treatment of calcinosis with infliximab in a patient with systemic sclerosis/myositis overlap syndrome. Rheumatology (Oxford). 2014;53(5):960-61.

43. de Paula DR, Klem FB, Lorencetti PG, et al. Rituximab-induced regression of CREST-related calcinosis. Clin Rheumatol. 2013;32(2):281-83.

44. Carsons SE, Vivino FB, Parke A, et al. Treatment Guidelines for rheumatologic manifestations of sjögren's syndrome: use of biologic agents, management of fatigue, and inflammatory musculoskeletal pain. Arthritis Care Res (Hoboken). 2017;69(4):517-27.

45. Puéchal X, Gottenberg JE, Berthelot JM, et al. Rituximab therapy for systemic vasculitis associated with rheumatoid arthritis: results from the autoimmunity and rituximab registry. Arthritis Care Res (Hoboken). 2012;64(3):331-9.

46. Puéchal X, Miceli-Richard C, Mejjad O, et al. Anti-tumour necrosis factor treatment in patients with refractory systemic vasculitis associated with rheumatoid arthritis. Ann Rheum Dis. 2008;67(6):880-4.

47. Carvajal Alegria G, Uguen A, Genestet S, et al. New onset of rheumatoid vasculitis during abatacept therapy and subsequent improvement after rituximab. Joint Bone Spine. 2016;83(5):605-6.

Chapter 19

Adverse Effects of Biologics: Feared or Real?

Sunil Dogra, Manju Daroach

INTRODUCTION

Biologic therapies are molecules that target specific proteins implicated in immune-mediated disease. The use of biologic therapies in treatment of chronic skin diseases has led to improved prognosis, control of symptoms and better quality of life. With the widespread use of these agents, the associated adverse effects should be more thoroughly evaluated. Biologic therapies have led to more effective therapeutic response but are also associated with many adverse effects including some rare serious side effects. This chapter summarizes the side effects seen with biologic therapy commonly used in various dermatological disorders.

DEFINITION

An adverse drug reaction is defined as "an appreciably harmful or unpleasant reaction, resulting from an intervention related to the use of a medicinal product, which predicts hazard from future administration and warrants prevention or specific treatment, or alteration of dosage regimen, or withdrawal of the product".[1] In 1972, the World Health Organization (WHO) also defined it as "a response to a drug which is noxious and unintended, and which occurs at doses normally used in man for the prophylaxis, diagnosis, or therapy of disease, or for the modifications of physiological function".

ADVERSE DRUG REACTION TO BIOLOGICS

For better understanding of the adverse effects of biologics, some key differences between small molecule drugs and biologics should be known. Most drugs are small compounds with molecular weights less than 1 kDa, while biologic agents are larger sized proteins that are designed to be structurally similar to autologous proteins with molecular weights much greater than 1 kDa.[2] Drugs are synthetic compounds, whereas biologic agents are produced with molecular genetic technique and purified from engineered cells.[2] The metabolism of drugs is thought to sometimes yield immunogenic intermediates. On the other hand, biologic agents do undergo processing but are not metabolized. Finally, biologic agents have inherent immune-mediated effects as they originate from foreign non-self-proteins, which are typically not expected to be seen with drugs because they are smaller synthetic compounds.[2,3]

CLASSIFICATION OF ADVERSE DRUG REACTIONS[4]

The adverse reactions to drugs can be classified according to their action. One such classification scheme categorizes adverse reactions to drugs in types A through E.[4,5]

1. *Type A reactions*: These correspond to the drug's pharmacologic activity, are dose dependent and are predictable.
2. *Type B reactions*: These are not related to the drug's pharmacologic activity, are unpredictable and include immune-mediated side effects and hypersensitivity reactions.
3. *Type C reactions*: These are due to the chemical structure of the drug and its metabolism.
4. *Type D reactions*: These are delayed reactions that appear many years after the treatment.
5. *Type E reactions*: These reactions are those that occur after withdrawal of a specific drug.

Another classification of adverse drug reactions given by Pichler and modified by Hausmann and colleagues is given in Table 19.1.[4]

Table 19.1: Proposed classification of adverse reactions to the biologic agents.[3]

Type	Mechanism	Example of reaction	Causative medication
α	Overstimulation	Cytokine release syndrome (cytokine storm)	Muromonab, TGN1412
β	Hypersensitivity	Common acute infusion reactions	Rituximab
		Delayed infusion reactions	Etanercept, adalimumab
		Anaphylaxis	Muromonab, cetuximab, omalizumab
γ	Cytokine or immune imbalance	Immunodeficiency Increased risk of tuberculosis	Anti-tumor necrosis factor (TNF) agents
		Hypogammaglobulinemia	Rituximab
		Autoimmunity: Systemic lupus erythematosus or vasculitis	Interferon-gamma (IFN-γ)
		Atopic disorders: Atopic dermatitis	Anti-TNF agents
δ	Cross-reactivity	Acne from anti-EGFR	Cetuximab
ε	Nonimmunologic	Neuropsychiatric side effects including confusion or depression	IFN-α

Table 19.2: Commonly used biologics in dermatology.

Disease group	Category of biologic used	Examples
Autoimmune bullous dermatoses	Anti-CD20 monoclonal antibody	Rituximab
Psoriasis	T cell activation inhibitors	Alefacept, abatacept
	Tumor necrosis factor-alpha (TNF-α) antagonists	Infliximab, adalimumab, etanercept
	Interleukin (IL)-12/23 antibodies	Ustekinumab
	Anti-IL-23 inhibitors	Tildrakizumab, guselkumab
	IL-17/IL-17R inhibitors	Secukinumab, ixekizumab, brodalumab
	Anti-CD6 antibody	Itolizumab
Hidradenitis suppurativa	TNF-α antibody	Adalimumab
Connective tissue disorders		Infliximab, etanercept rituximab
Urticaria	Anti-immunoglobulin E (IgE) antibody	Omalizumab

ADVERSE DRUG REACTIONS OF BIOLOGICS: COMMONLY USED IN DERMATOLOGY

Biologics which are commonly used in various disorders in dermatology are mentioned in Table 19.2.

SIDE EFFECTS OF INDIVIDUAL DRUGS

Rituximab[6]

Early Adverse Events

1. *Infusion-related reactions*: Infusion-related reactions occur most commonly during initial 30 minutes to 2 hours of infusion. These occur in around 10% of patients receiving rituximab. For prevention of this reaction, patient should be premedicated with antihistaminics and hydrocortisone. Various manifestations which can occur are:
   - Fever and chills
   - Rash
   - Headache and nausea
   - Pruritus or urticaria
   - Hypotension, bronchospasm and angioedema

In this situation, rituximab infusion must be stopped for 30 minutes. Hydrocortisone and antihistaminics can be reinstituted. Infusion can be restarted at half the previous rate.

Delayed reactions are also seen with rituximab with mean duration of 7 days postinfusion presenting as serum sickness like reaction manifesting commonly as fever, arthralgia and rash.

2. *Cytokine-release syndrome*: Cytokine-release syndrome is rare in patients of pemphigus treated with rituximab. This occurs commonly in patients of lymphoproliferative disorders, during the initial 90 minutes of infusion. The mechanism behind this syndrome is altered level of cytokines in body and increased levels of cytokines like interleukin (IL)-8, interferon-gamma (IFN-γ) and tumor necrosis factor-alpha (TNF-α) due to rapid infusion of drug. In severe cytokine-release syndrome, elevation of liver enzymes, D-dimer levels and prolonged prothrombin time can occur. This is clinically characterized by dyspnea, fever, chills, urticaria and pulmonary insufficiency and is associated with considerable mortality. These patients may be treated with aggressive hydration and anti-inflammatory drugs and lesser doses of subsequent therapy.[7]

Late Adverse Events

1. *Infections*: The incidence of serious infections is 5.3/100 patient-years and most of them occur within 7 months of infusion.[8] And infections are the major cause of death. Various infective complications include:
   - Community acquired pneumonia
   - *Pneumocystis carinii* pneumonia (PCP)
   - Cytomegalovirus (CMV) gastritis
   - Sepsis
   - Pyelonephritis
   - Upper respiratory tract infections, nasopharyngitis, urinary tract infections, bronchitis and sinusitis
   - Viral infections, including progressive multifocal leukoencephalo-pathy (PML).

2. *Cardiac side effects*: Sinus tachycardia, dysrhythmia and myocardial ischemia can occur in patient receiving rituximab. These are more common in patients with pre-existing cardiac disorders. These patients require monitoring during infusion of rituximab.

3. *Immune/autoimmune adverse events*: Uveitis, optic neuritis, systemic vasculitis, pleuritis, lupus-like syndrome, serum sickness, polyarticular arthritis and vasculitis with rash are the immune-mediated adverse reactions seen with rituximab.

4. *Hypogammaglobulinemia*: Hypogammaglobulinemia can occur in patients receiving rituximab. This is common in patients who receive

maintenance doses of rituximab. In a study, mean interval to document this was after 1.2 years of rituximab infusion.[9] This may be associated with increased risk of infections. Prophylactic antibiotics are not effective in prevention of infections. Rituximab-induced hypogammaglobulinemia may persist for years but usually is not symptomatic. Patients with infections may be considered for intravenous immunoglobulin (IVIg) treatment.[4]

5. *Neoplasia*: Disease progression of Kaposi's sarcoma in human immuno-deficiency virus (HIV) patients has occurred with rituximab.

6. *Gastrointestinal side effects*: In patients receiving rituximab in combination with chemotherapy, bowel obstruction and perforation can occur. In postmarketing reports, the mean time documented for gastrointestinal perforation was 1–77 days in patients with non-Hodgkin's lymphoma (NHL).

7. *Pulmonary side effects*: Fatal interstitial lung disease and fatal bronchiolitis obliterans can also occur with rituximab. There are also reports of deep vein thrombosis and pulmonary embolism after infusion.

8. *Hematological side effects*:
   - *Late-onset neutropenia (LON)*: It is defined as unexplained neutropenia in the absence of an alternative explanation, usually of grade 3 or 4 starting at least 28 days after the last dose of rituximab.[10] The incidence of LON is generally reported to be in the range of 3–27%.[11] An increased risk of LON is seen in patients with stem cell transplant, lymphoma, with multiple doses and rarely in patients with autoimmune diseases. Also, there are reports of LON in pemphigus patients occurring after 19 weeks of exposure.[12] A multifactorial etiology is likely to underlie the blood dyscrasia. This may occur 1 month to 1 year post rituximab with prevalence of around 8% in lymphoma patients.[13] Several mechanisms have been suggested for LON; which include direct toxic effect of rituximab on the bone marrow,[11] immune-mediated neutropenia[14] and apoptosis of neutrophils by Fas-Fas ligand secretion by infiltrated granular lymphocytes in the bone marrow[15] but, none of them have been proven. In some patients, treatment with granulocyte colony-stimulating factor has been required.
   - *Prolonged neutropenia*: It is defined as neutropenia that has not resolved between 24 days and 42 days after the last dose of rituximab treatment.

9. *Cutaneous side effects*:
   - *Urticaria*: It is commonly seen in patients treated with rituximab with the incidence ranging from 3% to 14% in nonrandomized trials.[16]
   - *Severe mucocutaneous reactions*: The onset of these reactions has varied from 1 week to 13 weeks following rituximab exposure and

there are rare reports of occurrence. These reactions include Stevens-Johnson syndrome,[17] lichenoid dermatitis, vesiculobullous dermatitis and paraneoplastic pemphigus.

- *Other cutaneous side effects*: Rash, exfoliation, vasculitis have also been reported with rituximab infusion.

Infliximab

1. *Infusion-related reactions*: With infliximab, infusion-related reactions are common to occur, generally mild to moderate in up to 20% of patients, usually within initial 2 hours of infusion. Infusion reactions are common in patients with neutralizing antibodies. Common manifestations include urticaria, pruritus, rash, headache, flushing, fever, chills, nausea, tachycardia or dyspnea.[18] Severe reactions like anaphylaxis and hypotension occur in less than 1% patients receiving infliximab.

2. *Cutaneous side effects*:
   - *Cutaneous vasculitis*: Infliximab has been associated with paradoxical development of leukocytoclastic vasculitis due to increased inflammatory activity.
   - Drug rash
   - *Others*: Erythema nodosum, Sweet's syndrome, bullous eruptions, necrotizing fasciitis, cutaneous ulcerations, eczematid-like purpura of Doucas and Kapetanakis, atopic dermatitis, nevi, etc.[18]

3. *Infections*: Infliximab receiving patients are at high risk of acquiring infections so cautious use is advised. Patients with mycobacterial and deep fungal infections are a contraindication for its use. There is increased risk of viral [human herpesvirus (HHV)-8, CMV, herpes zoster, molluscum], bacterial (pneumococcal, legionella, moraxella) and fungal (histoplasmosis, cryptococcosis, PCP, aspergillosis) infections in patients receiving infliximab. Tuberculosis has been most closely linked to use of infliximab. Patients are prone to get extrapulmonary mycobacterial infection and disseminated infections as well. Patients need to be screened for tuberculosis before infliximab, to prevent reactivation of latent tuberculosis. If infliximab is required in patients positive for latent tuberculosis infection, then they should be started on isoniazid prophylaxis before infliximab.

4. *Cardiovascular disease*: Tumor necrosis factor exerts negative inotropic effects and can promote fibrosis, hypertrophy and cardiomyopathy in animal models. There is an evidence of worsening heart failure with infliximab so caution should be exercised in patients with moderate to severe congestive heart failure.

5. *Demyelinating diseases*: Infliximab infusion has been associated with rare development of demyelinating disorders like sclerosis, optic neuritis

and Guillain-Barré syndrome. Caution should be exercised in patients with pre-existing demyelinating disorders.

6. *Lupus-like syndrome*: Infliximab has been reported to induce lupus-like syndrome, which improves after discontinuation of the drug. Reason for development of lupus is proposed to be increased level of autoantibodies after infliximab. The onset of symptoms ranges from less than 1 month to more than 4 years. Clinical features are most commonly cutaneous with reports of malar rash, pruritic rash, photosensitivity, purpura, discoid rash, mucosal ulcers and alopecia. Other features include constitutional symptoms, arthralgia, pericarditis, pleural or pericardial effusions, deep venous thrombosis, pneumonitis and neuritis. The mainstay of treatment is withdrawal of the offending drug. Symptoms generally resolve within 3 weeks to 6 months after withdrawal. However, many patients require traditional therapy for idiopathic systemic lupus erythematosus (SLE), including topical or systemic steroids, antimalarials and less frequently immunosuppressants.[19]

7. *Autoantibodies*: It has been seen in various studies, that there is development of antinuclear antibodies (ANAs) and anti-dsDNA antibody in patients receiving infliximab, which is a transient phenomenon.[20] ANA positivity is seen in around 60% patients receiving infliximab.

8. *Immunogenicity*: Neutralizing antibodies are seen in around 10% of patients and these patients are more likely to get infusion reactions.

9. *Malignancy*: Non-Hodgkin's lymphoma—There are case reports and case series showing increased risk of lymphoma in patients receiving infliximab but the linkage is not confirmed. The incidence of non-lymphoma cancers is not increased in patients receiving infliximab as compared to the control population.

10. *Other systemic complications*: Aseptic meningitis, polymyositis, pancytopenia, serum sickness, acute idiopathic pancreatitis, cholestatic liver disease, transaminitis, anaphylactic-like reactions, etc.[18]

Etanercept[18]

1. *Injection site reactions*: Injection site bleeding and bruising has been seen commonly with etanercept. These occur in around 37% cases and last an average of 3–5 days and eventually tolerance develops to these reactions. The mechanism of these reactions is suggested to be a delayed-type hypersensitivity reaction that is T cell mediated, which wanes over time due to induction of tolerance.

2. *Infections*: Upper respiratory tract infections are commonly associated with etanercept treatment. Reports of multifocal septic arthritis and osteomyelitis are also there. Other rare reports of orbital myositis, viral pneumonia, histoplasmosis, toxoplasmosis and aspergillosis are

documented with etanercept. Reactivation of latent tuberculosis is seen with etanercept treatment. The chances of reactivation are however lesser than infliximab. Tubercular tonsillitis and peritonitis have also been reported.

3. *Lymphoma and other malignancies*: It is unclear that lymphoma risk increases with etanercept. Nonlymphoma cancers are not associated with etanercept.

4. *Cardiovascular complications*: It should be avoided in patients with severe congestive cardiac failure as worsening of heart failure may occur.

5. *Demyelinating disorders*: There are rare reports of development of demyelinating disorders after treatment with etanercept.

6. *Lupus-like syndrome*: Drug-induced lupus is seen with etanercept treatment. Subcutaneous lupus-like lesions can be commonly seen.

7. *Immunogenicity*: Around 5% of patients receiving etanercept develop antibodies but these are not related with the efficacy or adverse effects.

8. *Cutaneous side effects*: Cutaneous vasculitis can occur with etanercept. Other reported cutaneous adverse effects are erythema multiforme and toxic epidermal necrolysis.

9. *Other systemic complications*: Aplastic anemia, lung injury and silent thyroiditis have also been reported with infliximab rarely.

Adalimumab[21]

1. *Injection site reactions*: Injection site reactions are the most common side effect of adalimumab. These occur in the form of erythema, itching, pain and swelling. These are mild to moderate, which do not lead to discontinuation of drug and usually do not tend to recur.

2. *Infections*: Adalimumab increases the risk of nonserious infections marginally:
   - Upper respiratory tract infection
   - Sinusitis
   - Flu-like symptoms
   - Urinary tract infections.

   It also increases the risk of serious infections like:
   - *Tuberculosis*: Reactivation of latent tuberculosis is seen with adalimumab. Miliary, lymphatic, pulmonary and peritoneal tuberculosis have been seen with adalimumab treatment. Most cases occur in first 8 months.
   - *Deep fungal infections*: Adalimumab treatment also exposes the patient to risk of deep fungal infections like histoplasmosis, coccidioidomycosis, aspergillosis, nocardiosis, etc.

3. *Cardiovascular diseases*: It increases risk of congestive cardiac failure but lesser than infliximab. So, it should be avoided in severe congestive cardiac failure.

4. *Demyelinating disorders*: It increases the risk of demyelinating disorders. So, it should not be used in cases of multiple sclerosis and other demyelinating disorders and should be discontinued, if these develop.

5. *Lupus-like syndrome*: Lupus-like syndrome can occur with adalimumab which remits after discontinuation of drug.

6. *Immunogenicity*: Neutralizing antibodies are seen in patients receiving adalimumab and have a decreased efficacy in those with positive neutralizing antibodies.

7. *Lymphoma and other neoplasms*: Patients with psoriasis on adalimumab have two- to three fold increased risk of lymphoma but not solid organ malignancies.

8. *Cutaneous side effects*: Infectious skin complications like cellulitis, herpes zoster and erysipelas can be seen. Other skin complications include anaphylactoid reactions like urticaria, angioedema and pruritus.

9. *Systemic complications*: Pancytopenia and transaminitis can be seen with adalimumab which warrants intermittent laboratory monitoring.

Secukinumab

In the ERASURE study, during the 12-week of induction period, 55.1% patients had at least one adverse event in the 300 mg secukinumab group and most common were upper respiratory tract infection, nasopharyngitis and headache. In FIXTURE study also nasopharyngitis, headache and diarrhea were commonly seen, which were common in induction as well as the entire treatment period.

Various side effects seen with secukinumab are listed here.[22-24]

1. Nasopharyngitis
2. Diarrhea
3. Dizziness
4. Headache
5. *Neutropenia*: IL-17A stimulates the neutrophil trafficking and granulopoiesis. So neutropenia is important adverse event and must be considered in patients for secukinumab. Rich et al.[23] have reported neutropenia in 19 patients in the 12-week induction phase and in 30 patients in the maintenance phase (weeks 12–32). Dosing was not interrupted or withheld as no clinically significant adverse events were associated with the development of neutropenia. The neutropenia resolved during the course of the study in all cases.
6. *Infections and infestations*:
   • Upper respiratory tract infections
   • Candida infection is commonly seen. This can be treated with standard therapy and does not lead to discontinuation of therapy.
   • Oral herpes, tinea pedis and otitis externa have also been seen.

7. Treatment emergent anti-secukinumab antibodies—very uncommonly formed. In the FIXTURE study, 0.4% patients developed these antibodies, but had no relation with loss of efficacy or adverse events.
8. Mucocutaneous adverse effects—urticaria can occur.
9. Ophthalmological adverse effects—conjunctivitis.

Omalizumab

Serious adverse effects are very uncommon with omalizumab.[25] Various side effects seen with omalizumab are listed here.
1. Injection site reactions—the most common
2. Upper respiratory tract infections
3. Headache
4. Pharyngitis
5. Fatigue, arthralgia, dizziness, pruritus, dermatitis, earache
6. *Anaphylaxis*: The mechanism of anaphylaxis with omalizumab is poorly understood. Suggested mechanism is because omalizumab is composed of 5% mouse polypeptide, it is possible that immunoglobulin E (IgE)-mediated reactions may occur against the murine sequences. It has a very low incidence and occurs during the first 2 hours of infusion. In a postmarketing trial during the first three injections, these reactions occur after 1 hour of injection and during further injections within 30 minutes. So recommended time for monitoring during initial injections is 2 hours and subsequent injections is 30 minutes. Another recommendation is to educate patients about signs and symptoms and prescribing them epinephrine autoinjectors.
7. No significant laboratory abnormalities are seen with omalizumab, so no routine monitoring is recommended.

▌ SAFETY PROFILE OF BIOLOGICS IN PSORIASIS

Most commonly biologics are used in treatment of moderate to severe psoriasis which is not responding to conventional therapies or conventional therapies are contraindicated. In German, psoriasis registry "PsoBest" on long-term outcome and safety of systemic treatment and biologics found no significant difference in adverse events with respect to infections, major cardiac events, malignancies, etc.[26] Based on PSOLAR registry data through 2013, no safety concerns were observed with infliximab for all-cause mortality, major cardiac events or malignancy; however, association was noted with serious infections.[27] Compared with nonbiologic therapy, the use of biologic agents was not a significant predictor of death, major cardiac events or malignancy in psoriasis or psoriatic arthritis.[28,29] In a meta-analysis, it was found that biologics are superior as long-term therapy compared to placebo.

No differences were seen between adalimumab, etanercept or infliximab versus placebo with respect to the safety parameters, also the efficacy of secukinumab and infliximab was found superior to etanercept while that of infliximab was better than methotrexate in psoriasis.[29] A systematic review and meta-analysis has shown that the anti-ILs are amongst the best-tolerated agents, while anti-T cells increased events such as withdrawals and infections.[30] In patients with previous history of malignancies, there has been no increased risk of solid organ malignancies after biological treatment of psoriasis.[31] Most common dermatological side effect encountered in psoriasis patients with biologics was pruritus.[31] In future, biologics will gain a very popular role in the treatment of dermatological disorders. Biologics targeting a particular cytokine, leading to an efficient control of the disease with minimal side effects will be a boon to the treatment of several skin diseases. Hence, it is of utmost importance for all dermatologists to be well versed with the use of biologics and their potential safety concerns.

▌ REFERENCES

1. Edwards IR, Aronson JK. Adverse drug reactions: definitions, diagnosis and management. Lancet. 2000;356:1255-9.
2. Aubin F, Carbonnel F, Wendling D. The complexity of adverse side-effects to biological agents. J Crohn's Colitis. 2013;7:257-62.
3. Pichler WJ. Adverse side-effects to biological agents. Allergy Eur J Allergy Clin Immunol. 2006;61:912-20.
4. Patel SV, Khan DA. Adverse reactions to biologic therapy. Immunol Allergy Clin North Am. 2017;37:397-412.
5. Naisbitt DJ, Gordon SF, Pirmohamed M, et al. Immunological principles of adverse drug reactions: the initiation and propagation of immune responses elicited by drug treatment. Drug Saf. 2000;23:483-507.
6. Feldman RJ, Ahmed AR. Relevance of rituximab therapy in pemphigus vulgaris: analysis of current data and the immunologic basis for its observed responses. Expert Rev Clin Immunol. 2011;7:529-41.
7. Kulkarni HS, Kasi PM. Rituximab and cytokine release syndrome. Case Rep Oncol. 2012;5:134-41.
8. Tony HP, Burmester G, Schulze-Koops H, et al. Safety and clinical outcomes of rituximab therapy in patients with different autoimmune diseases: experience from a national registry (GRAID). Arthritis Res Ther. 2011;13(3):R75.
9. Casulo C, Maragulia J, Zelenetz AD. Incidence of hypogammaglobulinemia in patients receiving rituximab and the use of intravenous immunoglobulin for recurrent infections. Clin Lymphoma Myeloma Leuk. 2013;13:106-11.
10. Hincks I, Woodcock BE, Thachil J. Is rituximab-induced late-onset neutropenia a good prognostic indicator in lymphoproliferative disorders? Br J Haematol. 2011;53:411-3.
11. Wolach O, Bairey O, Lahav M. Late-onset neutropenia after rituximab treatment: case series and comprehensive review of the literature. Medicine (Baltimore). 2010;89:308-18.

12. Goh MS, McCormack C, Dinh HV, et al. Rituximab in the adjuvant treatment of pemphigus vulgaris: a prospective open-label pilot study in five patients. Br J Dermatol. 2007;156:990-6.
13. Salmon JH, Cacoub P, Combe B, et al. Late-onset neutropenia after treatment with rituximab for rheumatoid arthritis and other autoimmune diseases: data from the Autoimmunity and Rituximab registry. RMD Open. 2015;1(1):e000034.
14. Voog E, Morschhauser F, Solal-Céligny P. Neutropenia in patients treated with rituximab. N Engl J Med. 2003;348(26):2691-4; discussion 2691-4.
15. Papadaki T, Stamatopoulos K, Stavroyianni N, et al. Evidence for T-large granular lymphocyte-mediated neutropenia in rituximab-treated lymphoma patients: report of two cases. Leuk Res. 2002;26:597-600.
16. Bremmer M, Deng A, Gaspari A. A mechanism-based classification of dermatologic reactions to biologic agents used in the treatment of cutaneous disease: Part 2. Dermatitis. 2009;20:243-56.
17. Lowndes S, Darby A, Mead G, et al. Stevens-Johnson syndrome after treatment with rituximab. Ann Oncol. 2002;13(12):1948-50.
18. Scheinfeld N. A comprehensive review and evaluation of the side effects of the tumor necrosis factor alpha blockers etanercept, infliximab and adalimumab. J Dermatolog Treat. 2004;15:280-94.
19. Sehgal VN, Pandhi D, Khurana A. Biologics in dermatology: adverse effects. Int J Dermatol. 2015;54:1442-60.
20. Bobbio-Pallavicini F, Alpini C, Caporali R, et al. Autoantibody profile in rheumatoid arthritis during long-term infliximab treatment. Arthritis Res Ther. 2004;6:R264-72.
21. Scheinfeld N. Adalimumab: a review of side effects. Expert Opin Drug Saf. 2005;4:637-41.
22. Papp KA, Langley RG, Sigurgeirsson B, et al. Efficacy and safety of secukinumab in the treatment of moderate-to-severe plaque psoriasis: a randomized, double-blind, placebo-controlled phase II dose-ranging study. Br J Dermatol. 2013;168:412-21.
23. Rich P, Sigurgeirsson B, Thaci D, et al. Secukinumab induction and maintenance therapy in moderate-to-severe plaque psoriasis: a randomized, double-blind, placebo-controlled, phase II regimen-finding study. Br J Dermatol. 2013;168:402-11.
24. Langley RG, Elewski BE, Lebwohl M, et al. Secukinumab in plaque psoriasis: results of two phase 3 trials. N Engl J Med. 2014;371:326-38.
25. Chia J, Mydlarski PR. Omalizumab in dermatology: a review of the literature. J Am Acad Dermatol. 2015;72:AB210.
26. Reich K, Mrowietz U, Radtke MA, et al. Drug safety of systemic treatments for psoriasis: results from the German Psoriasis Registry PsoBest. Arch Dermatol Res. 2015;307:875-83.
27. Gottlieb AB, Kalb RE, Langley RG, et al. Safety observations in 12,095 patients with psoriasis enrolled in an international registry (PSOLAR): experience with infliximab and other systemic and biologic therapies. J Drugs Dermatol. 2014;13:1441-8.
28. Spehr C, Reich K, Mrowietz U, et al. PsoBest: drug safety in systemic treatments for psoriasis and psoriatic arthritis. J Invest Dermatol. 2015;135:S19.
29. Nast A, Jacobs A, Rosumeck S, et al. Efficacy and safety of systemic long-term treatments for moderate-to-severe psoriasis: a systematic review and meta-analysis. J Invest Dermatol. 2015;135:2641-8.

30. Baker EL, Coleman CI, Reinhart KM, et al. Safety of biologic treatments for moderate to severe plaque psoriasis: a systematic review, basic meta-analysis and Bayesian mixed treatment comparison. Pharmacotherapy. 2011;31:327e-8e.
31. Van Lümig PP, Driessen RJ, Berends MA, et al. Safety of treatment with biologics for psoriasis in daily practice: 5-year data. J Eur Acad Dermatol Venereol. 2012;26:283-91.

Chapter 20

Management of Latent Tuberculosis Infection

Bhushan Madke, Swetalina Pradhan

▌ INTRODUCTION

Anti-tumor necrosis factor-α (anti-TNF-α) agents are being increasingly used in the management of moderate-to-severe psoriasis. Therapy with anti-TNF-α agents is being fraught with reactivation of latent tuberculosis infection (LTBI). This chapter addresses the intricate relation between latent TB infection and anti-TNF-α agents and provides working guidelines for screening of LTBI and its management before prescribing anti-TNF-α therapy in patients with psoriasis.

The incidence of tuberculosis (TB) was 10.4 million globally in 2015, (ranging from 8.7 million to 12.2 million), equivalent to 142 cases per 1,00,000 population. Most of the estimated number of cases in 2015 occurred in Asia (61%) and the World Health Organization (WHO) African region (26%); smaller proportions of cases occurred in the Eastern Mediterranean region (7%), the Euroαpean region (3%) and the region of the Americas (3%).[1] The 30 high TB burden countries accounted for 87% of all estimated incident cases worldwide. The six countries that stood out as having the largest number of incident cases in 2015 were (in descending order) India, Indonesia, China, Nigeria, Pakistan, and South Africa (combined, 60% of the global total). Of these, China, India, and Indonesia alone accounted for 45% of global cases in 2015.[1] An estimated 11% of the incident TB cases in 2015 were among people living with human immunodeficiency virus (HIV). Approximately 1.4 million (ranging from 1.2 million to 1.6 million) people who were HIV-negative died from TB in 2015 and an additional 0.39 million (ranging from 0.32 million to 0.46 million) HIV-positive people died from TB. TB is one of the top 10 causes of death worldwide and it caused more deaths than HIV/AIDS in 2015.[1,2]

According to WHO Strategic and Technical Advisory Group for TB (STAG-TB), amongst all high burden country list (HBC) India has been included in the list of high TB-burden countries, high TB/HIV-burden countries and high MDR-TB-burden countries. Approximately 40% of Indians are latently infected with TB.[3]

▌PATHOGENESIS OF TUBERCULOUS INFECTION

Mycobacterium tuberculosis (*M. tuberculosis*)/tubercle bacilli are carried in airborne particles, called droplet nuclei, of 1–5 μ sized in diameter generated from the person having active respiratory TB (lung or laryngeal). After inhalation of the droplet nuclei containing *M. tuberculosis*, the infectious bacilli traverse the mouth or nasal passages, upper respiratory tract and bronchi to reach the alveoli of the lungs.

Within 2–8 weeks, special immune cells called macrophages ingest and surround the tubercle bacilli. The cells form a barrier shell, called a granuloma, that keeps the bacilli contained and under control leading to establishment of LTBI.

Persons with LTBI have *M. tuberculosis* in their bodies, but do not have TB disease and cannot spread the infection to other susceptible host. However, in some infected individuals, the tubercle bacilli overcome the cellular immune system and multiply, resulting in progression from LTBI to TB disease. The progression from LTBI to TB disease may occur at any time, from soon to many years later. Hence, detection of LTBI is of utmost important in cases where chance of iatrogenic immunosuppression persists. Currently, LTBI can be screened by using either tuberculin skin test (TST) or an interferon-gamma release assay (IGRA). It usually takes about 2–8 weeks interval period for the body's immune system to be able to react to tuberculin and for the infection to be detected by the TST or IGRA. Within weeks after infection, the immune system is usually able to halt the multiplication of the tubercle bacilli, preventing further progression.

Biologics are protein molecules, which target the specific points in the immunopathogenesis of the diseases. They are produced by recombinant DNA technology. These molecules target specific pathogenetic pathways in a disease. Because of this specific action on immune system they have very less side effects compared to other immunosuppressives having broader action. In the current era, biologics have revolutionized the treatment of various diseases and specifically dermatological conditions.

The biological drugs are divided into three groups:[4]
1. Recombinant human cytokines and growth factors
2. Monoclonal antibodies
3. Fusion antibody proteins.

Out of these three groups, monoclonal antibodies have been used frequently in various dermatological diseases. Out of monoclonal antibodies anti-TNF-α drugs like infliximab, adalimumab, certolizumab, and golimumab have been used commonly in various autoimmune and inflammatory conditions, i.e. psoriasis vulgaris, psoriatic arthropathy, pustular psoriasis, sarcoidosis, Crohn's disease, ulcerative colitis, rheumatoid arthritis, ankylosing spondylitis, hidradenitis suppurativa, subcorneal pustular dermatosis, pyoderma gangrenosum, toxic epidermal necrolysis, Behçet's syndrome, and SAPHO syndrome. Monoclonal antibodies like omalizumab, efalizumab, and rituximab have been found useful in various other conditions like atopic dermatitis, urticaria, dermatomyositis, discoid lupus erythematosus (DLE), lichen planus, CD20+ non-Hodgkin B-cell lymphoma, paraneoplastic pemphigus, urticarial vasculitis, systemic lupus erythematosus (SLE), cutaneous B-cell lymphoma, epidermolysis bullosa acquisita (EBA) and recalcitrant pemphigus.[5-18]

After monoclonal antibodies next commonly used biologicals are fusion proteins amongst which etanercept and alefacept have been Food and Drug Administration (FDA) approved for treatment of rheumatoid arthritis, ankylosing spondylitis, psoriatic arthropathy and plaque psoriasis (moderate-to-severe).[6-7]

Though there have been several indications of different biological drugs in dermatological diseases, out of them anti-TNF-α agents have been widely used and psoriasis has been the most common disease to be studied as an indication.

PSORIASIS, ANTI-TNF THERAPY AND LATENT TUBERCULOSIS INFECTION

The incidence of psoriasis is 0.5–3% of the world's population. The pathogenesis of psoriasis is multifactorial and is considered to be the result of combination of genetic susceptibility, immune dysregulation and environmental factors.[8] Key cytokines involved in the pathogenesis of psoriasis are tumor necrosis factor-alpha (TNF-α) and interleukins (IL-12, IL-17, IL-22, IL-23).[9] Due to advances in the understanding of the immunopathogenesis of psoriasis, more specific/targeted drugs are being used for the treatment of the same. In the last three decades, anti-TNF-α biological therapy has revolutionized the treatment of moderate-to-severe plaque psoriasis. There are five biologic therapies for moderate-to-severe plaque psoriasis currently approved by the US FDA and the European Medicines Agency (EMA). These include three TNF-α antagonist (adalimumab, etanercept, and infliximab), one IL-12/IL-23 p40 inhibitor (ustekinumab), and a recently approved IL-17A inhibitor (secukinumab).

However, various studies have confirmed that anti-TNF-α therapy is associated with 25 times risk of activation of LTBI, depending on the clinical setting and the anti-TNF agent used.[10,11]

Therefore, it is logical that psoriatic patients planned for anti-TNF-α therapy should be proactively screened for LTBI and if found to be positive preemptive antituberculosis treatment should be instituted prior to the initiation of biological treatment.

Latent Tuberculosis Infection: Who Needs Investigation?

Latent tuberculosis infection, defined as a state of persistent immune response to prior-acquired *M. tuberculosis* antigens without evidence of clinically manifested active TB. The lifetime risk of reactivation of TB in person with documented LTBI is 5–10%, with risk being maximum in first five years of acquiring infection.[12] Risk of reactivation depends on immunological status of the host. Testing for LTBI should be performed only in individuals who have high-risk of reactivation of TB and those who will benefit from treatment.

These high-risk groups as per current WHO guidelines are:
- People living with HIV
- Children less than 5 years who are in close contact with people suffering from TB
- Patients initiating anti-TNF-α treatment
- Patients receiving dialysis
- Patient preparing for organ or hematologic transplantation
- Patients with silicosis.[13]

Testing for LTBI should be performed only after clinical evaluation has ruled out active TB.

Screening for Latent Tuberculosis Infection

Tuberculin skin test and interferon gamma release assays (IGRAs) are being currently done for diagnosis of LTBI. The diagnosis of LTBI is traditionally based on TST positivity in the absence of active TB.[14] However, TST has a low sensitivity and specificity in patients with prior *Mycobacterium bovis* infection and Bacillus Calmette-Guérin (BCG) vaccination and hence loses its relevance. Therefore, IGRAs have been introduced to compensate for the drawback of TST in detecting LTBI.[15,16] It must be borne in mind that IGRAs are to be used for screening of LTBI and not for diagnosis of active TB.[17] Diagnosis of active TB requires different set of investigations. All patients with psoriasis who are considered as a potential candidate for receiving anti-TNF-α therapy should receive HIV testing independent of screening for LTBI.

Tuberculin Skin Test

Tuberculin skin test is one of the widely used investigations used for diagnosis of TB since the 19th century. Targeted tuberculin testing for LTBI has been considered as a strategic component of TB control by the Centers for Disease Control and Prevention (CDC, Atlanta, USA) which specifically identifies individuals at high-risk for developing TB and would benefit by the treatment of LTBI, if detected.

Tuberculin skin test administration: Tuberculin skin test is commonly done by intradermal injection, called the Mantoux technique (after Charles Mantoux), who described the technique in the early part of the 20th century. A standardized product called PPD-S (purified protein derivative-standardized) prepared from *M. tuberculosis* is used for this purpose. There are also various types of PPD of nontuberculous (i.e. atypical) Mycobacterium like PPD-A is (*M. avium*), PPD-G (gause strain of scotochromogen), PPD-B (nonphotochromogen Battey bacilli), PPD-F (rapid grower *M. fortuitum*), and PPD-Y (yellow photochromogen *M. kansasii*).

Tuberculin skin test is performed by injecting 0.1 mL of PPD into the inner surface of the forearm. The injection is given intradermally with a tuberculin syringe (plastic body with a less-than-half-inch needle, either 26 or 27 gauge), with the needle bevel facing upward. The injection should produce a pale elevation of the skin (a wheal) 6–10 mm in diameter when placed correctly. Subcutaneous administration will result in rapid "washout" from the area without time for the development of a reaction while very superficial placement will result into leakage of reagent through the skin. Hence, a highly trained laboratory professional should be delegated the task of TST administration. If the injection is unsuccessful and not able to raise a desired wheal, it may be repeated immediately, usually on the other forearm.

Reading of tuberculin skin test: The reaction should be read between 48 and 72 hours after administration.

The reaction is measured in millimeters of the induration (palpable, raised, hardened area, or swelling) across the forearm (perpendicular to the long axis). The induration and not the erythema measurement is done in the test.[18,19] The physician should particularly stress on measurement of the indurated area rather than accepting the reading as "positive" or "negative" as this will allow any future comparisons (Tables 20.1 and 20.2).

Interpretation of tuberculin skin test: Skin test interpretation depends on the below-mentioned two factors.
1. Measurement in millimeters of the induration
2. Person's risk of being infected with TB and of progression to disease if infected.

Boosted reaction: The ability to react to tuberculin may decrease over time in some persons infected with *M. tuberculosis* leading to a false-negative reaction. In such cases, two-step testing is done where second TST is given after an initial negative test. The initial TST may stimulate the immune system, causing a positive or boosted reaction to subsequent tests. The

Table 20.1: Classification of the tuberculin skin test reaction.

An induration of 5 mm or more is considered positive in:	An induration of 10 mm or more is considered positive in:	An induration of 15 mm or more is considered positive in:
• HIV-infected persons • A recent contact of a person with TB disease • Persons with fibrotic changes on chest radiograph consistent with prior TB • Patients with organ transplants • Persons who are immunosuppressed due to other reasons (e.g. taking the equivalent of >15 mg/day of prednisone for 1 month or longer, taking TNF-α antagonists, etc.)	• Recent immigrants (<5 years) from high-prevalence countries • Injection drug users • Residents and employees of high-risk congregate settings • Mycobacteriology laboratory personnel • Persons with clinical conditions that place them at high-risk • Children <4 years of age • Infants, children, and adolescents exposed to adults in high-risk categories	• Any person, including persons with no known risk factors for TB. However, targeted skin testing programs should only be conducted among high-risk groups

(HIV: Human immunodeficiency virus; TB: Tuberculosis; TNF-α: Tumor necrosis factor-α).

Table 20.2: Comparison between false-positive and false-negative reactions.

False-positive reactions	False-negative reactions
• Infection with nontuberculous mycobacteria • Previous BCG vaccination • Incorrect method of TST administration • Incorrect interpretation of reaction • Incorrect antigen bottle used	• Cutaneous anergy (anergy is the inability to react to skin tests because of a weakened immune system) • Recent TB infection (within 8–10 weeks of exposure) • Very old TB infection (many years) • Very young age infection (less than 6 months old) • Recent live virus vaccination (e.g. measles and smallpox) • Overwhelming TB disease • Some viral illnesses (e.g. measles and chicken pox) • Incorrect method of TST administration • Incorrect interpretation of reaction

(BCG: Bacillus Calmette-Guérin; TST: Tuberculin skin test; TB: Tuberculosis).

second boosted reading is the correct one, i.e. the result that should be used for decision-making or future comparison. Boosting is maximal if the second test is placed between 1 and 5 weeks after the initial test, and it may continue to be observed for up to 2 years.

Mantoux conversion: Conversion is defined as a change (within a 2-year period) of Mantoux reactivity, which meets either of the following criteria:[20]

- A change from a negative to a positive reaction
- An increase of greater than or equal to 10 mm
- Conversion has been associated with an annual incidence of TB disease of 4% in adolescents or 6% in contacts of smear-positive cases.

Conversion is the development of new or enhanced hypersensitivity due to infection with tuberculous or nontuberculous mycobacteria; including BCG vaccination which is opposite of boosting that occurs due to recall of the hypersensitivity response in the absence of new infection.

Therefore, when testing TB contacts for conversion, the second tuberculin test is done 8 weeks after the date of last contact with the source case.

Bacillus Calmette-Guérin vaccine and the Mantoux test: According to the US recommendation, TST is not contraindicated for BCG-vaccinated persons and also prior BCG vaccination should not influence the interpretation of the test.

A diagnosis of LTBI and treatment for the same is considered for any BCG-vaccinated person whose skin test is 10 mm or greater, under any of the following circumstances:

- History of contact with another person with infectious TB
- Was born or has lived in a high TB prevalence country
- Continuous exposure to populations where TB prevalence is high.

Disadvantages of tuberculin skin test: The disadvantages are mentioned below:

- Poor inter-reader reliability
- False-positives/specificity (nontuberculous mycobacterial infection or prior BCG vaccination)
- Poor positive predictive value in low prevalence region.

Interferon Gamma Release Assay

Background of IGRA: Various subsets of immune cells (e.g. macrophages, T lymphocytes) are involved in the immune response directed against the bacilli after being infected with *M. tuberculosis*. These cells do not fully eradicate the bacilli, but rather contain the infection.[21] Macrophages have an important role in the first-line of defense against the infection by ingesting and subsequently killing the organisms. However, *M. tuberculosis* bacilli escape the immune system and have the ability to persist within macrophages, thereby averting the attack by these host cells.[22,23] The cytokine interferon-gamma (IFN-γ) plays an important role in the elimination of *M. tuberculosis* by activating the production of reactive oxygen and nitrogen intermediates in the macrophages, which cause destruction of bacterial pathogens. CD4 T cells recognizing *M. tuberculosis* antigens produce IFN-γ causing activation of *M. tuberculosis* infected macrophages and kill the bacilli and control their growth.[24,25]

Interferon gamma release assays are blood-based tests assessing the presence of effector and memory immune responses directed against the *M. tuberculosis* antigens. They predominantly measure the presence of *M. tuberculosis* specific effector memory T cells, the presence of which is considered indicative of previous in vivo exposure to the bacilli. These tests measure the presence of an adaptive immune response to *M. tuberculosis* antigens, and are thus an indirect measure of *M. tuberculosis* exposure.[26,27]

Types of interferon gamma release assays: Two types of IGRAs that have been approved by the US FDA (Table 20.3).
- QuantiFERON®-TB Gold In-Tube test (QFT-GIT)
- T-SPOT®.TB test (T-Spot)

QuantiFERON®-TB Gold In-Tube test: Interferon gamma release assays are performed on fresh blood specimens. The QFT-GIT is performed by drawing 1 mL of blood into one of each of the three manufacturer precoated, heparinized tubes. The tubes are then incubated for 16–24 hours at 37°C within 16 hours of blood collection. The plasma is harvested after centrifugation and used to assess the concentration of IFN-α by enzyme-linked immunosorbent assay (ELISA) test. Results are interpreted according to the manufacturer's recommendations.[28]

Table 20.3: Comparison between QuantiFERON®-TB Gold In-Tube test (QFT-GIT) AND T-SPOT®.TB test.

	QFT-GIT	T-SPOT
Initial process	Process whole blood within 16 hours	Process peripheral blood mononuclear cells (PBMCs) within 8 hours, or if T-Cell Xtend® is used, within 30 hours
M. tuberculosis antigen	Single mixture of synthetic peptides representing ESAT-6, CFP-10 and TB7.7	Separate mixtures of synthetic peptides representing ESAT-6 and CFP-10
Measurement	IFN-γ concentration	Number of IFN-γ producing cells (spots)
Possible results	Positive, negative, and indeterminate	Positive, negative, indeter-minate, and borderline

(IFN-γ: Interferon necrosis-gamma).

T-SPOT.*TB test*: 8 mL of blood is required and the assay is performed within 8 hours of blood collection (using heparinized tubes). Alternatively, the manufacturer also provides a reagent (T-Cell Xtend) which extends processing time to 32 hours after blood collection. The T cell containing peripheral blood mononuclear cell (PBMC) fraction is separated from whole blood and distributed to the microtiter plate wells (2,50,000 cells/ well) provided in the T-SPOT®.TB assay kit. Following 16–20 hours (at 37°C with 5% CO_2) incubation, the number of IFN-γ-secreting T cells (represented as spot-forming units) can be detected by enzyme-linked immunospot (ELISPOT) assay. Results are interpreted according to the manufacturer's recommendations.[29]

Benefits of interferon gamma release assays: The benefits are listed below:
• Single visit
• Not affected by prior BCG vaccination status
• Not dependent on observer (erythema or induration unlike TST)
• Can be used for follow-up as it does not result in boosted reaction unlike TST.

Disadvantages of interferon gamma release assays: The disadvantages are listed below.
• *Cost*: It is an expensive test, as compared to TST. Hence, WHO guidelines suggest that IGRA should not replace TST in low and middle income countries for detection of LTBI.
• False positive and poor positive predictive value in low prevalence region.
• Blood samples must be processed within 8–30 hours after collection while white blood cells are still viable.
• Errors in collecting or transporting blood specimens or in running and interpreting the assay can decrease the accuracy of IGRAs.

WHICH TEST TO USE AND HOW TO USE?

It is imperative to screen patients for LTBI before patients are considered for anti-TNF-α agents, as it significantly increases risk of reactivation of TB. First step in screening for LTBI is to rule out active TB by history, clinical examination and if required necessary investigation (chest radiograph and sputum examination for acid-fast bacilli). All potential candidates should be asked about symptoms of active pulmonary TB (cough, hemoptysis, fever, night sweats, weight loss, chest pain, and shortness of breath).

Test for LTBI should be administered only when active TB is reasonably ruled out because if patient with active TB is treated as LTBI with monotherapy, it will be inadequate treatment and will lead to development of resistance. Diagnosis of active TB disease needs culture studies, nucleic acid-based tests and detection of acid-fast bacilli from appropriate clinical material. All psoriasis patients should be enquired for significant exposure to a source of tuberculosis (pulmonary or laryngeal) in the family and close contacts.

World Health Organization guidelines suggest use of either TST or IGRA (not both) for detection of LTBI. We propose following steps for detection of LTBI based on relevant literature and cost-effectiveness in our scenario. IGRAs should not replace TST in resource poor settings.

- TST should be used as first test for detection of LTBI.
- IGRA should be done:
  - When results from TST are indeterminate
  - When TST is positive and there is need to increase the acceptability of treatment
  - To follow-up patient who are on biological therapy, when TST is of limited value.
- In case, a patient is positive for TST or IGRA, chest X-ray should be done and any abnormality should prompt evaluation for treatment of active tuberculosis. A computed tomography scan can be ordered if chest X-ray reveals any tuberculous foci.

▌TREATMENT OF LATENT TUBERCULOUS INFECTION

Treatment options available for treatment of LTBI as per WHO guidelines are as follows:

- 6 months of isoniazid (INH) monotherapy
- 9 months of INH monotherapy[30]
- 3 months regimen of weekly rifapentine and isoniazid
- 3–4 months isoniazid and rifampicin
- 3–4 months of rifampicin monotherapy.

Pyrazinamide containing regimens are not used for treatment of LTBI because of unacceptable hepatotoxicity.

There are not enough studies to support or refute superiority of one regimen over another for treatment of LTBI. However, longer treatment has higher risk of hepatotoxicity and compliance issues. Hence, 3 months of rifampicin and isoniazid regimen is probably safer as compared to 6–9 months of isoniazid monotherapy.

American Thoracic Society (ATS) and CDC guidelines suggest use of INH daily for 9 months for treatment of LTBI as first-line therapy.[31]

The World Health Organization and National Institute of Health, United Kingdom recommend 6 months of INH as acceptable treatment for LTBI.

ADVERSE EVENT MONITORING

Patients having LTBI are not sick and are usually in good condition. Hence, it should be kept in mind to minimize the adverse effects due to treatment. The adverse effects are ususlly drug specific and include elevation of liver enzymes, peripheral neuropathy, and hepatotoxicity due to isoniazid. Rifamycin group of drugs usually cause cutaneous reactions, flu-like illness, gastrointestinal intolerance and hepatotoxicity. Out of these adverse reaction hepatotoxicity is alarming and should always be paid attention.

In a systematic review of national guidelines, it was concluded that individuals receiving treatment for LTBI should be monitored clinically on a regular monthly basis to find out any adverse effcets. The patients should be explained regarding the disease process, rationale of treatment and importance of treatment completion. If the patient is unable to consult the healthcare provider at the time of onset of symptoms, treatment should be stopped immediately.[32,33]

CONCLUSION

Anti-TNF-α therapy has already surpassed the conventional line of treatment for moderate-to-severe psoriasis in most of the developed countries of the world and soon will be an affordable therapeutic option in the Indian subcontinent. Tuberculosis being an endemic health concern in the Indian subcontinent and further reactivation by use of anti-TNF-α agents warrants existence of region specific guidelines for screening psoriatic patients, which are potential candidates for receiving anti-TNF-α agents. We hope that this chapter will guide the Indian dermatologist in starting anti-TNF-α therapy with certitude.

REFERENCES

1. www.who.int/tb/publications/global_report/en/ [Accessed November, 2016].
2. http://www.who.int/tb/publications/global_report/high_tb_burdencountrylists2016-2020.pdf [Accessed November, 2016].
3. Chadha VK. Tuberculosis epidemiology in India: A review. Int J Tuberc Lung Dis. 2005;9:1072-82.
4. Stern DK, Tripp JM, Ho VC, et al. The use of systemic immune moderators in dermatology. In: Maclean DI, Maddin WS (Eds). Dermatologic Clinics. Elsevier; 2005. p. 275.
5. Tzu J, Krulig E, Cardenas V, Kerdel FA. Biological agents in the treatment of psoriasis. G Ital Dermatol Venereol. 2008;143:315-27.
6. Zachariae C, Mørk NJ, Reunala T, et al. The combination of etanercept and methotrexate increases the effectiveness of treatment in active psoriasis despite inadequate effect of methotrexate therapy. Acta Derm Venereol. 2008;88: 495-501.

7. Gottlieb AB, Casale TB, Frankel E, et al. CD4+T -cell-directed antibody responses are maintained in patients with psoriasis receiving alefacept: Results of a randomized study. J Am Acad Dermatol. 2003;49:816-25.

8. Mitra A, Fallen RS, Lima HC. Cytokine-based therapy in psoriasis. Clin Rev Allergy Immunol. 2013;44:173-82.

9. Raychaudhuri SP. Role of IL-17 in psoriasis and psoriatic arthritis. Clin Rev Allergy Immunol. 2013;44:183-93.

10. Askling J, Fored CM, Brandt L, et.al. Risk and case characteristics of tuberculosis in rheumatoid arthritis associated with tumor necrosis factor antagonists in Sweden. Arthritis Rheum. 2005; 52:1986-92.

11. Wolfe F, Michaud K, Anderson J, et al. Tuberculosis infection in patients with rheumatoid arthritis and the effect of infliximab therapy. Arthritis Rheum. 2004; 50:372-9.

12. Comstock GW, Livesay VT, Woolpert SF. The prognosis of a positive tuberculin reaction in childhood and adolescence. Am J Epidemiol. 1974;99:131-8.

13. Pai M, Rodrigues C. Management of latent tuberculosis infection: An evidence-based approach. Lung India. 2015;32:205-7.

14. Ponce de León D, Acevedo-Vásquez E, Sánchez-Torres A, et al. Attenuated response to purified protein derivative in patients with rheumatoid arthritis: study in a population with a high prevalence of tuberculosis. Ann Rheum Dis. 2005;64:1360-1.

15. Pai M, Riley LW, Colford JM Jr. Interferon-gamma assays in the immunodiagnosis of tuberculosis: A systematic review. Lancet Infect Dis. 2004;4:761-76.

16. Pai M, Zwerling A, Menzies D. Systematic review: T-cell-based assays for the diagnosis of latent tuberculosis infection: an update. Ann Intern Med. 2008;149:177-84.

17. Jiang W, Shao L, Zhang Y, et al. High-sensitive and rapid detection of *Mycobacterium tuberculosis* infection by IFN-gamma release assay among HIV-infected individuals in BCG-vaccinated area. BMC Immunol. 2009; 10:31.

18. American Thoracic Society. The tuberculin skin test, 1981. Am Rev Respir Dis. 1981;124:346-51.

19. Targeted tuberculin testing and treatment of latent tuberculosis infection. American Thoracic Society MMWR Recomm Rep. 2000;49:1-51.

20. Nayak S, Acharjya B. Mantoux test and its interpretation. Indian Dermatol Online J. 2012;3:2-6.

21. Tufariello JM, Chan J, Flynn JL. Latent tuberculosis: mechanisms of host and bacillus that contribute to persistent infection. Lancet Infect Dis. 2003;3:578-90.

22. Russell DG. *Mycobacterium tuberculosis*: here today, and here tomorrow. Nat Rev Mol Cell Biol. 2001;2:569-77.

23. Vergne I, Chua J, Singh SB, et al. Cell biology of *Mycobacterium tuberculosis* phagosome. Annu Rev Cell Dev Biol. 2004;20:367-94.

24. Caruso AM, Serbina N, Klein E, et al. Mice deficient in CD4 T-cells have only transiently diminished levels of IFN-gamma, yet succumb to tuberculosis. J Immunol. 1999;162:5407-16.

25. Nathan CF, Murray HW, Wiebe ME, et al. Identification of interferon-gamma as the lymphokine that activates human macrophage oxidative metabolism and antimicrobial activity. J Exp Med. 1983;158:670-89.

26. Mack U, Migliori GB, Sester M, et al. Latent tuberculosis infection or lasting immune responses to *M. tuberculosis*? A TBNET consensus statement. Eur Respir J. 2009;33:956-73.

27. Lange C, Pai M, Drobniewski F, et al. Interferon-gamma release assays in the diagnosis of active tuberculosis: sensible or silly? Eur Respir J. 2009;33: 1250-3.

28. Cellestis.com. (2007). QuantiFERON-TB Gold In-Tube Results Interpretation Guide. Available from: http://www.cellestis.com/IRM/Company/ShowPage. aspx?CPID=1215. [Accessed 2007].

29. Oxford Immunotec (2009). T-SPOT.TB technical handbook.[online]. Available from: http://www.oxfordimmunotec.com/UK%20Technical%20Handbooks [Accessed 2009].

30. Ziakas PD, Mylonakis E. Four months of rifampin compared with 9 months of isoniazid for the management of latent tuberculosis infection: a meta-analysis and cost-effectiveness study that focuses on compliance and liver toxicity. Clin Infect Dis. 2009;49:1883-9.

31. American Thoracic Society and Centers for Disease Control and Prevention. Targeted tuberculin testing and treatment of latent tuberculosis infection. MMWR Recomm Rep. 2000;49:1-51.

32. Public Health Agency of Canada. Canadian Tuberculosis Standards, 7th edition. Canadian Thoracic Society and The Public Health Agency of Canada, 2014.

33. Schaberg T, Bauer T, Castell S, et al. Recommendations for therapy, chemo-prevention and chemoprophylaxis of tuberculosis in adults and children. German Central Committee against Tuberculosis (DZK), German Respiratory Society (DGP). Pneumologie. 2012;66(3):133-71.

Chapter 21

Adult Immunization Prior to Initiation of Biologic Therapy

Ankan Gupta

▌INTRODUCTION

Immunization is the process through which a person is made immune to an infectious agent, typically by the administration of a vaccine which stimulates the body's own immune system to protect him against subsequent exposure to that particular agent.[1] The concept is based on immunological memory where exposing the foreign molecules which are "nonself", orchestrate an immune response, which develops the ability to quickly respond to a subsequent encounter. Immunization is a proven tool for controlling and eliminating life-threatening infectious diseases and is estimated to avert between 2 and 3 million deaths each year.[1,2] Immunization in pediatric age group has been quite successful in our country, but adult "at risk" population is still vulnerable.[3] Patients with autoimmune diseases (AID) are arguably the most neglected group surprisingly in this respect knowing the fact that immunizing them helps in a long-term in a multifactorial way.

- Vaccinating them prevents from acquiring infections which would otherwise worsen the morbidity and mortality due to the immuno-suppressive nature of the disease [most noticeable in atopic dermatitis, complement deficiency in systemic lupus erythematosus (SLE), etc.] and the drug therapy used for its management.[4-8]
- There is an increased risk not only of infection in rheumatic diseases but also of infections being more severe.[5,6]
- *Malignancies*: These patients are also "at risk" of developing infection-induced malignancies, e.g. human papilloma virus (HPV) causing squamous cell carcinoma and hepatitis B virus (HBV) causing liver cancer.
- Infection itself is one of the most consistent factors in etiopathogenesis of AID. Making them immunosuppressed would initiate a vicious cycle of infection-relapse-drugs-immunosuppression-infection.[7]

With obvious benefits of immunizing such a patient, convincing them or their relatives is still a difficult task with reports of serious adverse events like paralysis, encephalomyelitis, and demyelinating disorders making rounds in social media and with internet doctors.[8] Vaccination in itself can trigger the disease theoretically,[9] making the entire exercise controversial; but the present evidence does not indicate that it increases the clinical or laboratory parameters of disease activity in AID.[10,11]

USE OF BIOLOGICS IN DERMATOLOGY

Psoriasis, autoimmune vesiculobullous disorders, hidradenitis suppurativa, alopecia areata, vitiligo, lupus erythematosus, dermatomyositis, scleroderma, and chronic urticaria are some of the well-established indications for the use of biologics in dermatology. All these share a common set of cytokine dysregulation and therefore a similar approach to management, which is using the traditional immunosuppressants or the biologics.[12]

IMMUNOSUPPRESSION

Immunosuppressants commonly used in dermatology are corticosteroids, azathioprine, mycophenolate mofetil, cyclosporine, methotrexate, cyclophosphamide, and biologics such as rituximab, interleukin (IL)-17 A blockers, and tumor necrosis factor alpha inhibitors (TNFi). There are several other newer smaller molecules that are getting launched each day to add to their ever increasing number. Most of these are being interchangeably used as an off-label indication for a disease, which has its own approved biologic. The inherent immunosuppressive properties of these diseases, various molecules having a different length and depth of immunosuppression and different doses and duration of the same molecule make it arduous for the experts to make protocols for immunization. What constitutes immunosuppression is also debated with common agreement presently dictating that drugs like biologics, cyclophosphamide, cyclosporine, leflunomide, and mycophenolate mofetil cause immune suppression at any dose while corticosteroids, methotrexate, and azathioprine increase the risk of infection in dose-dependent manner.[13,14] A concept of "low-dose immunosuppression" has been put forward which is defined as:

- Low-dose corticosteroid (<20 mg/day of prednisone or equivalent)
- Glucocorticoid replacement therapy in adrenal insufficiency
- Topical steroids or intra-articular, intrabursa, or intratendon steroid injection
- Low-dose methotrexate (<0.4 mg/kg/week or <20 mg/week)
- Low-dose azathioprine (<3 mg/kg/day)
- Low-dose 6-mercaptopurine (<1.5 mg/kg/day).

Adults receiving prednisolone in doses more than 20 mg/day for more than 2 weeks and children receiving more than 2 mg/kg/day for more than 1 month also constitute immunosuppression.[15]

Old age in itself is considered a state of immunosuppression with the concept of immune senescence defining it as "changes that reduce the protection of the vaccines as a result of aging and the effects of aging on natural and acquired immunities".[16] In the present text, we have not limited ourselves to the role of vaccines with biologics, but expanded to include vaccination with traditional immunosuppressants and vaccination in old age.

Table 21.1: Live vaccines and inert or the killed or inactivated vaccines.

Live vaccines	Killed vaccines
Oral polio	Pneumococcal[+]
BCG[*+]	Influenza[+]
MMR[*+]	Diphtheria[*]
Human papilloma virus[+]	Pertussis[*]
Yellow fever	Tetanus[*]
Herpes zoster[+]	Injectable polio[*]
	Hepatitis B[+]
	Hepatitis A
	Japanese encephalitis
	Meningococcal
	Tick-borne encephalitis

*Routinely given as per the National Program.
+Increased risk in the individuals with autoimmune diseases.
(BCG: Bacillus Calmette-Guérin; MMR: Measles, mumps, rubella).

▊ VACCINES

The available vaccines can be categorized into live vaccines and inert or the killed or inactivated vaccines as shown in Table 21.1.

General Principles of Vaccination in Autoimmune Diseases[17,18]

- Vaccination status of patients must ideally be assessed at the moment of diagnosis of an AID.
- Vaccination should ideally be completed before starting any immunosuppressant. A catch-up vaccination may be considered for missed vaccinations that are recommended for the general population. If the therapy has already been initiated, vaccines should be administered in the period of the lowest level of disease activity and the lowest dose of immunosuppressive therapy.
- Live vaccines are contraindicated in immunosuppressed individuals and pregnancy, but nonlive vaccines can safely be given.
  - Live vaccines should be administered ideally at least 4 weeks before starting any immunosuppressant or after cessation of immunosuppressive therapy.
  - Nonlive vaccines can be safely administered during immunosuppressant treatment; however, 2 weeks are required for the development of an immune response to inactivated vaccines. Therefore, if possible, inactivated vaccines should be administered at least 2 weeks before the commencement of immunosuppressive therapy without delaying the treatment.

- The safe time intervals for the administration of live vaccines after cessation of immunosuppressive therapy is:
  - 5 half-lives after the administration of biological agents or disease-modifying drugs (3–12 months)
  - 4 weeks after high-dose corticosteroid therapy ($\geq$ 20 mg/day prednisone or equivalent, for longer than 2 weeks)
  - 4 weeks after etanercept and 3 months after other TNFi (infliximab and adalimumab)
  - 4–12 weeks after the doses of more than equal to 0.4 mg/kg/week or more than equal to 20 mg/week of methotrexate
  - 6–12 months after rituximab (if possible, live vaccines should be canceled until the B-cell count returns to normal levels)
  - 2 years after leflunomide
  - For 6 months for other immunosuppressants not mentioned above
  - *Vaccination with intravenous immunoglobulin (IVIg)*: Inactivated vaccines and IVIg products may be administered simultaneously or within any time interval. An exception to this is the hepatitis A vaccine, which like other live vaccines should be administered either 2 weeks before the IVIg therapy or should be delayed for 3–11 months after the therapy. If a need for IVIg therapy arises within 14 days after the vaccination, the vaccine should be readministered 3–11 months after the IVIg therapy in patients without serological evidence of an antibody response.
- Live vaccines can be administered during sulfasalazine and hydroxychloroquine therapies.
- Vaccination of close contacts should be strongly considered in certain situations. Few live vaccines should not be given to immunocompromised hosts or their household contacts, e.g. oral polio and rotavirus; though measles, mumps, rubella (MMR), herpes zoster, and bacillus Calmette-Guérin (BCG) are safe for household contacts.[13,19] Conversely, if a patient cannot be vaccinated because of certain reasons, people who are in close contact with the patient can be vaccinated to reduce the risk of infection.
- Severe allergic reaction to the previously administered same vaccine is a contraindication for further vaccination.
- Increased interval between doses of a multidose vaccine does not diminish vaccine effectiveness; therefore, it is not necessary to restart the vaccine series or add doses to the series because of an extended interval between doses.
- If not administered on the same day, separate live vaccines by at least 28 days.

Efficacy of a Vaccine

It should ideally be demonstrated through clinical endpoints, e.g. incidence of infection, hospitalization, and death; however, most research is based on demonstration of B-cell generated antibodies as a surrogate marker for vaccination-induced protection, antibody titers, as well as the quality of the antibody response in terms of binding avidity and bactericidal or neutralizing activity of antibodies.

Essential Vaccines

Pneumococcal Vaccine

This is probably the most controversial and researched vaccination in individuals with immunosuppression or with acquired immune deficiency syndrome (AIDS).[20] There are two vaccines available in the market for pneumococcus.

- The 23-valent pneumococcal polysaccharide vaccine (PPSV23) which contains antigens of the 23 most common pneumococcal strains. It is effective against approximately 90% of all pneumococcal infections.
- The more effective 13-valent pneumococcal conjugate vaccine (PCV13). The cost of PCV13 in India is around 3 times that of PPSV23.

Though the Advisory Committee on Immunization Practices (ACIP) recommendations are succinct to guide us in different clinical scenarios, the few points not to be forgotten include:

- Only a single dose of PCV13 vaccine is recommended in adult life.
- There should be at least 1 year gap between the administrations of PCV13 and PPSV23.

Preferred dosing schedule is to start vaccination with PCV13, administer PPSV23 at least 1 year (8 weeks in few special situations) after PCV13 and repeat PPSV23 at least 5 years after the previous PPSV23 dose. All adults who already received PPSV23 should receive a dose of PCV13 more than equal to 1 year after receipt of PPSV23. Revaccinations with PPSV23 should occur 5 years after the last dose. A caution is warranted when planning pneumococcal vaccine in patients with Behçet's disease because of a theoretical risk of flaring up of the disease.

Lower efficacy with or without shorter seroprotection period has been reported in SLE patients, in other AID being treated with methotrexate and rituximab, but not with TNFi.[21,22]

Influenza Vaccine

The risk of hospital admission for influenza is higher in elderly patients (≥65 years) with AIDS or vasculitis, compared with the ones with no underlying medical condition.[23]

- *Preferred dosing schedule*: Yearly anti-influenza vaccination is recommended to all patients regardless of current therapy including pregnant women. It is not contraindicated in those with allergy to eggs.

The efficacy of concurrent immunosuppressants has been contradictory with reports of lower immunogenicity with steroids above 20 mg, azathioprine, mycophenolate, rituximab, and methotrexate but in most studies, neither disease-modifying antirheumatic drugs (DMARDs) nor biologics hampered humoral immune responses to influenza vaccination.[24,25] A list of currently available influenza vaccines is available at www.cdc.gov/flu/protect/vaccine/vaccines.htm.

Herpes Zoster Vaccine

Immunosuppressed patients have a higher risk of severe rash, visceral dissemination, or death, and hence, the prevention is desirable. Treatment with immunosuppressive drugs, except etanercept and methotrexate, increases this risk.[26] Herpes zoster vaccine is a live vaccine and it bears the potential risk of invasive infection in susceptible individuals. Center of Disease Control and Prevention Advisory Committee on Immunization Practices Recommendations (CDC-ACIP) and the American College of Rheumatology (ACR) suggest consideration of its use in patients more than 60 years-old, who are on "low-dose immunosuppressive therapy". Although the risk-benefit of the vaccine must be individually assessed, it is best avoided with:

- Treatment with all biologics, cyclosporine, cyclophosphamide, leflunomide, and higher doses of corticosteroids, methotrexate, and azathioprine
- Active leukemia, lymphoma, and malignant neoplasm affecting bone marrow or lymphatics
- Acquired immune deficiency syndrome or human immunodeficiency virus (AIDS or HIV) patients and those with CD4 lymphocyte counts less than 200 per mm^3
- Clinical or laboratory evidence of cellular immunodeficiency
- Pregnancy and severe acute illness.

Tetanus and Diphtheria (Td) Vaccines

- *Preferred dosing schedule*: Administer a single dose of Tetanus toxoid, diphtheria, and acellular pertussis (TdaP) followed by booster dose with Td every 10 years; however, passive immunization with tetanus Ig is required in cases of history of rituximab infusion in the past 24 weeks due to a possible reduction in immunogenicity due to rituximab. Though the literature does not suggest doing it in pemphigus but the authors recommend following this protocol in patients with autoimmune bullous disorders where raw skin is culture media for the microbe.

Adults with an unknown or incomplete history of a 3-dose primary series in childhood with tetanus and diphtheria toxoid-containing vaccines should complete the primary series followed by 10 yearly Td boosters. Pregnant women should receive 1 dose of TdaP during each pregnancy, preferably during 27–36 weeks, regardless of prior history of receiving TdaP.

Hepatitis B Vaccine

It is recommended for all patients with negative serology [hepatitis B surface antigen (HBsAg), anti-HB core antigen (HBc), and anti-HBs negative].

- *Preferred dosing schedule*: To be given in 3 doses at 0, 1–2 and 6 months and to measure the Anti-HBs titers at month 8 to assess the response. Seroprotection is defined as a serum titer more the equal to 10 IU/L and if it is not achieved, revaccination should be considered. Treatment with immunosuppressants can be started after first 2 doses.

Disease-modifying antirheumatic drugs (DMARDs) do not have a negative influence on the response to hepatitis B vaccination but TNFi and the combination of TNFi and methotrexate produce lesser immunogenicity. The effect of the newer biologics remains to be investigated.[27]

Human Papilloma Virus Vaccine

Human papilloma virus infection is of relevance in young girls suffering from SLE as there is a higher incidence, florid presentation, and lower rate of spontaneous clearance of infection in women affected with SLE.[28] Hence, HPV vaccination is recommended in women with SLE until the age of 26 years. An increased venous thromboembolism risk was observed with the quadrivalent vaccine, which has now been refuted by European League Against Rheumatism (EULAR).[29]

- *Preferred dosing schedule*: To be given in 3 doses at 0, 1–2, and 6 months.

There is no indication for BCG vaccine in adults as most of the tuberculosis cases in adulthood are due to the activation of latent tuberculosis cases. BCG vaccine cannot be administered to persons older than 6 years of age even if has not been administered before.

Vaccines for Travelers

Patients with severe immunosuppression should avoid travelling in yellow fever endemic countries. If it is mandatory to travel in endemic area or when yellow fever vaccination is mandatory, temporary discontinuation of treatment with immunosuppressive drugs is required in combination with rigorous mosquito protection measures. A complete destination-wise list can be referred to at https://wwwnc.cdc.gov/travel/destinations/list.

Safety of Vaccines

Autoimmune diseases are known to coexist. Their etiology is still not clear but environmental factors are considered to be important triggers which are not evident unless an environmental factor produces an overt expression. The term autoimmune inflammatory syndrome induced by adjuvants (ASIA) is a clinical condition of autoimmune nature, which is induced by the exposure to an environmental factor which may include vaccines and the adjuvants which are used to increase the immunogenicity.[30,31] Vaccine use has been associated with onset of AID, especially in patients already suffering from an AID, e.g. Guillain-Barré syndrome (GBS) with Td, polio and measles vaccine, autoimmune thrombocytopenia with MMR, development of multiple sclerosis with HBV vaccine, and autism with measles vaccine. However, practically the risk-to-benefit ratio is overwhelmingly in favor of vaccination and any untoward effect, though cannot be ignored still warrants a detailed evaluation to establish the causality.

Individuals who might be susceptible to develop vaccination-induced ASIA include patients with prior postvaccination autoimmune phenomena,[32] patients with a medical history of autoimmunity, or a history of atopy.[33]

Vaccination Schedule for Adults[34]

The vaccination schedule for adults has been given in Table 21.2.

Table 21.2: Vaccination schedule for adults.			
Vaccine	Schedule	Age group	Contraindications
Pneumococcus: • PCV13 • PPSV23	• Single dose • Every 5 years	Adults aged >65 years or aged 19–64 years with immunosuppression	
Influenza	Annually	All age groups	History of GBS within 6 weeks after previous vaccination Relative C/I: Egg allergy other than hives, e.g. angioedema, respiratory distress, lightheadedness, or recurrent emesis; or required epinephrine or another emergency medical intervention
Herpes zoster	Single dose	Adults aged >60 years or aged 19–64 years with immunosuppression	

Contd...

Contd...

Vaccine	Schedule	Age group	Contraindications
Td	Every 10 years booster	All age groups	GBS within 6 weeks after a previous dose of tetanus toxoid History of Arthus-type hypersensitivity reaction
Hepatitis B	3 doses (0, 1–2 and 6 months)	All age groups	
Human papillomavirus (HPV)	3 doses (0, 1–2, and 6 months)	Between 9–26 years in girls and preferably completed before the start of sexual activity Up to 21 years of age in males	Receipt of acyclovir or congeners 24 hours before vaccination (avoid use of these antiviral drugs for 14 days after vaccination)

(PCV13: 13-valent pneumococcal conjugate vaccine; PPSV23: 23-valent pneumococcal polysaccharide vaccine; GBS: Guillain-Barré syndrome; Td: Tetanus, Diphtheria).

CONCLUSION

Every dermatologist and especially the ones, who wish to dwell in the world of biologics, should understand the importance of vaccination in patients with AID and should use the first visit as an opportunity to inquire about the vaccination status of the individual. The immunization should start prior to the initiation of immunosuppressants. As of now scientific data regarding vaccination efficacy before biologic therapy for dermatological indications is scarce, but extrapolating the evidence from rheumatology literature should be a good first step. In Indian population, influenza, pneumococcal, and hepatitis B vaccines are safe and generally sufficiently immunogenic; whereas, HPV and herpes zoster vaccination might be considered in select subgroups of patients.

REFERENCES

1. World Health Organization. 2017. Immunization. [online] Available from: http://www.who.int/topics/immunization/en/. [Accessed December, 2017].
2. Plotkin SA. Vaccines: correlates of vaccine induced immunity. Clin Infect Dis. 2008;47(3):401-9.
3. Gluck T, Muller-Ladner U. Vaccination in patients with chronic rheumatic or autoimmune diseases. Clin Infect Dis. 2008;46(9):1459-65.
4. Lindegard B. Diseases associated with psoriasis in a general population of 159,200 middle-aged, urban, native Swedes. Dermatologica. 1986;172(6):298-304.

5. Doran MF, Crowson CS, Pond GR, et al. Frequency of infection in patients with rheumatoid arthritis compared with controls: a population-based study. Arthritis Rheum. 2002;46(9):2287-93.

6. Blumentals WA, Arreglado A, Napalkov P, et al. Rheumatoid arthritis and the incidence of influenza and influenza-related complications: a retrospective cohort study. BMC Musculoskelet Disord. 2012;13:158.

7. Doria A, Zampieri S, Sarzi-Puttini P. Exploring the complex relationships between infections and autoimmunity. Autoimmun Rev. 2008;8(2):89-91.

8. Conti F, Rezai S, Valesini G. Vaccination and autoimmune rheumatic diseases. Autoimmun Rev. 2008;8(2):124-8.

9. Takayama K, Satoh T, Hayashi M, et al. Psoriatic skin lesions induced by BCG vaccination. Acta Derm Venereol. 2008;88(6):621-2.

10. Wraith DC, Goldman M, Lambert PH. Vaccination and autoimmune disease: what is the evidence? Lancet. 2003;362(9396):1659-66.

11. Chen RT, Pless R, Destefano F. Epidemiology of autoimmune reactions induced by vaccination. J Autoimmun. 2001;16(3):309-18.

12. Kuek A, Hazleman BL, Ostor AJ. Immune-mediated inflammatory diseases (IMIDs) and biologic therapy: a medical revolution. Postgrad Med J. 2007; 83(978):251-60.

13. Bernatsky S, Hudson M, Suissa S. Anti-rheumatic drug use and risk of serious infections in rheumatoid arthritis. Rheumatology (Oxford). 2007;46(7):1157-60.

14. Schneeweiss S, Korzenik J, Solomon DH, et al. Infliximab and other immuno-modulating drugs in patients with inflammatory bowel disease and the risk of serious bacterial infections. Aliment Pharmacol Ther. 2009;30(3):253-64.

15. Auerbach PS. The Immunocompromised Traveller. An Advisory Committee Statement (ACS). Can Commun Dis Rep. 2007;33(ACS-4):1-24.

16. Lang PO, Govind S, Michel JP, et al. Immunosenescence: Implications for vaccination programmes in adults. Maturitas. 2011;68(4):322-30.

17. Tanrıöver MD, Akar S, Türkçapar N, et al. Vaccination recommendations for adult patients with rheumatic diseases. Eur J Rheumatol. 2016;3(1):29-35.

18. Murdaca G, Orsi A, Spanò F, et al. Influenza and pneumococcal vaccinations of patients with systemic lupus erythematosus: current views upon safety and immunogenicity. Autoimmun Rev. 2014;13(2):75-84.

19. Kroger AT, Atkinson WL, Marcuse EK, et al. General recommendations on immunization: recommendations of the Advisory Committee on Immunization Practices (ACIP). MMWR Recomm Rep. 2006;55:1-48.

20. Coulson E, Saravanan V, Hamilton J, et al. Pneumococcal antibody levels after pneumovax in patients with rheumatoid arthritis on methotrexate. Ann Rheum Dis. 2011;70(7):1289-91.

21. Mease PJ, Ritchlin CT, Martin RW, et al. Pneumococcal vaccine response in psoriatic arthritis patients during treatment with etanercept. J Rheumatol. 2004;31(7):1356-61.

22. Elkayam O, Ablin J, Caspi D. Safety and efficacy of vaccination against strepto-coccus pneumonia in patients with rheumatic diseases. Autoimmun Rev. 2007; 6(5):312-4.

23. Nichol KL, Wuorenma J, von Sternberg T. Benefits of influenza vaccination for low-, intermediate-, and high-risk senior citizens. Arch Intern Med. 1998; 158(16):1769-76.

24. Fomin I, Caspi D, Levy V, et al. Vaccination against influenza in rheumatoid arthritis: The effect of disease modifying drugs, including TNF alpha blockers. Ann Rheum Dis. 2006;65(2):191-4.

25. Gelinck LB, van der Bijl AE, Beyer WE, et al. The effect of anti-tumour necrosis factor alpha treatment on the antibody response to influenza vaccination. Ann Rheum Dis. 2008;67(5):713-6.

26. Smitten AL, Choi HK, Hochberg MC, et al. The risk of herpes zoster in patients with rheumatoid arthritis in the United States and the United Kingdom. Arthritis Rheum. 2007;57(8):1431-8.

27. Kuruma KA, Borba EF, Lopes MH, et al. Safety and efficacy of hepatitis B vaccine in systemic lupus erythematosus. Lupus. 2007;16(5):350-4.

28. Tam LS, Chan AY, Chan PK, et al. Increased prevalence of squamous intraepithelial lesions in systemic lupus erythematosus: association with human papillomavirus infection. Arthritis Rheum. 2004;50(11):3619-25.

29. Naleway AL, Crane B, Smith N, et al. Absence of venous thromboembolism risk following quadrivalent human papillomavirus vaccination. Vaccine Safety Datalink, 2008-2011. Vaccine. 2016;34(1):167-71.

30. Shoenfeld Y, Agmon-Levin N. 'ASIA'—autoimmune/inflammatory syndrome induced by adjuvants. J. Autoimmun. 2011;36(1):4-8.

31. Perricone C, Colafrancesco S, Mazor RD, et al. Autoimmune/inflammatory syndrome induced by adjuvants (ASIA): Unveiling the pathogenic, clinical and diagnostic aspects. J. Autoimmun. 2013;47:1-16.

32. Lee SH. Detection of human papillomavirus L1 gene DNA fragments in post-mortem blood and spleen after Gardasil® vaccination—A case report. Adv Biosci Biotechnol. 2012;3(8):1214-24.

33. Soriano A, et al. Predicting post-vaccination autoimmunity: Who might be at risk? Pharmacol Res. 2015;92:18-22.

34. US Department of Health and Human Services. (2017). Recommended Immunization Schedule for Adults Aged 19 Years or Older, United States, 2017. [online] Available from: https://www.cdc.gov/vaccines/schedules/downloads/adult/adult-combined-schedule.pdf. [Accessed December 2017].

Chapter 22

Cost-effectiveness and Quality of Life with Biologic Therapy

Shekhar Neema, Ankan Gupta

INTRODUCTION

Chronic skin diseases result in significant economic burden to patients and society. It can limit daily activities, require frequent hospital visits and admissions and result in loss of productivity. The cost incurred can be divided into direct medical cost which includes cost of the medicine, investigations and hospitalizations; and indirect medical costs due to absence from work, early mortality and time contributed by caregivers.

Biologics are new group of drugs which provide better quality of life and superior clinical outcomes in terms of faster and sustained improvement and prevention of long-term morbidity as compared to the traditional immunosuppressant. Treatment with biologics, though expensive initially, does decrease the indirect medical costs over a period of time. Whether the superior clinical outcome or improvement in quality of life is worth the cost difference is debatable and a subjective determinant but the authors feel that every patient should be given an option of the available therapeutic options. The following chapter is an effort to compare the treatment costs with available therapeutics in the field of dermatology. Indirect cost is difficult to calculate and varies from person to person and is not considered for summation. We have also not included the cost of hospitalizations as it is difficult to predict its duration and frequency. The dosage, schedule and monitoring protocols are based on standard guidelines. Consultation charges and day care costs are chosen arbitrarily and cost of investigations is based on a popular private laboratory available in most cities in the country.

In countries, where the treatment is neither funded by government, nor covered by the insurance companies consistently, pharmacoeconomic studies are needed to assess the cost of various therapeutic options. Till there is conclusive answer, the option of using biologics should be a personal preference for the patient and the treating physician.

PSORIASIS

Psoriasis is a common, chronic, immune-mediated skin disorder affecting 1–2% of general population. Almost 20–30% of those who are affected have moderate to severe disease requiring systemic therapy. Psoriasis severely impairs quality of life and results in economic burden to those who are affected and society at large.[1] Systemic treatment options for psoriasis include phototherapy, methotrexate, cyclosporine, hydroxyurea, and fumaric acid esters. Biologics give better clinical outcome in terms of faster and sustained reduction in psoriasis area severity index (PASI) and health-related quality of life (HRQoL) indices.[2]

COST ANALYSIS FOR SYSTEMIC THERAPY IN PSORIASIS

For the purpose of this chapter, we have attempted to calculate only the direct costs of available treatment options for one year cycle. The cost of treatment for 2nd year and afterwards is expected to be much lesser than the 1st year with the biologics because of their infrequent dosing in maintenance regimens (Tables 22.1 and 22.2).

Table 22.1: Cost analysis for systemic therapy in psoriasis for one year of therapy.

Drug	Cost of medicine	Schedule of treatment	Total cost for 1 year	Consul-tation	Investi-gations	Total cost
Metho-trexate Folic acid	₹ 20/- (15 mg) ₹ 2 (5 mg)	15 mg/ week 5 mg/ week	₹ 1040/- ₹ 104/-	Initial, after 15 days for the 1st month and monthly – Total cost = 14 × 500 = 7,000	Initial* = ₹ 5400/- Monitor-ing = ₹ 4320/- Cost of liver biopsy/ fibroscan = ₹ 5,000/-	₹ 22,864/-

a. Initial investigations include complete blood count (CBC), blood urea, serum creatinine, liver function test (LFT), blood sugar fasting and post prandial, chest X-ray, Mantoux or interferon-gamma release assays (IGRA), blood borne virus screening.
b. Monitoring includes CBC and SGOT, SGPT—after 7 days, 15 days, monthly for three months and three monthly thereafter.
c. A baseline liver biopsy or a fibroscan is indicated in all patients after cumulative dose of 1.5 gm.

| Cyclos-porine | ₹ 75 (100 mg) | 300 mg/ day – 1 month 250 mg/ day – 1 month 200 mg/ day – 10 months | ₹ 57,150 | Initial, after 15 days and monthly – Total cost = 14 × 500 = 7,000 | Initial – ₹ 2,000/- Monitoring – ₹ 18,000/- | ₹ 84,150/- |

Contd...

Contd...

Drug	Cost of medicine	Schedule of treatment	Total cost for 1 year	Consul-tation	Investi-gations	Total cost

a. Initial investigations include CBC, blood urea nitrogen, serum creatinine (twice in gap of one day), urinalysis, lipid profile, LFTs, serum potassium, magnesium and uric acid level

b. Monitoring test to be done every 15 days for one month and monthly thereafter. It includes CBC, LFT, urea, creatinine, triglycerides, cholesterol, uric acid, magnesium and potassium

c. Dose has been calculated as step down approach for 60 kg individual with normal renal function – 5 mg/kg for one month, 4 mg/kg for 1 month and 3 mg/kg for rest of the duration. Cyclosporine is generally continued as a single drug for not more than 3–6 months and is rotated with some other drug like acitretin. However, for ease of understanding and simplify the calculation, it has been shown to be used as monotherapy for 12 months.

Drug	Cost of medicine	Schedule of treatment	Total cost for 1 year	Consul-tation	Investi-gations	Total cost
Acitretin	₹ 60/- (25 mg)	50 mg once a day	₹ 43,800/-	Initial and monthly – Total cost = 12 × 500 = 6,000	Initial – ₹ 1200/- Monitoring ₹ 7,200/- Cost of X-ray wrist joint – ₹ 300	₹ 32,950/-

a. Initial investigations include CBC, LFT, lipid profile, renal function test, pregnancy test in women of child-bearing potential

b. Monitoring—monthly for three months and three monthly thereafter. Includes CBC, LFT, lipid profile, renal function test, pregnancy test

c. Yearly X-ray of wrist or symptomatic joints in patient in long-term retinoid therapy

d. Dose can be used as 25, 50 or 75 mg once a day. Psoriasis area severity index (PASI) – 75 is reached in 75 % of patient on higher doses of retinoids than those who are on 25 mg (46 %). 50 mg once a day has been used in calculation as it is effective in majority of cases on monotherapy with acitretin.

Drug	Cost of medicine	Schedule of treatment	Total cost for 1 year	Consul-tation	Investi-gations	Total cost
Narrow-band ultravio-let B (NBUVB) therapy	₹ 300/-	Start with 300 mJ and increase as per guidelines	₹ 300 × 54 = ₹ 16,200/-	Initial and monthly – Total cost = 12 × 500 = 6,000	–	₹ 22,200/-

a. Initial induction thrice weekly for 12 weeks, maintenance dose – twice a month. Total sessions 54 in a year

b. Psoralen and ultraviolet-A (PUVA) is more effective than NBUVB for management of psoriasis, however, it is more cumbersome to use. The cost of therapy will also increase, if we use psoralen.

Table 22.2: Cost analysis for biologics and biosimilar drugs for one year of therapy.

Drug	Cost of medicine	Schedule of treatment	Total cost	Consul-tation	Investi-gations	Total cost
Etaner-cept	₹ 17,170/- (MRP) PSP – First 6 pen – 60,000, then every pen 6,000 (50 mg)	50 mg twice weekly for three months 50 mg once a week for 9 months = 60 injections	3,84,000	Initial, after 15 days, month and then 3 monthly 500 × 7 = 3500	Initial - 5400 Monitoring – ₹ 400 × 3 = 1200	₹ 3,94,100/-
Biomi-mic – Intacept (Intas)	₹ 10,000 (MRP) 5833 (PSP)	Same as above	₹ 3,49,980	Same	Same	₹ 3,60,080/-
Biomi-mic – Etacept (Cipla)	₹ 6700/- (MRP) for 25 mg injection ₹ 3000 (reduced price)	Same	₹ 3,60,000/-	Same	Same	₹ 3,70,100/-

a. Dose used is 50 mg twice weekly for three months and 50 mg/ week thereafter. With this dose psoriasis area and severity index (PASI)-75 reached in 50% patients at the end of 12 weeks.
b. Maintenance dose can be reduced to 50 mg once a week or even 50 mg once every two weeks, thereby reducing the cost.
c. Initial investigations to be done are same as before initiating methotrexate, monitoring investigations are complete blood count (CBC), liver function test (LFT) every three monthly
d. Psoriasis area and severity index (PASI)-75, immunogenicity and remission data for etanercept biomimics are not available
e. Median time to relapse after achieving remission with originator molecule is 84 days and drug can be discontinued for three months in a year, which will further reduce the cost of therapy.

Inflixi-mab		•				
Remi-cade (original mole-cule)	₹ 41,000 (MRP) for 100 mg vial PSP - 17500 (100 mg vial)	5 mg/ kg 0, 2, 6 weeks and 8 weekly thereafter	₹ 4,20,000	Initial, after 15 days for first infusion, after 2 weeks	Initial = 5400 Monitoring = 3200	₹ 4,44,600

Contd...

Contd...

Drug	Cost of medicine	Schedule of treatment	Total cost	Consul-tation	Investi-gations	Total cost
		3 mg/kg	₹ 2,80,000	for second infusion, after 4 weeks and 8 weekly Total 8 × 2,000 = 16000		₹ 3,04,600
Bio-similar Infimab (Sun pharma)	₹ 32,000 (MRP) for 100 mg vial 12,000 (PSP)	Same	₹ 2,88,000 (3 mg/kg 1,92,000/-)	Same	Same	3,12,600 2,16,600

a. Dose has been calculated for 60 kg patient at the rate of 5 mg/kg. PASI- 75 response is seen in 80 percent patients with this dose.
b. 3 mg/kg dose can also be used, which results in PASI-75 response in almost 70% patients and result in significant reduction in cost.
c. Cost of consultation is higher as patient is required to be admitted in day care center for infusion
d. Initial investigations are same as which are done for methotrexate except baseline antinuclear antibodies (ANA) needs to be done, monitoring requires CBC and LFT before every infusion.

Drug	Cost of medicine	Schedule of treatment	Total cost	Consul-tation	Investi-gations	Total cost
Adali-mumab						
Biosimi-lar Exemp-tia (Zydus) Biomi-mics– Adfrar P (Torrent) Adalirel (Reliance)	₹ 25,000 (MRP) PSP – ₹ 11,000/-	80 mg loading dose. 40 mg week 1 and 40 gm once every two weeks	25 × 11,000 = 2,75,000	Initial, after 15 days, after one month and the 3 monthly 6 × 500 = 3000	Initial – 5400 Monitoring – 400 × 3 = 1200	₹ 2,84,600

a. Initial investigations are same as other TNF alpha blockers, monitoring requires CBC and LFT every three months.
b. Scheduled dose results in PASI-75 improvement in almost 80% patients
c. Originator molecule of adalimumab (Humira) is not available in India. Exemptia is most well-studied biosimilar, while other two molecules are intended copies (biomimics) while cost almost remains same for all three.

Contd...

Contd...

Drug	Cost of medicine	Schedule of treatment	Total cost	Consul-tation	Investi-gations	Total cost
Secuki-numab Origina-tor mole-cule, no bio-similar	₹ 14,500 (150 mg vial)	300 mg on week 0, 1, 2, 3, 4 and monthly thereafter.	4,64,000 (32 × 14500)	Initial, after 15 days, one month and 3 monthly	Initial – 5400 Monitoring – 400 × 3 = 1200	4,73,600
		150 mg	2,32,000	6 × 500 = 3000		2,41,600
Itolizu-mab	₹ 7950 (25 mg vial) (MRP) PSP - 5300	1.6 mg/kg every two weeks for 12 week and once in 4 weeks till 24 weeks (for 70 kg –5 vial)	30 vials in induction and 15 vials in main-tenance 45 × 5300 = 2,38,500	Initial, every two weeks for 12 weeks and once in 4 weeks for three months and three monthly = 9 × 2000 = 18000 (infusion) 2 × 500 = 1000 (Follow-up)	Initial – 5400 Moni-toring – 400 × 3 = 1200	₹ 2,64,100

a. Dose is administered for 6 months and patient to be observed without therapy, assuming that patient will maintain remission for next 6 months else cost of therapy could increase.
b. Initial and monitoring investigations are same as TNF alpha blockers
c. Cost of consultation is high as it requires infusion
d. Psoriasis area and severity index (PASI) -75 response was seen in almost 45% patients

COMPARISON OF COST AND EFFICACY OF SYSTEMIC AND BIOLOGIC THERAPY FOR PSORIASIS (TABLE 22.3)

Psoriasis area severity index-75 is the meaningful end point for management of psoriasis as less than 75% reduction in severity does not lead to improvement in quality of life.[14]

Table 22.3: Comparison of cost and efficacy of systemic and biologic therapy for psoriasis.

Drug	Efficacy			Cost in ₹ (For one year therapy)	Approximate cost of the therapy, 2nd year onwards
	Psoriasis area severity index (PASI)-75	PASI-90/100	Studies		
Metho-trexate	35% 60%	40%	CHAMPION (2008)[3] Heydendael VM (2003)[4]	22,864	6,304
Cyclospo-rine (5 mg/kg)	97% 88.6%	– –	IMSGCP (1993)[5] Laburte (1994)[6]	84,150	–
Acitretin	53%	–	Dogra (2013)[7]	32,950	46,200
Photo-therapy	55%	–	Dawe RS (2003)[8]	22,200	22,200
Enbrel	50%	–	Leonardi CL (2003)[9]	3,94,100	3,12,000
Intacept	–	–	No peer review publication till May 17	3,60,080	3,03,316
Etacept	–	–		3,70,100	3,12,000
Remicade (5 mg/kg)	80%	57%	Reich K (2005)[10]	4,44,600	3,41,250
Remicade (3 mg/kg)	70%	37%	Menter A (2007)[11]	3,04,600	2,04,750
Infimab	–	–	No data available	3,12,600	2,05,700
Adalimu-mab	75%	51%	CHAMPION (2008)[3] Study done on origi-nator molecule. No studies in psoriasis available for bio-similar	2,84,600	2,62,600
Itolizumab	45.5%	–	Krupashankar DS (2014)[12]	2,64,100	
Secukinu-mab	81%	59.6%	Langley RJ (2014)[13]	4,73,600	3,48,000 (300 mg) 1,74,000 (150 mg)

- Reduction in cost of therapy in second year for most biologics is because of not using induction therapy in these patients.

Out of available systemic therapy for psoriasis, narrowband ultraviolet B (NBUVB) appears to be most cost-effective as PASI-75 is achieved in almost 55% patients and therapy is relatively free of adverse effects. If available, NBUVB is a reasonable first line therapy for management of chronic plaque psoriasis. Methotrexate is very efficacious for management of psoriasis and is cost-effective, though requires frequent monitoring for adverse effect. Acitretin monotherapy can also be used for management of psoriasis, however it may result in dose limiting adverse effect when used in dose of 50 mg/day. Cyclosporine is extremely effective for management of psoriasis and result in PASI-75 in almost 90% patients; however it is more expensive as compared to other first line treatments and cannot be used for longer periods. Cyclosporine is generally used as crisis buster drug and used intermittently to manage exacerbations.

In biologic therapy, adalimumab appears to be most cost effective as it leads to PASI-75 response in 75% patients and PASI-90 response in 51% patients. Adalimumab is followed by infliximab (3 mg/kg), as it leads to PASI-75 improvement in 70% patients and PASI-90 improvement in 37% patients. However, infliximab is given as infusion and requires repeated visits to health care establishment. This is followed by itolizumab, however for itolizumab PASI-75 is achieved at 28 weeks. Secukinumab achieves PASI-75 and 90 response in maximum patients and results in rapid improvement. Infliximab (5 mg/kg) also achieves PASI-75 and 90 in significant number of patients, however it turns out to be more expensive than secukinumab for similar PASI achieved. Etanercept appears to be least cost-effective among biologicals, as it leads to PASI-75 response in 50% patients and is more expensive than adalimumab and infliximab (3 mg/kg) with much less number of patients achieving PASI-75.

National Institute of Clinical Excellence, UK (NICE) guidelines (2012) suggest that biologics should be used when first line conventional therapy is not able to control the disease. 2017 NICE guidelines for use of biologics in psoriasis suggest that adalimumab should be first line of biological treatment especially when psoriatic arthritis is present. Secukinumab can also be used as first line biological therapy irrespective of arthropathy. Infliximab should be reserved for patients with very severe disease or when other biologics have failed.[15]

Various studies have been conducted to understand cost-effectiveness of biologicals. A study was conducted on economic impact of high need psoriasis before and after introduction of biologics in Netherlands in 2010. Study concluded that patient during biologic treatment resulted in decrease in direct cost despite high treatment cost, this reduction in direct costs results from decrease in medical consultation and hospitalisation.[16] Study conducted by Fonia et al. in London had similar findings that while cost of treatment increases significantly after introduction of biologics, however this cost reduces due to change in pattern of healthcare delivery in patients using biologics.[17] Nelson et al. conducted a cost-effectiveness study of biologics based on literature review. In this study, outcomes which were considered were PASI-75 and dermatology life quality index (DLQI) minimally important difference (MID). PASI-75 is defined as 75% improvement in PASI score from baseline while five point change in DLQI from baseline represents DLQI MID. As per this study, most cost-effective medication in terms of cost per patient achieving DLQI MID was found to be etanercept 25 mg subcutaneous weekly followed by infliximab 3 mg/kg for three infusion. Most cost-effective medication in terms of cost per patient achieving PASI-75 scores was found to be infliximab 3 mg/kg three infusion followed by adalimumab 40 mg subcutaneous every other week.[18] This study did not include drugs like ustekinumab and secukinumab as these drugs were not available when study was conducted. Introduction of new biologics in those patients who have failed or respond poorly to one biologic appears to be cost-effective alternative and improves the quality of life in patients with severe psoriasis.[19]

▌PEMPHIGUS

Pemphigus is defined as a group of blistering disorders characterized by acantholysis resulting in intraepithelial blisters in skin and mucosa.[20] The different forms of pemphigus are distinguished by their clinical features and associated autoantigens and pemphigus vulgaris represents the most common form. The incidence rate in a German study has been postulated to be 0.1–0.5 per 100,000,[21] however there is no such data for Indian subcontinent.

Pemphigus usually occurs in adults, with an average age of onset at 40–60 years,[22] making it a high socioeconomic burden for the patient as well as the family, both in terms of direct and indirect costs. The initial treatment for pemphigus group of diseases involve initiation of systemic steroids at 1–2 mg/kg body weight/day which is universally accepted, however the choice of the steroid sparing agent for treatment of the refractory cases and maintenance of remission is still an area of argument. Use of intravenous immunoglobulin (IVIg) as an emergency measure in nonresponsive cases which is a norm in west is seldom practised in India because of the high cost. Steroid sparing immunosuppressants, such as azathioprine (Aza), mycophenolate mofetil (MMF), methotrexate and cyclophosphamide (Cyc) are popularly used to minimize the risk of adverse effects of long-term steroids and are prescribed either at the onset or subsequently in the treatment course.[23] Rituximab (Rtx) which was traditionally reserved for refractory pemphigus is now routinely prescribed in nonrefractory cases too.

COST ANALYSIS FOR SYSTEMIC THERAPY IN PEMPHIGUS

Widespread loss of skin barrier leads to hypoproteinemia, blood and fluid loss along with electrolyte imbalances and increased risk for local and systemic infections which warrants supportive management and adds to the cost of the therapy which cannot be quantified and will not be discussed further in the chapter. The topical steroids and calcineurin inhibitors with daily antiseptic baths and dressings are also mandatory and their cost depends upon the percentage body area involved, and hence incalculable.

Management of pemphigus vulgaris will be discussed hereafter for a reference of pharmacoeconomic aspect of all vesiculobullous disorders. The scoring system used to measure the severity of pemphigus is pemphigus disease activity (PDAI) score but is seldom used in most studies. Instead definitions used for disease extent, severity and remission are used according to the widely accepted consensus statement.[24]

Although published literature does not support one therapeutic modality over another;[25] in author's experience, Rtx is a far more superior therapy for pemphigus, especially when used early in the disease for early control and sustained remission of the disease process. The adjuvants discussed here would include Aza, MMF, Cyc and (Rtx) (Tables 22.4 and 22.5). The general toxicity of Cyc makes it a lesser favorable option and most literature on treatment aspect of pemphigus suggests avoidance of Cyc as a steroid sparing agent as far as possible.[26-28] Another popular therapy conceptualized in India and widely practised is dexamethasone-cyclophosphamide or dexamethasone pulse.[29] The rationale of the duration and dosage of therapy

Table 22.4: Cost analysis for systemic therapy in pemphigus.

Drug	Cost of medicine	Schedule of treatment	Total cost	Consultation	Investigations	Total cost
Azathioprine (2.5 mg/kg)	50 g for 9.50/-	2.5 mg/kg for 12 weeks followed by tapering by 0.5 mg every 6–8 weeks	4250/-	Every 2 weeks for first 2 months and every 2 months thereafter 14 × 500 = 7000/-	a. 2,600/- b. 900 × 14 = 12,600/-	19,450/-

a. Initial investigations which are not done as a part of presteroid work up include liver function test (LFT) and thiopurine methyltransferase activity.
b. Monitoring includes LFT every 2 weeks for first 2 months and every 2 months thereafter.

Contd...

Contd...

Drug	Cost of medicine	Schedule of treatment	Total cost	Consul-tation	Investi-gations	Total cost
Myco-phenolate mofetil	500 g for 62/-	1-3 g/day	18,350/- to 55,000/-	Every two weeks during the first two months, once monthly thereafter 500 × 18 = 9,000	a. 1100/- b. 1100 × 18 = 19,800/-	48,250 to 84,900/-

a. Initial extra investigations include LFT and renal function test (RFT).
b. Monitoring includes LFT and RFT every two weeks during the first two months, once monthly within the first year, and every three months thereafter

Drug	Cost of medicine	Schedule of treatment	Total cost	Consul-tation	Investi-gations	Total cost
Cyclopho-sphamide	50 mg for 4/-	1–3 mg/ kg/day	1,160/- to 3,480/-	Every two weeks during the first two months, once monthly thereafter 500 × 18 = 9,000	a. 1100/- b. 1100 × 18 = 19,800/-	31,060 /- to 33,380/-

a. Initial extra investigations include LFT and RFT.
b. Monitoring includes LFT and RFT every two weeks during the first month followed by monthly for as long as on the drug.

Drug	Cost of medicine	Schedule of treatment	Total cost	Consul-tation	Investi-gations	Total cost
Rituximab	500 g for 37,675 /-	Schedule A 1g on days 1 and 14	1,50,700/-	Every month for the first 3 months and quarterly thereafter 500 × 6 = 3000/-	12,500/-	1,66,200/-
		Schedule B 500 g on days 1 and 14	75,350	Same as above	Same as above	90,850/-

a. Initial extra investigations include blood borne virus screening along with Hepatitis-B core antigen, high resolution CT thorax with quantiferon Tb gold, echocardiography (ECHO) with echocardiogram (ECG).
b. Monitoring includes no investigations particularly.

Contd...

Contd...

Drug	Cost of medicine	Schedule of treatment	Total cost	Consul-tation	Investi-gations	Total cost
Dexame-thasone-cyclo-phosp hamide pulse	Dexame-thasone injection for 75/- Cyclo-phospha-mide injection for 75/- Dextrose for 35/- Daily Tab Cyclo-phospha-mide 50 mg for 3.79	Dexame-thasone 100 mg on day 1, 2 and 3 in 5% of 500 mL dextrose Cyclophos-phamide 500 mg on day 2 Daily cyclopho-sphamide at 50 mg/day	₹ 6133/-	Every month in a day-care facility for 3 days 3,000 × 12 = 36,000/-	2280 × 12 = 27,360	69,493/-

a. Daily ECG and serum electrolytes on all 3 days of pulse and urinalysis prior to and after the 2nd day is practiced in most centers.
b. The regimen does not include daily steroids and that cost may be deducted from the other regimens mentioned above which include continuous use of steroids.
c. The cost of consultation is higher as it includes 3 days of day-care admission also.

Table 22.5: Cost analysis for adjuctive drugs in pemphigus for one year of therapy.

The adjunctive drug	Cost in ₹ (For one year therapy)
Azathioprine	19,450/-
Mycophenolate mofetil	48,250/-
Cyclophosphamide	31,060/-
Rituximab	90,850/- (Schedule B)
Dexamethasone-cyclophosphamide (DCP) pulse	69,493/-

is poorly understood and outcome data with regards to attainment of early and late end points (Murrell et al.) is unavailable.

To complicate things, the timing of the introduction of the second drug is also controversial. Few dermatologists introduce them at the start of the treatment along with systemic steroids or use them in treatment resistant cases or when disease flares and some introduce them later in the course of the illness after decreasing the doses of steroids, to avoid profound immunosuppression at once; as increase in doses of steroids rather than adding an adjuvant, all of which are slow acting drugs, helps more in the disease control process.[30] For the purpose of a fair calculation, we assume a 60 kg adult male with no comorbidities who is started on systemic steroids alone in the beginning and the adjuvant is introduced later in the disease when the steroid has been tapered to 40 mg/day (0.66 mg/kg/day). Like psoriasis, indirect cost of disease and cost of hospitalization is not calculated and the cost of a 10-month treatment period is chosen as that (8–12 months) has been found to be the average period after which a pemphigus patient achieves complete remission on therapy.[31-34]

The calculations are based on the premise that the treatment with the adjuvant was given till the patient achieved complete remission on therapy which hypothetically is 10 months on an average, which of course is not the case in every patient and is created to have a logical comparison.

We would fail in our duties if we do not mention that the total amount of steroid needed is much less and an average duration to achieve initial and eventual clinical remission is far lesser with Rtx as compared to the other options which brings down the indirect costs of the therapy by a huge amount. The studies used to calculate the average duration of treatment also mentions failure cases which are least with rituximab. Though the difference between Aza and Rtx with this calculation is a lot, it would be interesting to calculate it in a real life prospective study, which should be much lesser according to author's opinion. The initial one-time expense is a limiting factor in Indian population that usually deters the clinician and patient to opt for Rtx but the overall treatment cost would not be much different and the consultation should encourage the use of Rtx which has been a game changer in management of vesiculobullous disorders according to most experts.

COST ANALYSIS FOR BIOLOGICS AND BIOSIMILAR DRUGS OF RITUXIMAB

The cost of the Ristova, the biologic and the biomimics like Reditux, Ikgdar, Rituxirel and Mabtas is almost the same but most biomimics are available at 50% the cost price in most institutes which brings the cost for Rtx therapy down. Although there are no head to head trials between the biologic and biomimic for pemphigus in literature, the efficacy of biomimics has been proven beyond doubt.

CONCLUSION

Biologics are important addition to armamentarium of physicians managing chronic skin diseases. Biologics increases the direct cost of therapy and result in increased economic burden of the disease during the initial treatment period but the indirect cost comes down. The use of biologics only for treatment resistant cases just because of the cost is not justified and every patient should be foretold the treatment options and given a choice to choose the modality he prefers.

ADDENDUM

Authors have taken cost of investigations and drugs from prevailing market rates and have verified them to best of their knowledge. However, India is a huge and heterogeneous market and it is possible that rates of drugs may vary from place to place and time to time. These calculations have only been done to understand cost-effectiveness of various drugs in these diseases and do not have legal or financial implications.

REFERENCES

1. Parisi R, Symmons DP, Griffiths CE, et al. Global epidemiology of psoriasis: a systematic review of incidence and prevalence. J Invest Dermatol. 2013; 133(2):377-85.
2. Merola JF, Lockshin B, Mody EA. Switching biologics in the treatment of psoriatic arthritis. Semin Arthritis Rheum. 2017;47(1):29-37.
3. Saurat JH, Stingl G, Dubertret L, et al. Efficacy and safety results from the randomized controlled comparative study of adalimumab vs. methotrexate vs. placebo in patients with psoriasis (CHAMPION). Br J Dermatol. 158(3):558-66.
4. Heydendael VM, Spuls PI, Opmeer BC, et al. Methotrexate versus cyclosporine in moderate-to-severe chronic plaque psoriasis. N Engl J Med. 2003;349(7): 658-65.
5. Cyclosporin versus etretinate: Italian multicenter comparative trial in severe plaque-form psoriasis. Italian Multicenter Study Group on Cyclosporin in Psoriasis. Dermatology. 1993;187 (Suppl. 1):8-18.
6. Laburte C, Grossman R, Abi-Rached J, et al. Efficacy and safety of oral cyclosporin A (CyA; Sandimmune++) for long-term treatment of chronic severe plaque psoriasis. Br J Dermatol. 1994;130:366-75.
7. Dogra S, Jain A, Kanwar AJ. Efficacy and safety of acitretin in three fixed doses of 25, 35 and 50 mg in adult patients with severe plaque type psoriasis: a randomized, double blind, parallel group, dose ranging study. J Eur Acad Dermato Venereol. 2013;27(3):e305-11.
8. Dawe RS. A quantitative review of studies comparing the efficacy of narrow-band and broad-band ultraviolet B for psoriasis. Br J Dermatol. 2003;149(3): 669-72.
9. Leonardi CL, Powers JL, Matheson RT, et al. Etanercept as monotherapy in patients with psoriasis. N Engl J Med. 2003;349(21):2014-22.
10. Reich K, Nestle FO, Papp K, et al. Infliximab induction and maintenance therapy for moderate-to-severe psoriasis: a phase III, multicentre, double-blind trial. Lancet. 2005;366(9494):1367-74.
11. Menter A, Feldman SR, Weinstein GD, et al. A randomized comparison of continuous vs. intermittent infliximab maintenance regimens over 1 year in

the treatment of moderate-to-severe plaque psoriasis. J Am Acad Dermatol. 2007;56(1):31.e1-15.

12. Krupashankar DS, Dogra S, Kura M, et al. Efficacy and safety of itolizumab, a novel anti-CD6 monoclonal antibody, in patients with moderate to severe chronic plaque psoriasis: results of a double-blind, randomized, placebo-controlled, phase-III study. J Am Acad Dermatol. 2014 Sep;71(3):484-92.

13. Langley RG, Elewski BE, Lebwohl M, et al. Secukinumab in plaque psoriasis—results of two phase 3 trials. N Eng J Med. 2014;371(4):326-38.

14. Reich K, Griffiths CE. The relationship between quality of life and skin clearance in moderate-to-severe psoriasis: lessons learnt from clinical trials with infliximab. Arch Dermatol Res. 2008;300(10):537-44.

15. Smith CH, Jabbar Lopez ZK, Yiu ZZ, et al. British Association of Dermatologists guidelines for biologic therapy for psoriasis 2017. Br J Dermatol. 2017;177(3):628-36.

16. Driessen RJ, Bisschops LA, Adang EM, et al. The economic impact of high need psoriasis in daily clinical practice before and after the introduction of biologics. Br J Dermatol. 2010;162(6):1324-9.

17. Fonia A, Jackson K, Lereun C, et al. A retrospective cohort study of the impact of biologic therapy initiation on medical resource use and costs in patients with moderate to severe psoriasis. Br J Dermatol. 2010;163(4):807-16.

18. Nelson AA, Pearce DJ, Fleischer AB, et al. Cost-effectiveness of biologic treatments for psoriasis based on subjective and objective efficacy measures assessed over a 12-week treatment period. J Am Acad Dermatol. 2008;58(1):125-35.

19. Sawyer LM, Wonderling D, Jackson K, et al. Biological therapies for the treatment of severe psoriasis in patients with previous exposure to biological therapy: a cost-effectiveness analysis. Pharmacoeconomics. 2015;33(2):163-77.

20. Mihai S, Sitaru C. Immunopathology and molecular diagnosis of autoimmune bullous diseases. J Cell Mol Med. 2007;11(3):462-81.

21. Kneisel A, Hertl M. Autoimmune bullous skin diseases. Part 1: Clinical manifestations. J Dtsch Dermatol Ges. 2011;9(10):844-56.

22. Joly P, Litrowski N. Pemphigus group (vulgaris, vegetans, foliaceus, herpetiformis, brasiliensis). Clin Dermatol. 2011;29(4):432-6.

23. Bystryn J, Steinman NM. The Adjuvant Therapy of Pemphigus. An Update. Arch Dermatol. 1996;132(2):203-12.

24. Murrell DF, Dick S, Ahmed AR, et al. Consensus statement on definitions of disease, end points, and therapeutic response for pemphigus. J Am Acad Dermatol. 2008;58(6):1043-6.

25. Martin LK, Werth VP, Villaneuva EV, et al. A systematic review of randomized controlled trials for pemphigus vulgaris and pemphigus foliaceus. J Am Acad Dermatol. 2011;64(5):903-8.

26. Zhao CY, Murrell DF. Pemphigus vulgaris: an evidence-based treatment update. Drugs. 2015;75(3):271-84.

27. Vanstreels L, Alkhateeb A, Megahed M. Pemphigus vulgaris. Therapy with cyclophosphamide. Hautarzt. 2013;64(5):330-2.

28. Ruocco E, Wolf R, Ruocco V, et al. Pemphigus: associations and management guidelines: facts and controversies. Clin Dermatol. 2013;31(4):382-90.

29. Kanwar AJ, De D. Pemphigus in India. Indian J Dermatol Venereol Leprol. 2011;77:439-49.

30. Atzmony L, Hodak E, Leshem YA, et al. The role of adjuvant therapy in pemphigus: A systematic review and meta-analysis. J Am Acad Dermatol. 2015;73(2):264-71.
31. Chams-Davatchi C, Mortazavizadeh A, Daneshpazhooh M, et al. J Eur Acad Dermatol Venereol. 2013;27(10):1285-92.
32. Cummins DL, Mimouni D, Anhalt GJ, et al. Oral cyclophosphamide for treatment of pemphigus vulgaris and foliaceus. J Am Acad Dermatol. 2003;49(2):276-80.
33. Almugairen N, Hospital V, Bedane C, et al. Assessment of the rate of long-term complete remission off therapy in patients with pemphigus treated with different regimens including medium- and high-dose corticosteroids. J Am Acad Dermatol. 2013;69(4):583-8.
34. Joly P, Maho-Vaillant M, Prost-Squarcioni C, et al. French study group on autoimmune bullous skin diseases. First-line rituximab combined with short-term prednisone versus prednisone alone for the treatment of pemphigus (Ritux 3): a prospective, multicentre, parallel-group, open-label randomised trial. Lancet. 2017;389(10083):2031-40.

Chapter 23

Biologics in Children: Which, When, Why?

Tanumay Raychaudhury

▌ INTRODUCTION

The experience with biologics in pediatric population is majorly from their use in juvenile idiopathic arthritis (JIA) and inflammatory bowel diseases. These drugs provide better disease control without cumulative toxicity to the end organs and prevent/retard damage from active disease. The same principle is extended to pediatric psoriasis and psoriatic arthritis which is more common in type 1 or early onset psoriasis.

Periodic fever syndromes, certain autoimmune bullous disorders, juvenile collagen vascular diseases, extensive and refractory alopecia areata, and chronic refractory urticaria are among other entities in dermatology which are treated with biologics.

We will dwell on available biologics for various indications and their efficacy and safety in children based on available literature.

▌ PSORIASIS

Etanercept

In November 2016, Food and Drug Administration (FDA) approved etanercept for management of psoriasis in pediatric population (4–17 years), making it first biologic to be approved for management of pediatric psoriasis. It is FDA approved for management of JIA in children older than 2 years. Dose to be used is 0.8 mg/kg/week, maximum being 50 mg/week. Etanercept is safe, effective, and has sustained benefit up to 5 years in management of psoriasis.

A randomized double blind placebo-controlled trial was conducted by Amy S Paller et al. on 138 patients. Etanercept was used in dose of 0.8 mg/kg (maximum 50 mg) weekly. Psoriasis Area and Severity Index (PASI) 50, PASI 75, and PASI 90 were achieved in 75%, 57%, and 27%, respectively in etanercept group at the end of week 12. PASI 50, PASI 75, and PASI 90 rates for placebo were 23%, 11%, and 7%, respectively.[1]

In an open label extension of this study, etanercept was found to be safe and effective till 264 weeks (5 years).[2]

Adalimumab

Adalimumab has been approved by European Medicines Agency (EMA) for management of moderate to severe psoriasis in children older than 4 years in 2015. It is not US-FDA approved yet for use in pediatric psoriasis; however, it is FDA approved for management of JIA in this age group.

A phase III, randomized, double blind study conducted by Kim Papp et al. in 114 children with severe psoriasis. Adalimumab was used in dose of 0.8 mg/kg (maximum 40 mg), 0.4 mg/kg (maximum 20 mg) every other week, and methotrexate 0.1–0.4 mg/kg/week. At the end of 16 weeks, 58% of patients in adalimumab 0.8 mg/kg group, 44% patients in 0.4 mg/kg group, and 32% in methotrexate group achieved PASI 75.[3]

Infliximab

Infliximab is FDA approved for management of Crohn's disease in children older than 6 years. It is not FDA approved for management of pediatric psoriasis. However, it has been used in few patients not responding to conventional biologic therapy and etanercept. Infliximab appears to be effective for management of pediatric psoriasis, however its safety is not established and should be used only if patient is not responding to other TNF-α blockers.[4] Dose used is 3–5 mg/kg at 0 week, 2 weeks, 6 weeks, and 8 weekly thereafter.

Secukinumab

Secukinumab has not been studied in pediatric age group. No data is available for its use in pediatric age group and hence it can not be recommended. A multicenter randomized control trial is underway for secukinumab in children aged 6–18 years.

Ustekinumab

Ustekinumab is interleukin (IL)-12/23 blocker and is not available in India as of now. It has been used in one case of 14-year-old boy with plaque psoriasis. Dose used were 45 mg subcutaneous once a month for 2 months and then every 12 weeks.[5] A phase III, randomized, placebo-controlled trial has been conducted in adolescent patients aged 12–17 years. Patients were given standard dose of ustekinumab (0.75 mg/kg <60 kg, 45 mg—60–100 kg, and 90 mg—>100 kg) or half of standard dose at week 0, 4, and every 12 weeks. At week 12, patient with standard dosing achieved PASI 75 and PASI 90 in 80.6% and 61.1%, respectively. In patients on half standard dosing achieved PASI 75 and PASI 90 in 78.4% and 54.1% patient, respectively. Treatment response was comparable to adults and was sustained for 1 year without any unexpected adverse events.[6]

Table 23.1: Monitoring and vaccinations of drugs used in psoriasis.

Drugs	Dose/route	Baseline tests	Follow-up tests	Vaccinations
Etanercept	0.8 mg/kg subcutaneous injection weekly	Mantoux test below 5 years; IRA above 5 years	Annual Mantoux test/IRA	Update vaccinations
Infliximab	3–5 mg/kg intravenous infusion at weeks 0, 2, 6, then every 8 weeks	Chest X-ray Complete blood counts LFT	LFT every 4–6 months (may require more frequent with infliximab)	Avoid live and live attenuated vaccines (e.g. varicella, MMR, oral typhoid, yellow fever, intranasal influenza, herpes zoster, BCG for up to 1 year post stopping drug)
Adalimumab	24 mg/m² subcutaneous injection (maximum 40 mg) every 2 weeks	HIV, if at risk HBsAg, HCV, if at risk Serum electrolytes	CBC Other monitoring will depend on situation	
Ustekinumab	0.75 mg/kg (for patients ≤60 kg; otherwise same dosage for adults) at week 0 and 4 then every 12 weeks			

(IRA: Interferon release assay; LFT: Liver function test; HIV: Human immunodeficiency virus; HBsAg: Hepatitis B surface antigen; HCV: Hepatitis C virus; CBC: Complete blood count; MMR: Measles, mumps, and rubella; BCG: Bacillus Calmette-Guérin).

Monitoring and Vaccinations

Monitoring and vaccinations of drugs used in psoriasis are given in Table 23.1.

▌OMALIZUMAB

Omalizumab is a recombinant humanized monoclonal antibody directed against immunoglobulin E (IgE). It is approved for chronic spontaneous urticaria (CSU) in individuals older than 12 years of age. In July 2016, FDA has approved omalizumab for management of moderate to severe persistent asthma in children older than 6 years of age (previously approved for more than 12 years of age).

Chronic Spontaneous Urticaria

It has been used for treatment of CSU not responding to antihistamines in children as young as 4 years of age. In this case series by Elena Netchiporouk et al., dose of omalizumab was based on total IgE level and baseline CD63 expression. Patients were given either 150 mg or 300 mg subcutaneously monthly.[7]

Atopic Dermatitis

Atopic dermatitis is an off-label indication for management of atopic dermatitis. It has been found to be variably effective in various studies. A placebo-controlled study conducted by Peter Maxmilian Heil et al. in adult patients with atopic dermatitis found omalizumab to be ineffective.[8] Another randomized, placebo-controlled trial in patients with severe refractory urticaria in patients with age group 4–22 years found that there is decrease in T helper type 2 (Th2) cytokines in treatment group, however the clinical improvement in treatment group did not differ significantly from control group.[9]

A study conducted by M Hotze et al. found omalizumab to be effective in a subset of adult patients with atopic dermatitis and absence of filaggrin mutation.[10]

There have been various case series involving management of refractory atopic dermatitis in pediatric age group using omalizumab. In a case series published by Joshua Lane et al. involving three patients in age group of 10–13 years found omalizumab to be effective. The dose used was 150–450 mg twice weekly in this case series.[11] Another case series published by JL Barrios et al., involving pediatric patients found that omalizumab is effective for management of severe atopic dermatitis. In this case series, patients age varied from 6 years to 19 years and omalizumab dose was based on IgE and body weight (same as asthma), maximum being 375 mg subcutaneous every 2 weeks.

The available literature suggest that omalizumab is effective for management of atopic dermatitis, however dose required is more than required for CSU and should be based on weight and serum IgE level. The subset of patients with absence of filaggrin mutation have better control of disease with omalizumab. Omalizumab is unlikely to be used for atopic dermatitis when newer molecules like dupilumab and nemolizumab, which have more specific action in atopic dermatitis, becomes available.

RITUXIMAB

Rituximab is an anti-CD20 monoclonal antibody approved for management of non-Hodgkin lymphoma, rheumatoid arthritis, Wegener's granulomatosis, and microscopic polyangiitis. Off-label dermatological indications include immunobullous disorders and autoimmune connective tissue diseases (AICTD). Rituximab is not approved for pediatric use. It has been sporadically used for management of steroid-resistant nephrotic syndrome and demyelinating disorders of central nervous system (CNS).

Systematic review conducted by Mahmoud et al. found rituximab safe and effective for management of pediatric systemic lupus erythematosus (SLE). Most common dose used was 375 mg/m^2 weekly.[12] It has also been used in management of juvenile dermatomyositis in children aged 10–17 years in similar dose.[13] Rituximab has also been used in successful management of recalcitrant juvenile pemphigus vulgaris, infantile bullous pemphigoid, and pemphigus foliaceus.[14,15] There are 17 case reports of pediatric pemphigus vulgaris treated with rituximab and youngest patient treated was 4 years old. Dose used is 375 mg/m^2 every week; however in some cases only two doses were given 15 days apart and patient responded.[16]

Although, rituximab is not approved for management of pediatric dermatological disorders, it can be used in refractory cases. Safety concerns, risk of infections, and dosing schedule have not been clearly defined in this age group till now.

▌CONCLUSION

Biologics are not considered safe in children due to risk of infections and interference with vaccination. Exclusion of pediatric patients from initial trial of biologics and subsequent poor availability of data has fuelled this concern. There is growing body of evidence that biologics are safe to use in pediatric age group and should be used, if necessary, keeping vaccination protocols in mind. FDA approval of etanercept and EMA approval of adalimumab for management of pediatric psoriasis exemplify this.

▌REFERENCES

1. Paller AS, Siegfried EC, Langley RG, et al. Etanercept treatment for children and adolescents with plaque psoriasis. N Engl J Med. 2008;358(3):241-51.
2. Paller AS, Siegfried EC, Pariser DM, et al. Long-term safety and efficacy of etanercept in children and adolescents with plaque psoriasis. J Am Acad Dermatol. 2016;74(2):280-7.
3. Papp K, Thaçi D, Marcoux D, et al. Efficacy and safety of adalimumab every other week versus methotrexate once weekly in children and adolescents with severe chronic plaque psoriasis: a randomised, double-blind, phase 3 trial. Lancet. 2017;390(10089):40-9.
4. Menter MA, Cush J. Successful treatment of pediatric psoriasis with infliximab. Pediatr Dermatol. 2004;21(1):87-8.
5. Fotiadou C, Lazaridou E, Giannopoulou C, et al. Ustekinumab for the treatment of an adolescent patient with recalcitrant plaque psoriasis. Eur J Dermatol. 2011;21(1):117-8.
6. Landells I, Marano C, Hsu MC, et al. Ustekinumab in adolescent patients age 12 to 17 years with moderate-to-severe plaque psoriasis: results of the randomized phase 3 CADMUS study. J Am Acad Dermatol. 2015;73(4):594-603.

7. Netchiporouk E, Nguyen CH, Thuraisingham T, et al. Management of pediatric chronic spontaneous and physical urticaria patients with omalizumab: case series. Pediatr Allergy Immunol. 2015;26(6):585-8.

8. Heil PM, Maurer D, Klein B, et al. Omalizumab therapy in atopic dermatitis: depletion of IgE does not improve the clinical course—a randomized, placebo-controlled and double blind pilot study. J Dtsch Dermatol Ges. 2010;8(12): 990-8.

9. Iyengar SR, Hoyte EG, Loza A, et al. Immunologic effects of omalizumab in children with severe refractory atopic dermatitis: a randomized, placebo-controlled clinical trial. Int Arch Allergy Immunol. 2013;162(1):89-93.

10. Hotze M, Baurecht H, Rodríguez E, et al. Increased efficacy of omalizumab in atopic dermatitis patients with wild-type filaggrin status and higher serum levels of phosphatidylcholines. Allergy. 2014;69(1):132-5.

11. Lane JE, Cheyney JM, Lane TN, et al. Treatment of recalcitrant atopic dermatitis with omalizumab. J Am Acad Dermatol. 2006;54(1):68-72.

12. Mahmoud I, Jellouli M, Boukhris I, et al. Efficacy and Safety of Rituximab in the Management of Pediatric Systemic Lupus Erythematosus: A Systematic Review. J Pediatr. 2017;187:213-9.e2.

13. Cooper MA, Willingham DL, Brown DE, et al. Rituximab for the treatment of juvenile dermatomyositis: a report of four pediatric patients. Arthritis Rheum. 2007;56(9):3107-11.

14. Connelly EA, Aber C, Kleiner G, et al. Generalized erythrodermic pemphigus foliaceus in a child and its successful response to rituximab treatment. Pediatr Dermatol. 2007;24(2):172-6.

15. Schmidt E, Herzog S, Bröcker EB, et al. Long-standing remission of recalcitrant juvenile pemphigus vulgaris after adjuvant therapy with rituximab. Br J Dermatol. 2005;153(2):449-51.

16. Kincaid L, Weinstein M. Rituximab Therapy for Childhood Pemphigus Vulgaris. Pediatr Dermatol. 2016;33(2):e61-4.

Chapter 24

Biologics in Presence of Hepatitis B and C Infection

D Banerjee, Shekhar Neema

▌ INTRODUCTION

Hepatitis B and C infections are common in Indian population. Hepatitis B virus (HBV) accounts for 15–30% of acute hepatitis in India while acute infection by hepatitis C virus (HCV) is usually asymptomatic. The transmission of these hepatotropic viruses is by blood transfusion, sexual route, perinatal transmission, intravenous drug abuse, and occupational exposure. The asymptomatic nature of infection mandates screening for these infections prior to administration of immunosuppressive medications, as immunosuppression can result in reactivation of virus and can result in acute liver damage.

▌ HEPATITIS B VIRUS

Hepatitis B virus infection is one of the most common infections in world. Approximately 2 billion people have been infected and 350 million are chronic carriers. India belongs to intermediate endemicity country with 4% of population is chronic hepatitis B carrier. Acute infection by HBV presents as hepatitis, but outcome of infection depends on age of the patient. Approximately 95% neonate, 20–30% of children aged 1–5 years and less than 5% of adults develop chronic carrier state. Immunization has resulted in decrease in prevalence of infection where immunization coverage is good.

Diagnosis of Hepatitis B Virus Infection

Diagnosis of HBV infection is based on serological markers and it is important for dermatologist to understand the variety of serological markers available and their significance. Serological markers available are hepatitis B surface antigen (HBsAg), hepatitis B surface antibody (anti-HBs), hepatitis B envelope antigen (HBeAg), hepatitis B envelope antibody (anti-HBe), anti-HBc IgM and IgG (core antigen) (Table 24.1).

Hepatitis B surface antigen is considered hallmark of HBV infection and persistence of HBsAg 6 months after acute infection defines chronicity. Anti-HBs results from immunity to HBV infection and is the only serological marker present in those who have acquired immunity by vaccination. HBeAg and anti-HBe represent infectivity and viral replication. Anti-HBc IgM and

Table 24.1: Serological markers available for diagnosis of hepatitis B virus infection.

HBsAg	Anti-HBs	Anti-HBc IgM	Anti-HBc IgG	HBeAg	Anti-HBe	Remarks
–	+	–	–	–	–	Vaccination Recovery from infection
+	–	+	–	+	–	Acute infection
+	–	–	+	+	+/–	Chronic carrier state
–	–	–	+	–	+/–	Isolated HBc Can result in reactivation on immunosuppression
–	+	–	+	–	+	Recovery from acute infection

(HBsAg: Hepatitis B surface antigen; Anti-HBs: Hepatitis B surface antibody; IgM: Immunoglobulin M; HBeAg: Hepatitis B envelope antigen; Anti-HBc: Hepatitis B core antibody; Anti-HBe: Hepatitis B envelope antibody; IgG: Immunoglobulin G).

IgG represents serological response to clinical infection. IgM corresponds to symptomatic phase and IgG persists during chronic infection.

Hepatitis B virus deoxyribonucleic acid (DNA) can be measured in blood by polymerase chain reaction (PCR) and is a direct measurement of viral load. The availability of this test has made HBeAg redundant as it is the most reliable marker of viral replication. Quantitative measurement of HBsAg is also available and can predict response to interferon therapy.[1,2]

Pathogenesis and Clinical Features

Hepatitis B virus is partially double stranded DNA virus and belongs to *Hepadnaviridae* family. Liver damage caused by virus is immune-mediated and depends on host immune response. Acute exacerbation of chronic hepatitis, fulminant hepatitis, glomerulonephritis, and vasculitis are immune-mediated phenomenon.

As we have already discussed symptoms and outcome depends on the age at which infection was acquired. Infection acquired in infancy and childhood is asymptomatic but has higher chances of chronic infection, while adults are mostly symptomatic but risk of development of chronic carrier state is less than 5%. Less than 1% of patients of acute HBV infection develop fulminant hepatic failure.

Patients who become chronic carrier develops initial phase of immune tolerance for years when patient is HBsAg, HBeAg positive, and has high HBV DNA levels but normal aminotransferases. Second phase is characterized by loss of immune tolerance and is known as immune clearance phase.

This is characterized by decrease in HBsAg and HBV DNA concentration but rise in aminotransferases. Ten to twenty percent of patients become HBeAg negative and develop anti-HBe. These seroconverted patients have low HBV DNA levels and normal aminotransferases, this phase is called as inactive phase and has good clinical outcome. Recurrent increase in aminotransferases and failure to achieve immune clearance increases risk of development of cirrhosis. Twenty to thirty percent of the patients who are HBeAg negative develops active disease with increase in aminotransferases and have high risk of development of cirrhosis.[1,2]

Treatment of Hepatitis B Virus Infection

Treatment includes general measure and specific pharmacologic therapy. General measures include regular monitoring and preventing use of hepatotoxic drugs and alcohol. Specific pharmacotherapeutic agents available for treatment of HBV infections are interferon α and nucleoside and nucleotide analogues. These are lamivudine, adefovir, tenofovir, entecavir, and telbivudine. These drugs should be prescribed by hepatologist and are outside of scope of this book.

Hepatitis B Infection and Biologics

We will discuss use of available biologics in presence of concurrent chronic HBV infection and monitoring of these patients while on biologics. Every patient in whom biologic therapy is planned should undergo appropriate screening for HBV infection. One should also be aware of window period of 2–10 weeks before appearance of HBsAg and development of symptoms after acquiring infection. It is also important to remember that HBsAg negative and anti-HBc IgG positive infection can also occur and it can result in reactivation of infection. If we take in to account poor quality control of test kits, false negative results from test, and risk of acquiring infection during therapy, this situation becomes more complex and mandates monitoring for liver function in patients who were found negative for infection at baseline.

Tumor Necrosis Factor-α Inhibitors

Tumor necrosis factor-α (TNF-α) inhibitors are contraindicated in patients with chronic hepatitis B infection for fear of reactivation. There are published reports where TNF-α blockers have been used successfully for management of psoriasis in presence of HBV infection. Zingarelli et al.[3] reported that 27 HBV infected patients were treated with anti-TNF agents and HBV reactivation was documented in 73% patients without HBV prophylaxis and 14% of patients who were given anti-HBV therapy.[4] A prospective study conducted by Vassilopoulos et al. on safety of anti-TNF-α agents in presence of HBV infection included patients who were vaccinated for HBV, resolved HBV infection, and chronic HBV infection. In 19 patients with resolved HBV infection, none of the patient developed reactivation of HBV infection or increase in transaminases. In 19 patients, who had postvaccination status, there was decrease in anti-HBs levels after therapy, but there was no evidence of reactivation. Fourteen patients with chronic HBV infection were included in study, eight patients were classified as inactive hepatitis [HBeAg—negative, normal alanine aminotransferase/aspartate aminotransferase (ALT/AST), and HBV DNA <2,000 IU/mL] and six as chronic hepatitis B (HBV DNA >2,000 IU/mL, ALT/AST—persistently elevated). These patients were treated with etanercept (n = 6), adalimumab (n = 4), infliximab (n = 4). All patients were treated with antiviral therapy along with anti-TNF therapy. One patient developed viral reactivation due to development of lamivudine resistant strain, while four patients developed transient increase in transaminases without increase in HBV DNA level.[5]

The available literature suggests that TNF inhibitors can be used in patient with chronic hepatitis B along with oral antiviral therapy. Patient should be regularly monitored for evidence of viral reactivation and ideally therapy should be monitored by hepatologist.

Secukinumab

Prescribing information suggests that patients should be screened for hepatitis B infection prior to administration of secukinumab. However, there is no data available for use of secukinumab in this subset of patients. IL-17 has been linked with development of fibrosis in patients of chronic hepatitis B. This coupled with the fact that TNF inhibitors have been used safely along with oral antivirals, it will be safe to assume that secukinumab can be used in this subset of patients along with oral antivirals in consultation with hepatologist. With the availability of literature guidelines about use of secukinumab in this setting may change at a later date.[6]

Rituximab

Chronic HBV infection is a contraindication for use of rituximab as it can lead to viral reactivation. Acute HBV reactivation can lead to acute liver failure in up to 25% of cases. Patients who are HBsAg positive are at highest risk, but those who are HBsAg negative and anti-HBc positive can also develop viral reactivation. The risk of reactivation in HBsAg positive patients can be up to 50%, while in HBsAg −/anti-HBc + subset it can be up to 20%. Ideally, patients in whom rituximab is planned should be screened for HBsAg and anti-HBc as risk of reactivation in patients who are HBsAg −/Anti-HBc + is quite high (Flowchart 24.1). Risk of reactivation in patients

Flowchart 24.1: Practical approach to patient in whom biological therapy is contemplated.[10,11]

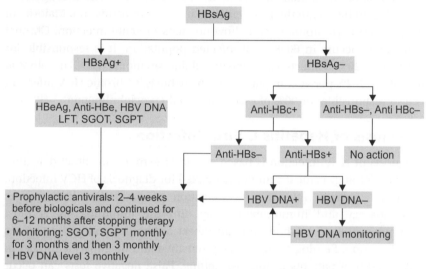

(HBsAg: Hepatitis B surface antigen; HBeAg: Hepatitis B envelope antigen; HBV: Hepatitis B virus; anti-HBc: Hepatitis B core antibody; DNA: Deoxyribonucleic acid; LFT: Liver function test; SGOT: Serum glutamic oxaloacetic transaminase; SGPT: Serum glutamic pyruvic transaminase).

who are treated with prophylactic antiviral therapy decreases substantially.[7] Antiviral therapy should be started within 1 week of administration of rituximab.[8]

Most of this data is from patients with lymphoproliferative malignancy which is quite different from dermatology patients of autoimmune blistering disorders. Patients with malignancy are administered rituximab for longer period of time (six cycles or more) and it is used in association with other chemotherapeutic agents. The extrapolation of this data to dermatology patients is not entirely correct. However, patient should be screened and patients who are positive should be treated with appropriate antivirals before starting rituximab. These patients should be followed up for risk of reactivation of HBV. The data of viral reactivation in dermatology patients is lacking, however it appears that risk of reactivation is lower as compared to malignancy patients and use of antiviral prophylaxis when appropriate can further reduce this risk.[9]

HEPATITIS C VIRUS

Hepatitis C virus is a single stranded ribonucleic acid (RNA) virus of *Flavivirus* family. The prevalence of HCV infection is approximately 2%.

Modes of transmission of HCV virus is through intravenous drug abuse, infected blood, perinatal, and sexual transmission. Intravenous drug abuse and infected blood are the most efficient mode of transmission. Majority of patients are asymptomatic and show no signs of acute infection. Chronic hepatitis C occurs in 60–85% of infected population. It is responsible for cirrhosis in 20% of infected and hepatocellular carcinoma (HCC) develops at the rate of 1–4% per year in patients with cirrhosis.[12] Chronic HCV infection is also responsible for 90% of essential mixed cryoglobulinemia.

Diagnosis of Hepatitis C Virus Infection

Diagnosis of HCV infection is based on either serology or direct detection of virus. Serology is most commonly utilized for diagnosis of HCV infection. There are various methods for detection of antibodies like enzyme immunoassay and immunoblot assay. Enzyme immunoassay is most commonly utilized method and can detect antibodies within 4–10 weeks after infection. Serological test is very sensitive and diagnosis is missed in only 0.5–1% of patients in low-risk setting. False negative tests can occur in immunocompromised patients and in patients with essential mixed cryoglobulinemia. Viral RNA can be detected using PCR and is utilized for assessing treatment response. Genotyping of virus helps in predicting outcome of therapy and influence choice of therapy.[13]

Treatment of Hepatitis C Virus Infection

Every patient with chronic HCV infection is a candidate for antiviral therapy. However, patients with normal aminotransferases and no histologic evidence of necroinflammatory changes have excellent prognosis even without treatment. Patients with raised aminotransferases level and mild histological changes can be followed up by liver biopsy every 3–5 years and regular aminotransferases measurement. Patients with persistently elevated aminotransferases and moderate to severe changes in liver biopsy are candidates for interferon therapy.

Availability of direct acting antivirals (DAA) has changed the treatment of HCV infection. These drugs can lead to sustained viral clearance after 12 weeks of therapy. These drugs are sofosbuvir, daclatasvir, simeprevir, ledipasvir, paritaprevir, ombitasvir, and dasabuvir. Many other drugs of same class are available and are being developed. Interferon free regimens are now available and has made treatment of HCV infection safe and effective.[14]

Hepatitis C Virus Infection and Biologics

Hepatitis C virus infection is listed as relative contraindication for use of biologics. We will discuss the available data on use of biologics in patients

Flowchart 24.2: Practical approach on management of patient with chronic HCV infection on whom biological therapy is planned.[10,11]

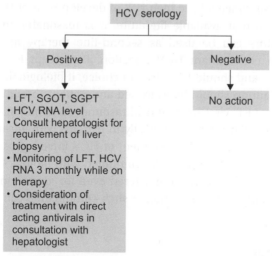

(HCV: Hepatitis C virus; LFT: Liver function test; SGOT: Serum glutamic oxaloacetic transaminase; SGPT: Serum glutamic pyruvic transaminase; RNA: Ribonucleic acid).

with concomitant HCV infection. Treatment options like methotrexate and other hepatotoxic drugs cannot be used. Cyclosporine can be used safely as it inhibits viral replication, but it has certain other problems associated with long-term use (Flowchart 24.2).

Tumor Necrosis Factor-α Inhibitors

The prescribing information on available TNF inhibitors state chronic HCV infection as one of the contraindications and prior testing for HCV is advised in all cases in whom biologics are planned. Hepatitis mediated by HCV is autoimmune in nature and TNF-α plays an important role in liver damage caused by virus. However, it is also known that TNF-α is essential for host defense against pathogen. There is a concern that use of these drugs can lead to reactivation of infection or can result in rapid end organ damage. In a systemic review, Caso et al. reported safe use of etanercept and adalimumab in patients of psoriatic arthritis with concomitant HCV infection. Most of these patients were not on any concomitant antiviral therapy. TNF-α inhibitors were found to be effective and there was no deterioration of liver function test (LFT) after therapy.[15] Another study conducted by Costa et al. on 15 patients with psoriatic arthritis reported that TNF-α inhibitors can be safely used in patients with concomitant HCV infection for up to 1 year.[16] Nuzzo et al. described two cases of psoriasis with advanced liver disease due to HCV infection treated with etanercept. These patients developed hepatocellular carcinoma (HCC) on long-term use of etanercept despite being on regular follow-up with α fetoprotein and transaminases. However, whether TNF-α inhibitors played any role in development of HCC is not known, as these patients have high risk of development of HCC.[17]

From the current available literature, it is reasonable to assume that TNF-α inhibitors can be used as second-line therapy in patients with psoriasis with concomitant HCV infection. Etanercept is the drug with maximum data and should be a drug of choice, if biologic therapy is being considered. Caution should be exercised and patient should be on regular follow-up with LFT, viral load, and ultrasound examination of liver to be performed at regular interval especially in patients with advanced disease.

The availability of DAA for treatment of HCV infection can change this scenario and antiviral drugs can be combined with biologics and possibly then biologics can be safely administered even for long-term in advanced disease. It remains to be seen whether such combination can be safely and effectively used.

Secukinumab

The data on availability of use of secukinumab in patients with hepatitis C infection is scarce. There is a case report where secukinumab has been used in conjunction with DAA and patient underwent remission at 12 weeks for psoriasis and had undetectable viral load.[18]

Due to paucity of available data, one should be cautious about using secukinumab in patients with HCV infection and hepatologist consultation should be sought along with frequent monitoring of liver functions and viral load while patient is on therapy.

Rituximab

Rituximab is an anti-CD20 monoclonal antibody. It is used for management of HCV associated cryoglobulinemia. The study done by Quartuccio et al. reported that rituximab is safe for management of HCV associated cryoglobulinemia. It does not lead to flare of HCV infection even without use of concomitant antivirals. It can be safely used for long-term therapy.[19] Rituximab associated HCV flares has been reported in oncology literature and has resulted in death or liver failure in some cases. However, these patients are on other immunosuppressive and hepatotoxic medications and not only on rituximab monotherapy. Risk of reactivation of HCV infection in rheumatology literature is scant. It has been successfully used in management of pemphigus with HCV infection without any deterioration of liver function or reactivation of HCV infection.[20]

The existing literature suggests that rituximab can be safely used for management of pemphigus in presence of HCV infection. However, one should always be aware of concomitant immunosuppressive medications like corticosteroid or azathioprine which can increase the risk of viral reactivation and hepatic damage. It is best to administer rituximab in this scenario in consultation with experienced hepatologist. It is also important to discuss use of DAA and regular monitoring of liver function and viral load.

CONCLUSION

The presence of chronic hepatitis B and C infection are considered contra-indications for use of biologic therapy. However, biologics are one of the most effective therapies for management of these diseases and lack of this therapeutic option makes management unsatisfactory. The available data suggest that biologics can be safely used for management of these diseases, however treating physician should be aware of diagnosis and management algorithm for chronic hepatitis B and C infection, need for regular follow-up in these patients and frequent consultation with hepatologist.

REFERENCES

1. Dienstag JL. Hepatitis B virus infection. N Engl J Med. 2008;359(14):1486-500.
2. Trépo C, Chan HL, Lok A. Hepatitis B virus infection. Lancet. 2014;384(9959): 2053-63.
3. Zingarelli S, Frassi M, Bazzani C, et al. Use of tumor necrosis factor-α-blocking agents in hepatitis B virus-positive patients: reports of 3 cases and review of the literature. J Rheumatolo. 2009;36(6):1188-94.
4. Papatheodoridis GV, Dimou E, Dimakopoulos K, et al. Outcome of hepatitis B e antigen-negative chronic hepatitis B on long-term nucleos(t)ide analog therapy starting with lamivudine. Hepatology. 2005;42(1):121-9.
5. Vassilopoulos D, Apostolopoulou A, Hadziyannis E, et al. Long-term safety of anti-TNF treatment in patients with rheumatic diseases and chronic or resolved hepatitis B virus infection. Ann Rheum Diss. 2010;69(7):1352-5.
6. Wang L, Chen S, Xu K. IL-17 expression is correlated with hepatitis B related liver diseases and fibrosis. Int J Mol Med. 2011;27(3):385-92.
7. Seto WK, Chan TS, Hwang YY, et al. Hepatitis B reactivation in patients with previous hepatitis B virus exposure undergoing rituximab-containing chemotherapy for lymphoma: a prospective study. J Clin Oncol. 2014;32(33): 3736-43.
8. Huang YH, Hsiao LT, Hong YC, et al. Randomized controlled trial of entecavir prophylaxis for rituximab-associated hepatitis B virus reactivation in patients with lymphoma and resolved hepatitis B. J Clin Oncol. 2013;31(22):2765-72.
9. Kanwar AJ, Vinay K, Heelan K, et al. Use of rituximab in pemphigus patients with chronic viral hepatitis: Report of three cases. Indian J Dermatol Venereol Leprol. 20141;80(5):422-6.
10. Bonifati C, Lora V, Graceffa D, et al. Management of psoriasis patients with hepatitis B or hepatitis C virus infection. World J Gastroenterol. 2016;22(28): 6444-55.

11. Tsutsumi Y, Yamamoto Y, Ito S, et al. Hepatitis B virus reactivation with a rituximab-containing regimen. World J Hepatol. 2015;7(21):2344-51.
12. Shepard CW, Finelli L, Alter MJ. Global epidemiology of hepatitis C virus infection. Lancet Infect Dis. 2005;5(9):558-67.
13. Lauer GM, Walker BD. Hepatitis C virus infection. N Eng J Med. 2001;345(1): 41-52.
14. Asselah T, Boyer N, Saadoun D, et al. Direct-acting antivirals for the treatment of hepatitis C virus infection: optimizing current IFN-free treatment and future perspectives. Liver Int. 2016;36(Suppl 1):47-57.
15. Caso F, Cantarini L, Morisco F, et al. Current evidence in the field of the management with TNF-α inhibitors in psoriatic arthritis and concomitant hepatitis C virus infection. Expert Opin Biol Ther. 2015;15(5):641-50.
16. Costa L, Caso F, Atteno M, et al. Long-term safety of anti-TNF-α in PsA patients with concomitant HCV infection: a retrospective observational multicenter study on 15 patients. Clin Rheumatol. 2014;33(2):273-6.
17. Di Nuzzo S, Boccaletti V, Fantini C, et al. Are anti-TNF-α agents safe for treating psoriasis in hepatitis C virus patients with advanced liver disease? Case reports and review of the literature. Dermatology. 2016;232(1):102-6.
18. Martinez-Santana V, Rodriguez-Murphy E, Smithson A, et al. Efficacy and safety of direct-acting antiviral agents when combined with secukinumab. Eur J Hosp Pharm. 2017;25(1):53-6.
19. Quartuccio L, Zuliani F, Corazza L, et al. Retreatment regimen of rituximab monotherapy given at the relapse of severe HCV-related cryoglobulinemic vasculitis: long-term follow up data of a randomized controlled multicentre study. J Autoimmun. 2015;63:88-93.
20. Amber KT, Kodiyan J, Bloom R, et al. The controversy of hepatitis C and rituximab: A multidisciplinary dilemma with implications for patients with pemphigus. Indian J Dermatol Venereol Leprol. 2016;82(2):182-3.

Chapter 25

Biologics in Special Situation

Shekhar Neema

▌INTRODUCTION

Biologics are a newer group of drugs and like all new drugs, trials are conducted and approval obtained in physiologically most robust population (adults—18-60 years). The pediatric and geriatric population, pregnant and lactating mothers are vulnerable population and are generally not included in drug trials. Inclusion of this population in trials is fraught with ethical issues and is generally avoided. This noninclusion results in inability to use drug freely in this population even when indications exist. With continuous use and anecdotal reports, evidence in this population builds up slowly and physicians develops more confidence in using new drugs (which are no longer new) in vulnerable populations. Etanercept was approved for management of chronic plaque psoriasis in adults in 2004, while approval for pediatric psoriasis was given in November 2016. This reflects fear of regulatory authorities and in the mind of physicians about using newer drugs in special population and situations. Biologics in pediatric age group has already been discussed in a separate chapter and in this chapter we will discuss other special situation and population.

▌BIOLOGICS IN PREGNANCY

Pregnancy is a complex physiological state, where maternal immune system undergoes changes and shift from T helper 1 (Th1) cell to Th2 response. This shift is required for immune tolerance toward developing fetus. Psoriasis is a Th1 mediated disease and approximately half of the patients improve while other half either reports no change or worsening of disease. Severity of psoriasis has been linked with poor pregnancy outcome due to immune dysregulation, other factors like drug intake, concomitant metabolic syndrome also adds to poor pregnancy outcome in patients with psoriasis.[1]

Pregnancy is a state in which any decision taken for patient have potential effect on two lives, one of them is unborn and is in developmental stage. The decision to administer any drug during pregnancy is difficult because of potential risk to fetus. The decision to give any drug to pregnant women is a fine balance between benefit to mother and risk of potential adverse effect in fetus, this algorithm gets further complicated by effect of untreated disease in mother on fetus, risk of progression of disease in mother causing severe morbidity or mortality and general reluctance on part of mother to take any drug to safeguard her unborn child.

Drugs used for management of psoriasis like cyclosporine is a pregnancy category C drug and methotrexate is category X drug, while most of the biologics in use are pregnancy category B drug and are considered reasonably safe.

The issues, which need to be discussed are:
- Inadvertent administration of biologic in an unplanned pregnancy
- Decision to give biologics in pregnant mother for treatment
- Effect on fetus and/or neonate.

The question, which one commonly comes across when patient in reproductive age group on biologics become pregnant, is teratogenicity. Should one continue pregnancy or terminate it because of the risk of congenital malformations? Current prescribing information recommends that antitumor necrosis factor-α (TNF-α) should be discontinued prior to conception (etanercept 3 weeks prior to conception and infliximab 6 months before conception). The data which is available is mostly from use in rheumatology and gastroenterology patients and registry data about pregnancy outcome and congenital malformation.

Antitumor Necrosis Factor-α Therapy

Risk of Adverse Fetal Outcome

There are various case series when pregnant women were exposed to infliximab. In infliximab safety database in 2004, outcome of 96 infliximab exposed pregnancy was reported. Rate of miscarriage was same as general population.[2] In Crohn's treatment registry, 117 patients had infliximab exposure during conception and first trimester period. The rate of miscarriage and neonatal complications were same as general population.[3] In another series of 42 patients who were exposed to infliximab (n-35) and adalimumab (n-7), reported 6 low-birth-weight babies and 7 preterm deliveries. These outcomes were not statistically significant as compared to controls.[4] It is prudent to be careful about infusion reaction and anaphylaxis, as it can precipitate labor in advanced pregnancy.

Teratogenicity

A systematic review has been published by European League against Rheumatism (EULAR) on use of disease modifying antirheumatic drugs in pregnancy. The registry data and systematic literature review supports use of anti-TNF-α treatment in first half of pregnancy. Carter et al. have reported association of anti-TNF drugs with vertebral, anal, cardiac, tracheoesophageal, renal, and limb (VACTERL) group of anomalies; however, this paper was criticized because of poor methodology. The current evidence suggests that there is no increased risk of congenital malformations in babies whose mother were exposed to anti-TNF therapy during conception and first half of pregnancy.[5,6]

Effect on Fetus or Neonate

As we have already discussed, use of anti-TNF drugs in first half appears to be safe. Use of this drug in second and third trimester can result in transplacental transfer. Since, IgG is actively transported from maternal to fetal circulation, fetal serum concentration can exceed that of maternal drug levels. Affinity of neonatal Fc receptor on trophoblast cell is highest for monoclonal antibodies (infliximab) and less for fusion protein (etanercept). Infliximab administered during third trimester can persists for 6–12 months in infant circulation.[7] To prevent neonatal exposure to these drugs, infliximab should be discontinued by 21–22 weeks period of gestation, adalimumab by 26–28 weeks while etanercept by 30–32 weeks.

All neonates who were exposed to anti-TNF therapy after 22 weeks of gestation should undergo complete immunization except live vaccines [Bacillus Calmette-Guérin (BCG) vaccine and rotavirus vaccine].[8]

Anti-interleukin-17 (IL-17) Blockers

Secukinumab

Secukinumab is likely to have low risk of adverse maternal and fetal outcome. However, human data is not available and it should be stopped 19 weeks before conception. In unplanned pregnancy, where pregnant women is exposed to secukinumab expert advice is recommended. Patient should be counseled about limited availability of human data and should be managed with fetomaternal medicine specialist.[9]

Rituximab

Pemphigus is an uncommon disease in pregnancy. Severe pemphigus requiring biologic therapy for management is rare. Prednisolone and IVIg are traditionally considered safe in pregnancy. Rituximab is a pregnancy category C drug. Its prescribing information states that contraception should be advised during and after 12 months of rituximab use in women in reproductive age group. British Society of Rheumatology (BSR) guidelines recommend that rituximab be stopped 6 months prior to conception. BSR registry data of 32 pregnant patients who were exposed to rituximab prior to conception reported that rate of live births and absence of congenital malformation were reassuring.[10]

Rituximab can cause neonatal cytopenia or B-cell depletion and can increase risk of infections in neonate.[8]

Omalizumab

Omalizumab is a pregnancy category B-drug. Prescribing information by manufacturer states that data on use in pregnancy is insufficient. There are various case reports of use of omalizumab in pregnancy for urticaria with successful treatment as well as favorable outcome of pregnancy.[11] Omalizumab pregnancy registry [Xolair Pregnancy Registry (EXPECT)] has been collecting data of safety of omalizumab in pregnancy. Pregnancy outcome was consistent with baseline outcome seen in asthma patients. No pattern of anomalies have been reported.[12] It should also be noted that second generation antihistamines like cetirizine, loratadine, and levocetirizine are pregnancy category B, while fexofenadine and desloratadine are pregnancy category C. Prednisolone and cyclosporine are pregnancy category C. This leaves us with little choice for urticaria in pregnancy (Table 25.1).

Table 25.1: Biologics use during pregnancy.

Drug	Pregnancy cat	Preconception	During pregnancy	Unplanned pregnancy	Neonate
Etanercept	B	• Limited data • Appears to be safe	• Safe in first and second trimester • Increase risk of maternal infection	• Can be continued • Increase maternal infection risk • No increase risk of congenital malformation	• Neonatal immuno-suppression, if used in third trimester • Should be stopped by 30–32 weeks • Avoid live vaccine for 6 months
Adalimumab	B	• Limited data • Appears to be safe	• Safe in first and second trimester • Risk of maternal infection	• Can be continued • No increase risk of congenital malformation	• Neonatal infection • Stop by 26–28 weeks • Avoid live vaccine for 6 months

Contd...

Contd...

Drug	Preg-nancy cat	Preconcep-tion	During pregnancy	Unplanned pregnancy	Neonate
Infliximab	B	• Limited data • Appears to be safe	• Safe in first and early second trimester • Risk of maternal infection	• Can be continued • No increase risk of congenital malforma-tion	• Neonatal infection • Stop by 20–22 weeks • Avoid live vaccine for 6–12 months
Secukinumab	B	• No data • Stop 19 weeks before concep-tion	• No data • Should not be used	• Specialist consul-tation • No human data	• No data • Stop 19 weeks before conception
Rituximab	C	Should be stopped 6 months prior to concep-tion	Should not be used during pregnancy	Specialist consultation of feto-maternal medicine expert required	• Neonatal infection • B cell depletion and lympho-cytopenia • Avoid live vaccine for 12 months after exposure
Omalizumab	B	• Limited data • Appears to be safe	Appears to be safe, can be used	• Can be continued • No increase risk of congenital malfor-mation	Appears to be safe

Biologics during Lactation

Most of the drugs administered to mother get secreted in breast milk. Quantity of drugs which gets secreted varies and they may or may not be harmful to baby. Biologics are IgG molecule while predominantly IgA is secreted in breast milk. These drugs are protein and likely to be metabolized in gastrointestinal system of infant. The available studies suggest that anti-TNF drug concentration in breast milk is minimal and unlikely to be of any clinical significance. In absence of large data, guidelines suggest that mother on anti-TNF therapy should be encouraged to breastfeed.[5]

There is no data on rituximab use in breastfeeding and should be avoided. Omalizumab is compatible with breastfeeding and breastfeeding should be encouraged in patients on breastfeeding.

Biologics in Geriatric Population

Elderly patients have special concerns. They are more prone to infections and are often on multiple drugs. Most of the trials which are conducted are on patients between 18 and 65 years, therefore safety and efficacy data in elderly population is scant. Most of the data in elderly patients are based on postmarketing case series and studies.

Antitumor Necrosis Factor-α and Interleukin-17 Blocker

A retrospective study conducted by Momose et al. in Japan reported that biologics are effective in patients older than 75 years. Biologics used in this study were infliximab, adalimumab, secukinumab, and ustekinumab. There was increased frequency of adverse events, which requires observation.[13] Another retrospective study conducted by Ikari et al. in elderly patients with rheumatoid arthritis (RA) reported that rate of discontinuation of biologics in elderly patients (>75 years) was significantly high.[14] The study conducted by Garber et al. compared safety and efficacy of biologics and conventional systemic agents for treatment of moderate-to-severe psoriasis in elderly (>65 years) and adults. They reported that there was no statistically significant difference in safety and efficacy of biologic agents in adult and elderly; however in elderly population, risk of adverse events with conventional therapy was found to be higher as compared to biologic therapy.[15]

Rituximab

The French rituximab registry with 2 years follow-up had patients in different age group. This registry data is mainly based on RA data and does not include pemphigus group of disorders. They reported that drug is less effective in patients older than 75 years and elderly were more prone to infections.[16] Available literature in dermatology suggests that rituximab is effective in treatment of elderly pemphigus patients. There is no data to suggest that it is less effective for management of pemphigus in elderly patients. However, caution should be exercised while administering rituximab in elderly patients as they are more prone to infections, cardiovascular events, and hematologic adverse effects. Vaccination should be completed to prevent infections.

Omalizumab

Omalizumab is approved for management of asthma in children older than 6 years and chronic spontaneous urticaria for children older than 12 years. There is no upper limit of age for administration of omalizumab; however, prescribing information states that data in elderly patients is scant. It has been used for management of uncontrolled asthma and chronic spontaneous urticaria in elderly patients effectively in various case series. The available data supports use of omalizumab for management of chronic spontaneous urticaria. However, higher than expected arterial thrombotic events have been reported in asthma patients on omalizumab.[17,18]

Biologics in Presence of Other Comorbidities

Chronic Renal Failure

Psoriasis is associated with metabolic syndrome in 30–40% patients. These patients are at high risk of development of chronic renal failure. Psoriasis per se can increase risk of renal dysfunction; however, exact mechanism of this is not known. Drugs like cyclosporine are nephrotoxic and can lead to renal dysfunction. Drugs and their active and inactive metabolites get excreted by kidneys, thereby complicating treatment algorithms in presence of organ dysfunction. It is important to be aware of this risk, while managing psoriasis and patient at risk should be followed-up for development of renal dysfunction, especially when patient is on cyclosporine and nonsteroidal anti-inflammatory drug (NSAID). The physician should also be able to manage psoriasis in presence of established chronic kidney disease.

Management of psoriasis in presence of renal dysfunction remains challenging as conventional systemic therapy like cyclosporine is nephrotoxic and kidney is primary route of elimination for methotrexate precluding their use. Phototherapy may not be feasible because of frequent hospital visit that it requires. Biologics are protein molecules and are metabolized by proteolysis; fragments are excreted in bile and urine. Pharmacokinetic data of biologics in presence of renal dysfunction is not available as this group of population has not been studied. Studies conducted by Gisondi and Girolomoni reported that glomerular filtration rate in patients on etanercept does not change.[19] There are various case reports of successful use of anti-TNF therapy for management of psoriasis in presence of end stage renal disease (ESRD) on hemodialysis.[20,21] Similar data on secukinumab is not available. Infliximab should be used with caution as it can lead to fluid overload in these patients. Patients with ESRD have impaired host defenses and careful monitoring for infections is required in these patients.

Rituximab is used in management of kidney disease of autoimmune etiology [antineutrophil cytoplasmic antibodies (ANCAs) associated renal vasculitis, antiglomerular basement membrane (anti-GBM) disease, and lupus nephritis]. Rituximab can be used for management of autoimmune blistering diseases in presence of impaired renal function; however, it should be used in consultation with nephrologist. High risk of infection and fluid overload should be addressed in these patients.

The guidelines for management of chronic spontaneous urticaria suggest use of second generation antihistamines as first-line therapy and omalizumab in cases in which patient is not responding to fourfold increase in dose of antihistamines. Commonly used antihistaminics like levocetrizine, desloratidine and fexofenadine requires dose adjustment in presence of renal failure. The availability of literature for use of omalizumab in chronic urticaria in presence of renal dysfunction is scant. However, omalizumab is an IgG molecule and metabolized by proteolysis. There is no evidence of renal toxicity of omalizumab in pharmacokinetic studies. As per available literature, omalizumab can be used if indicated.

Chronic Liver Disease

Psoriasis is associated with increased risk of nonalcoholic fatty liver disease and use of hepatotoxic drug like methotrexate, acitretin, and azathioprine for longer duration further increase the risk of development of chronic liver disease. As psoriasis is a common disease, it can also coexist with chronic liver disease of various etiology. Treatment of psoriasis in presence of chronic liver failure can be challenging as hepatotoxic drugs and drugs which are primarily metabolized in liver have to be used with caution. Pharmacokinetic data of biologics in presence of chronic liver failure is not available. This is further complicated by fact that TNF-α blockers have been linked to drug induced liver injury (DILI). Median latency period before development of DILI was 13 weeks.[22] The etiological evaluation of chronic liver disease should be done prior to starting any biologic therapy as hepatitis B and C induced chronic liver disease requires specialist consultation before treatment with biologics is contemplated.

There are various case series and individual case report of successful use of TNF inhibitors for management of psoriasis with chronic liver disease resulting from various etiologies. Data of secukinumab use in presence of cirrhosis of liver is scant and no recommendation is available, author has used secukinumab in two patients with cirrhosis of liver and found it to be safe and effective (unpublished observation). Large safety data of biologic use in this setting is not available. Etanercept is biologic with maximum available literature in this setting, risk of development of autoimmune hepatitis is minimal unlike monoclonal antibodies (infliximab and adalimumab) and is safe in presence of hepatitis C virus (HCV) infection. The available literature suggests that etanercept is preferable drug in this setting.

Autoimmune blistering diseases are rare diseases and coexistent chronic liver disease with this group of disorders is quite rare. Screening of concomitant hepatitis B and hepatitis C infection should be done prior to initiation of rituximab as reactivation of hepatitis B and C can occur and thus rituximab is contraindicated. However, it can be used with careful consideration in consultation with hepatologist.

Rituximab is used for management of HCV associated cryoglobulinemia. Since hepatitis C-induced liver damage is immune mediated in nature and liver function also tends to improve in these patients. There are case reports of successful treatment of pemphigus with concomitant HCV infection; however, reactivation of HCV infection can occur and treatment should be done in consultation with hepatologist.[23]

Chronic hepatitis B infection has a significant risk of worsening or reactivation on administration of rituximab. Complete serological evaluation and HBV DNA level should be done. Antiviral therapy (lamivudine, entecavir, and tenofovir) should be started in consultation with hepatologist. Rituximab should be used after adequate viral suppression has been achieved and antiviral should be continued for 6–12 months after last dose of rituximab to prevent late reactivation.[24]

Cardiac Disease

Psoriasis is associated with increased risk of ischemic heart disease and cardiovascular risk factors. The risk of cardiovascular events is significantly reduced with anti-TNF-α therapy or methotrexate. Anti-TNF therapy significantly reduces the risk of myocardial infarction and major adverse cardiac event but not heart failure.[25] The circulating TNF may induce or exacerbate the development of cardiac failure, blocking TNF should improve heart failure but various trials have suggested otherwise. Anti-TNF therapy is contraindicated in patients with advanced congestive heart failure (CHF) [New York Heart Association III or IV (NYHA III or IV)]; however, it can be used in mild-to-moderate CHF (NYHA I or II).[26]

The data regarding reduction in risk of cardiovascular events or exacerbation of heart failure with anti-IL-17 antibodies (secukinumab) and anti-IL-12/23 antibodies (ustekinumab) is scant and these drugs should be used cautiously in presence of advanced CHF.

Various case reports of myocardial infarction, coronary spasm, and ventricular tachycardia have been reported with rituximab. It generally occurs after first infusion but can occur in subsequent infusion also. Ischemic events generally occur in patient with underlying cardiovascular risk factors but it may occur in patients without any risk factors.[27] In patient with underlying risk factors, cardiologist consultation should be obtained prior to starting rituximab. Infusion should be done where facilities for cardiopulmonary resuscitation is available especially in patients with underlying heart disease.

Cancer

There are two issues which need to be discussed in this heading. First is increased risk of malignancy associated with use of biologicals which has been discussed in detail in adverse effect chapter. Second issue which needs to be discussed is use of biologics in patients with current or treated malignancy. Patient with current or treated cancer can have associated moderate-to-severe psoriasis requiring systemic therapy. The decision to treat such patients can be quite challenging as one has to choose between conventional systemic therapy or biological agents. There is an unknown risk of cancer recurrence in patients on immunosuppressive medications and definite guidelines for treatment in such situations is scarce.

There are various systematic reviews, which suggest that there is an increased risk of nonmelanoma skin cancer in patients treated with anti-TNF therapy; however, there has been no significant increase in risk of solid malignancy. There are studies which have compared relative risk of development of malignancy in patients treated with disease modifying antirheumatic drugs (DMARD) or biologics in cancer survivors. The available data suggests that there is no increase in risk of cancer recurrence in patient treated with biologic as compared to conventional systemic therapy; however, the available data is limited and is confounded by various other factors. Till the time more robust evidence emerges in this group of population, it is recommended that patient should be informed about possible increase in risk of recurrence of cancer in patient being treated with biologic therapy.[25,28]

▍CONCLUSION

Biologics are relatively new drugs and their use in special situations is not yet clear. Despite being an effective therapy, there is some hesitation on part of treating physician in such situations. This hesitation stems from the fact that data in these scenarios are scant. We have tried to provide current data available but it leaves lot to be discussed and their usage will attain clarity as more and more data becomes available.

▍REFERENCES

1. Bobotsis R, Gulliver WP, Monaghan K, et al. Psoriasis and adverse pregnancy outcomes: a systematic review of observational studies. Br J Dermatol. 2016;175(3):464-72.

2. Antoni CE, Furst D, Manger B, et al. Outcome of pregnancy in women receiving remicade®(infliximab) for the treatment of crohn's disease or rheumatoid arthritis. Arthritis Rheum. 2001;44(9):S152.

3. Lichtenstein GR, Feagan BG, Cohen RD, et al. Serious infection and mortality in patients with Crohn's disease: more than 5 years of follow-up in the TREAT™ registry. Am J Gastroenterol. 2012;107(9):1409-22.

4. Schnitzler F, Fidder H, Ferrante M, et al. Outcome of pregnancy in women with inflammatory bowel disease treated with antitumor necrosis factor therapy. Inflamm Bowel Dis. 2011;17:1846-54.

5. Skorpen CG, Hoeltzenbein M, Tincani A, et al. The EULAR points to consider for use of antirheumatic drugs before pregnancy, and during pregnancy and lactation. Ann Rheum Dis. 2016;75(5):795-810.

6. Carter JD, Ladhani A, Ricca LR, et al. A safety assessment of tumor necrosis factor antagonists during pregnancy: a review of the Food and Drug Administration database. J Rheumatol. 2009;36(3):635-41.

7. Förger F. Treatment with biologics during pregnancy in patients with rheumatic diseases. Reumatologia. 2017;55(2):57-8.

8. Soh MC, MacKillop L. Biologics in pregnancy—for the obstetrician. The Obstetrician & Gynaecologist. 2016;18(1):25-32.

9. Rademaker M, Agnew K, Andrews M, et al. Psoriasis in those planning a family, pregnant or breast-feeding. The Australasian Psoriasis Collaboration. Australas J Dermatol. 2017. doi:10.1111/ajd.12641.

10. De Cock D, Birmingham L, Watson KD, et al. Pregnancy outcomes in women with rheumatoid arthritis ever treated with rituximab. Rheumatology (Oxford). 2017;56(4):661-3.

11. Pardo LB, Blanch MA, Radojicic C. Use of omalizumab for treatment of antihistamine and steroid resistant chronic idiopathic urticaria during pregnancy. J Allergy Clin Immunol. 2015;135(2):AB129.

12. Namazy J, Cabana MD, Scheuerle AE, et al. The Xolair Pregnancy Registry (EXPECT): the safety of omalizumab use during pregnancy. J Allergy Clin Immunol. 2015;135(2):407-12.

13. Momose M, Asahina A, Hayashi M, et al. Biologic treatments for elderly patients with psoriasis. J Dermatol. 2017;44(9)1020-3.

14. Ikari Y, Miwa Y, Yajima N. SAT0086 The association between elderly rheumatoid arthritis patients using biologics and adverse events: retrospective cohort study. Ann Rheum Dis. 2017;76(Suppl 2):801.

15. Garber C, Plotnikova N, Au SC, et al. Biologic and conventional systemic therapies show similar safety and efficacy in elderly and adult patients with moderate to severe psoriasis. J Drugs Dermatol. 2015;14(8):846-52.

16. Payet S, Soubrier M, Perrodeau E, et al. Efficacy and safety of rituximab in elderly patients with rheumatoid arthritis enrolled in a French Society of Rheumatology registry. Arthritis Care Res (Hoboken). 2014;66(9):1289-95.

17. Sussman G, Gonçalo M, Sánchez-Borges M. Treatment dilemmas in chronic urticaria. J Euro Acad Dermatol Venereol. 2015;29(S3):33-7.

18. Presa IJ, Rodríguez BN, Bareño BR, et al. Chronic urticaria in special populations: children, pregnancy, lactation and elderly people. 2016;3(4):423-38.

19. Gisondi P, Girolomoni G. Glomerular filtration rate in patients with psoriasis treated with etanercept. J Int Med Res. 2016;44(1 suppl):106-8.

20. Cassano N, Vena GA. Etanercept treatment in a hemodialysis patient with severe cyclosporine-resistant psoriasis and hepatitis C virus infection. Int J Dermatol. 2008;47(9):980-1.

21. Saougou I, Papagoras C, Markatseli TE, et al. A case report of a psoriatic arthritis patient on hemodialysis treated with tumor necrosis factor blocking agent and a literature review. Clin Rheumatol. 2010;29(12):1455-9.

22. Ghabril M, Bonkovsky HL, Kum C, et al. Liver injury from tumor necrosis factor-α antagonists: analysis of thirty-four cases. Clin Gastroenterol Hepatol. 2013;11(5):558-64.

23. Amber KT, Kodiyan J, Bloom R, et al. The controversy of hepatitis C and rituximab: a multidisciplinary dilemma with implications for patients with pemphigus. Indian J Dermatol Venereol Leprol. 2016;82(2):182-3.

24. Sena Nogueira Maehara L, Huizinga J, Jonkman MF. Rituximab therapy in pemphigus foliaceus: report of 12 cases and review of recent literature. Br J Dermatol. 2015;172(5):1420-3.

25. Roubille C, Richer V, Starnino T, et al. Evidence-based recommendations for the management of comorbidities in rheumatoid arthritis, psoriasis, and psoriatic arthritis: expert opinion of the Canadian Dermatology-Rheumatology Comorbidity Initiative. J Rheumatol. 2015;42(10):1767-80.

26. Heslinga SC, Sijl AM, De Boer K, et al. Tumor necrosis factor blocking therapy and congestive heart failure in patients with inflammatory rheumatic disorders: a systematic review. Curr Med Chem. 2015;22(16):1892-902.

27. Armitage JD, Montero C, Benner A, et al. Acute coronary syndromes complicating the first infusion of rituximab. Clin Lymphoma Myeloma. 2008;8(4):253-5.

28. Majewksi S, Kheterpal M, Nardone B, et al. First line biologic agent therapy for moderate-to-severe psoriasis in cancer survivors. J Am Acad Dermatol. 2016; 74(5):AB250.

Chapter
26

Tofacitinib

Sunil Kothiwala

INTRODUCTION

Tofacitinib (formerly known as CP-690,550, CP690550, tasocitinib) is a small molecule and novel selective immunosuppressant that inhibits Janus kinase 1 (JAK1)/JAK3, and to some degree JAK2 resulting in the interruption of intracellular signaling, suppression of immune cell activation and inflammation in T-cell mediated disorders. It was approved by the Food and Drug Administration (FDA) in 2012 for moderate-to-severe rheumatoid arthritis with an insufficient response or intolerance to methotrexate. Due to worries about the risk of infections, the drug failed to win approval as a rheumatoid arthritis therapy in Europe. FDA approval for using tofacitinib in psoriasis treatment is still on hold due to safety reasons.

JAK/STAT PATHWAY (FIG. 26.1)

The JAK-signal transducer and activator of transcription (JAK-STAT) pathway is utilized by cytokines including interleukins (ILs), interferons (IFNs), and other molecules to transmit signals from the cell membrane to nucleus via integral membrane proteins resulting in deoxyribonucleic acid (DNA) transcription and gene expression.[1] There are three major components of JAK-STAT Pathway: (1) a cell surface receptor, (2) a JAK and (3) a STAT protein. JAK family includes JAK1, JAK2, JAK3 and tyrosine kinase 2 (TYK2). Upon engagement of extracellular ligands, intracellular JAK proteins, which associate with type I/II cytokine receptors, become activated and phosphorylate STAT (STAT1, STAT2, STAT3, STAT4, STAT5a, STAT5b and STAT6) proteins, which dimerize and then translocate into the nucleus to directly regulate gene expression. This pathway induces cell proliferation, differentiation, migration, and apoptosis which are decisive for immune development. Mutations that affect the normal functioning of JAK signaling cause inflammatory diseases, erythrocytosis, gigantism and leukemia.[2] Tumor necrosis factor (TNF), IL-1, IL-17, IL-18, and transforming growth factor-beta (TGF-β) cytokines are independent of JAKs signaling.

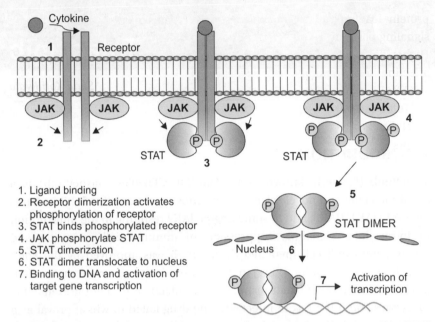

1. Ligand binding
2. Receptor dimerization activates phosphorylation of receptor
3. STAT binds phosphorylated receptor
4. JAK phosphorylate STAT
5. STAT dimerization
6. STAT dimer translocate to nucleus
7. Binding to DNA and activation of target gene transcription

Fig. 26.1: Janus kinase-signal transducer and activator of transcription (JAK-STAT) pathway. JAK inhibitors antagonize JAK protein function and prevent activation of the pathway.

PHARMACOLOGY

The molecular formula of free base of tofacitinib is $C_{16}H_{20}N_6O$ and it has a molecular weight of 312.4 daltons. The active substance is the citrate salt of tofacitinib has a molecular formula of $C_{16}H_{20}N_6O \cdot C_6H_8O_7$, the molecular weight of 504.5 daltons, and is currently available in the form of tablets. The absolute oral bioavailability is 74% and the peak plasma concentrations (C_{max}) of the drug are reached within 30–60 minutes after oral administration, but reduced by 32% when the drug is coadministered with a high-fat meal. The half-life of the substance is approximately 180 minutes.[3]

The plasma protein binding of the drug, predominantly to albumins, is 40%. In vitro studies indicate that tofacitinib is mainly metabolized by cytochrome P450 (CYP) 3A4 (CYP3A4) and CYP2C19. The drug has 70% hepatic clearance, while the remaining 30% is excreted through the kidneys. Tofacitinib is metabolized by oxidation of the pyrrolopyrimidine, piperidine rings, and the piperidine ring side-chain, demethylation, and glucuronidation.[4]

MECHANISM OF ACTION

Tofacitinib citrate is believed to be pan-JAK inhibitor with predominance for JAK1/JAK3 heterodimers and JAK2/JAK2 homodimers by competing with adenosine triphosphate (ATP) for the ATP binding site of the JAK protein leading to JAK inactivation which subsequently modulates the signaling pathway by preventing phosphorylation and activation of STATs.[5] Higher doses of the drug have predominance for inhibition of JAK2/JAK2 affecting the hematopoiesis, while lower doses predominantly inhibit JAK1/JAK3

Tofacitinib blocks γ-chain cytokines, including IL-2, IL-4, IL-7, IL-9, IL-15, IL-21 through JAK1/JAK3. It also inhibits activation of JAK1/JAK2/TYK2 which results in blocking of IL-6, IL-10, IL-11, IL-12, IL-20, IL-22, IL-23, IFN-α/β, IFN-γ.[6] To a lesser extent the drug blocks IL-3, IL-5, granulocyte/macrophage colony-stimulating factor (GM-CSF), erythropoietin (EPO), prolactin, leptin, growth hormone, and IFN-γ through JAK2/JAK2 homodimers.[4-6]

▌USES

FDA Approved
- Moderate to severe rheumatoid arthritis.

Off Label Indications[7-9]
- Psoriasis
- Alopecia areata (AA)
- Vitiligo
- Atopic dermatitis (AD)
- Nail dystrophy associated with AA.

Psoriasis

The pathogenesis of psoriasis involves various cytokines out of which IL-12 and IL-23 are the key mediators. IL-23 stimulates TH17 cells to produce IL-17, another important pathogenic molecule in psoriasis. Blockade of IL-23 using tofacitinib indirectly results in a decrease in IL-17.[10] To date, in dermatology, psoriasis has been the most heavily studied indication for JAK inhibitors. The FDA has yet to approve tofacitinib for this indication.

The efficacy and safety of tofacitinib 5 mg and 10 mg have been determined in phase 3 randomized controlled trials (RCTs) (Table 26.1) which demonstrated better improvement in Physician's Global Assessment (PGA) and Psoriasis Area and Severity Index (PASI) 75 in comparison to placebo.[11-13] Histopathological evaluation of tofacitinib treated lesions showed reduced cytokines, lower numbers of DC and T cells, and decreased IL-23/Th17 activity.[14] Increased weight and prior biologic treatment were associated with lower response rates.[15] It was also reported that withdrawal results in worsening of disease but recovered following retreatment and when tofacitinib 10 mg was given continuously, the improvement was maintained for 56 weeks.[16]

Table 26.1: Randomized controlled trials comparing tofacitinib, placebo and etanercept in patients with moderate-to-severe plaque psoriasis.

Reference/ Year	Type of study	No. of patients	Dosage/ Duration	Assessment scores used	Efficacy	Adverse effects
Tofacitinib versus placebo:						
Papp et al.[11]/2015	Two phase 3 RCTs	1,861	5 mg, 10 mg twice daily/16 weeks	Clear/almost clear PGA and PASI 75	Greater proportion of patients achieved PGA responses and high PASI 75 rates with tofacitinib than placebo	Herpes zoster (n = 12) in tofacitinib group. Nasopharyngitis
Bissonnette et al.[12]/2015	Phase 3 RCT	666	5 mg, 10 mg twice daily/24 weeks	Clear/almost clear PGA and PASI 75	PASI 75 rate: • Tofacitinib 5 mg versus placebo—56.2% versus 23.3% • Tofacitinib 10 mg versus placebo—62.3% versus 26.1% • After 16 weeks of retreatment, 48% and 72% regained PASI 75 response with tofacitinib 5 mg and 10 mg doses	Infections and infestations as nasopharyngitis, with no difference between the groups
Feldman et al.[13]/2016	Two phase 3 RCTs	1,861	5 mg, 10 mg twice daily/16 weeks	Patient-reported outcomes including DLQI, ISS, PtGA and JPA	All patient-reported outcomes were significantly improved in patients receiving tofacitinib in comparison with placebo. The greater effect was observed for the 10 mg dosage. The response was maintained for 52 weeks	–

Contd...

Contd...

Reference/ Year	Type of study	No. of patients	Dosage/ Duration	Assessment scores used	Efficacy	Adverse effects
Tofacitinib versus etanercept:						
Bachelez et al.[17]/2015	Phase 3 RCT	1,106	5 mg, 10 mg twice daily/ 12 weeks	Clear/almost clear PGA and PASI 75	PASI 75 responses were 39.5% (5 mg), 63.6% (10 mg) for tofacitinib treatment and 58.8% for etanercept treatment, and 5.6% for placebo	There was no difference in AEs between treatment versus placebo groups
Valenzuela et al.[18]/2016	Phase 3 RCT	1,101	5 mg, 10 mg twice daily/ 12 weeks	Patient-reported outcomes, including DLQI, ISS and PtGA	Improvement of DLQI score showed similar rates between tofacitinib 10 mg and etanercept of 47.3% and 43.6%, respectively. Itch was significantly reduced by tofacitinib compared with etanercept and placebo	

(RCT: Randomized controlled trial; PGA: Physician's Global Assessment; PASI: Psoriasis Area and Severity Index; DLQI: Dermatology Life Quality Index; ISS: Itch Severity Score, PtGA: Patient Global Assessment).

There are two RCTs which compared tofacitinib 10 mg twice daily and etanercept 50 mg subcutaneously twice weekly concluded noninferiority of tofacitinib to etanercept therapy.[17,18] Rates of adverse events appeared to be similar with both the 5 mg and 10 mg dosing regimens.

The use of topical tofacitinib (2% ointment) has been explored in psoriasis. Improvement in psoriasis was observed with topical tofacitinib;[19] however, the degree of improvement relative to controls was modest and not always statistically significant.[20]

Atopic Dermatitis

The pathogenesis of AD is complex but in part involves increased helper T cell type 2 (TH2) immunity driven by JAK-STAT signaling downstream of cytokines, such as IL-4, IL-5, and IL-13. The efficacy of oral tofacitinib 5 mg daily or twice daily was recently reported in patients with moderate to severe AD that previously failed all common treatments with 66.6% reduction in the severity scoring of AD index and a 69.9% reduction in pruritus and sleep loss scores.[21]

In a phase 2 study comparing topical tofacitinib 2% with vehicle, showing a more significant reduction in the area and severity of eczema in the tofacitinib group in comparison to placebo.[22]

Alopecia Areata

The pathogenesis of AA involves hair follicle attack by autoreactive CD8 T cells. In AA, JAK-STAT-dependent cytokines, including IFN-γ and IL-15, drive proliferation and activation of autoreactive T cells, suggesting that JAK inhibition might be an effective treatment.

Recently, a retrospective study including patients with either AA, alopecia totalis (AT), alopecia universalis (AU) with duration of current disease activity greater than 10 years or severe AA treated up to 18 months using tofacitinib reported some hair growth in 77%, greater than 50% improvement in severity of alopecia tool (SALT) score in 58% and greater than 90% improvement in 20% of patients.[23] In another study of adolescents (12–17 years old) with severe AA, AT, and AU, after a mean of 6.5 months of treatment with tofacitinib reported a 93% median change in SALT score from baseline.[24] In one trial, 3-month treatment period of tofacitinib 5 mg twice daily in severe AA, AT or AU has been showed some hair regrowth in nearly two-thirds of patients and 32% of patients achieved greater than 50% improvement in their SALT score.[25] Furthermore, tofacitinib 5 mg twice daily for 5–6 months in three patients with AU and nail dystrophy resulted in remission of nail dystrophy. As in AD, topical JAK inhibitors are under investigation in AA.[26]

Vitiligo

Vitiligo might be susceptible to treatment with JAK inhibitors because IFN-γ utilizes JAK-STAT pathway to mediate targeted destruction of melanocytes by CD8+ T cells. Generalized vitiligo showed near complete repigmentation of affected areas of the face, forearms, and hands over 5-month treatment with tofacitinib (5 mg every other day for 3 weeks followed by 5 mg daily). Following treatment discontinuation, however loss of repigmentation was observed.[27] The authors have proposed that JAK1/JAK2 is involved in IFN-γ signal transduction and that the use of the JAK1/3 inhibitor blocks the IFN-γ signaling and decreases C-X-C motif chemokine 10 (CXCL10) expression. The expression of CXCL10 in keratinocytes is induced by IFN-γ and it has been found to be an intermediate of depigmentation in vitiligo.

Other Dermatological Diseases

There are some case reports which showed efficacy of tofacitinib in chronic actinic dermatitis, dermatomyositis, erythema multiforme, hypereosinophilic syndrome, lupus erythematosus, palmoplantar pustulosis, polyarteritis nodosa.[7-9]

▌ BASIC INFORMATION[28]

Trade name: Xeljanz, Xeljanz XR

Developed and marketed by: Pfizer

Preparation: Tablet, 5 mg (equivalent to 8 mg tofacitinib citrate), 11 mg (Xeljanz XR) (equivalent to 17.77 mg tofacitinib citrate)

Route of administration: Oral

Dosage: 5 mg twice a day or 11 mg once a day

Pretreatment evaluation and investigations:
- History of any old or current infection like tuberculosis (TB), and infections caused by bacteria, fungi, or viruses, history of malignancy, history of gastric ulcer, diverticulitis or perforation.
- Complete hemogram
- Urine routine and microscopic examination
- Liver function tests (LFTs): including hepatitis B virus (HBV) and hepatitis C virus (HCV) panel
- Renal function test
- Fasting lipid profile
- Chest X-ray, Mantoux test, interferon-gamma release assay (IGRA) test for TB
- Human immunodeficiency virus (HIV).

During treatment:
- Complete blood count (CBC), LFTs
- Fasting lipid profile.

Table 26.2: Adverse effects of tofacitinib.

Cutaneous	Noncutaneous

• Herpes zoster
• Disseminated molluscum
• Reactivation of herpes simplex
• Eruptive squamous cell carcinoma
• DRESS syndrome
• Drug rash
	• Upper respiratory tract infections
	• Nasopharyngitis headache
	• Gastrointestinal perforation
	• Central nervous system (CNS): Headache, distal symmetric polyneuropathy
	• Enterovaginal fistula
	• Laboratory abnormalities:
	  ▪ Dose-dependent decrease in hemoglobin levels, RBCs, and neutrophil counts
	  ▪ Dose-dependent increase in creatinine phosphokinase (CPK), high-density lipoprotein (HDL), low-density lipoprotein (LDL), and total cholesterol level

ADVERSE EFFECTS

All the reported side effects can be divided in two groups: (1) cutaneous and (2) noncutaneous (Table 26.2). The clinical studies showed that percentages of safety events of special interest occurring in the study population, that include serious infections, herpes zoster, nonmelanoma skin cancer and major adverse cardiovascular events, were low (<1%), with a similar rate in comparison to all approved TNF inhibitors and other biologic disease-modifying antirheumatic drugs (DMARDs) in similar patient populations.[17,18] No cases of reactivation of TB were found in a systematic review of five RCTs with tofacitinib.[29] The influence of tofacitinib on hematologic values was dose-dependent. Longer studies are required to determine the further drug safety.

CONTRAINDICATION, WARNING AND PRECAUTIONS

- Absolute contraindication—none
- Known hypersensitivity
- Patients with old TB or active serious infections warranting systemic antibiotic therapy
- Patient with history of gastric ulcers, diverticulitis and perforations
- Patient with severe liver disease
- Patient with history of malignancy
- Concomitant administration of potent inhibitors of CYP3A4 and CYP2C19 like ketoconazole and fluconazole—the recommended dose is Xeljanz 5 mg once daily
- Coadministration of potent inducers of CYP3A4 with Xeljanz/Xeljanz XR is not recommended. Immunization with live vaccines not recommended. Do not start or continue tofacitinib in patients with a lymphocyte count

less than 500 cells/mm³, an absolute neutrophil count (ANC) less than 1,000 cells/mm³ or a hemoglobin level less than 9 g/dL.

- Use in combination with biologic DMARDs or with potent immunosuppressants such as azathioprine and cyclosporine is not recommended
- Grapefruit and grapefruit juice may interact with tofacitinib and lead to unwanted side effects.

SPECIAL SITUATION

Pregnancy and Lactation

Pregnancy Category C

There are no adequate and well-controlled studies in pregnant women. Tofacitinib has been shown to be fetecidal and teratogenic in rats and rabbits when given at exposures 146 times and 13 times, respectively, the maximum recommended human dose. It should be used during pregnancy only if the potential benefit justifies the potential risk to the fetus.

Tofacitinib was secreted in milk of lactating rats. It is not known whether tofacitinib is excreted in human milk.

Hepatitis B or C Infection

It is not known, if tofacitinib is safe and effective in people with hepatitis B or C.

Pediatric Population

It is not known, if tofacitinib is safe and effective in children.

CONCLUSION

Taken together all reported data on tofacitinib show that it hold promise as a new treatment modality by targeted inhibition of JAK-STAT pathway in pathogenesis of various skin disorders. The oral administration, financial issues in terms of cost-effectiveness compared to biologic agents and may be tofacitinib's advantages. Efficacy of tofacitinib in other challenging dermatoses like AD, AA and vitiligo seeks further larger studies. Notwithstanding serious adverse effects have been reported in patients taking higher dosages of tofacitinib, additional studies would have to investigate the drug safety. Based on the promising results so far and the large number of ongoing clinical trials, however, it is likely that tofacitinib and other JAK inhibitors will become an important part of the dermatologist's treatment in the future. Initial results in the treatment of psoriasis and AD with topical tofacitinib are not consistent, but the rapid itch reduction was noted. Further randomized, controlled studies on efficacy and safety of the topical formulations of tofacitinib and other JAK inhibitors would be of great value for psoriasis, AD, AA and localized vitiligo.

▌REFERENCES

1. Babon JJ, Lucet IS, Murphy JM, et al. The molecular regulation of Janus kinase (JAK) activation. Biochem J. 2014;462(1):1-13.
2. O'Shea JJ, Holland SM, Staudt LM. JAKs and STATs in immunity, immunodeficiency, and cancer. N Engl J Med. 2013;368(2):161-70.
3. Dowty ME, Lin J, Ryder TF, et al. The pharmacokinetics, metabolism, and clearance mechanisms of tofacitinib, a Janus kinase inhibitor, in humans. Drug Metab Dispos. 2014;42(4):759-73.
4. Food and Drug Administration. (2012). Pharmacology review(s). [online] Available from https://www.accessdata.fda.gov/drugsatfda_docs/nda/2012/203214Orig1s000PharmR.pdf. [Accessed December, 2017].
5. Ghoreschi K, Jesson MI, Li X, et al. Modulation of innate and adaptive immune responses by tofacitinib (CP-690,550). J Immunol. 2011;186(7):4234-43.
6. Frasor J, Barkai U, Zhong L, et al. PRL-induced ERalpha gene expression is mediated by Janus kinase 2 (Jak2) while signal transducer and activator of transcription 5b (Stat5b) phosphorylation involves Jak2 and a second tyrosine kinase. Mol Endocrinol. 2001;15:1941-52.
7. Kostovic K, Gulin SJ, Mokos ZB, et al. Tofacitinib, an oral Janus kinase inhibitor: perspectives in dermatology. Curr Med Chem. 2017;24(11):1158-67.
8. Damsky W, King BA. JAK inhibitors in dermatology: the promise of a new drug class. J Am Acad Dermatol. 2017;76(4):736-44.
9. Shreberk-Hassidim R, Ramot Y, Zlotogorski A. Janus kinase inhibitors in dermatology: a systematic review. J Am Acad Dermatol. 2017;76(4):745-53.
10. Teng MW, Bowman EP, McElwee JJ, et al. IL-12 and IL-23 cytokines: from discovery to targeted therapies for immune-mediated inflammatory disease. Nat Med. 2015;21(7):719-29.
11. Papp KA, Menter MA, Abe M, et al. Tofacitinib, an oral Janus kinase inhibitor, for the treatment of chronic plaque psoriasis: results from two randomized, placebo-controlled, phase III trials. Br J Dermatol. 2015;173:949-61.
12. Bissonnette R, Iversen L, Sofen H, et al. Tofacitinib withdrawal and retreatment in moderate-to-severe chronic plaque psoriasis: a randomized controlled trial. Br J Dermatol. 2015;172:1395-406.
13. Feldman SR, Thaçi D, Gooderham M, et al. Tofacitinib improves pruritus and health-related quality of life up to 52 weeks: results from 2 randomized phase III trials in patients with moderate to severe plaque psoriasis. J Am Acad Dermatol. 2016;75:1162-70.e3.
14. Krueger J, Clark JD, Suárez-Fariñas M, et al. Tofacitinib attenuates pathologic immune pathways in patients with psoriasis: a randomized phase 2 study. J Allergy Clin Immunol. 2016;137(4):1079-90.
15. Menter MA, Papp KA, Cather J, et al. Efficacy of tofacitinib for the treatment of moderate to severe chronic plaque psoriasis in patients subgroups from two randomized phase 3 trials. J Drugs Dermatol. 2016;15:568-80.
16. Griffiths CE, Vender R, Sofen H, et al. Effect of tofacitinib withdrawal and re-treatment on patient-reported outcomes: results from a phase 3 study in patients with moderate to severe chronic plaque psoriasis. J Eur Acad Dermatol Venereol. 2017;31(2):323-32.

17. Bachelez H, van de Kerkhof PC, Strohal R, et al. Tofacitinib versus etanercept or placebo in moderate-to-severe chronic plaque psoriasis: a phase 3 randomised non-inferiority trial. Lancet. 2015;386(9993):552-61.
18. Valenzuela F, Paul C, Mallbris L, et al. Tofacitinib versus etanercept or placebo in patients with moderate to severe chronic plaque psoriasis: patient-reported outcomes from a phase 3 study. J Eur Acad Dermatol Venereol. 2016;30(10):1753-9.
19. Ports WC, Khan S, Lan S, et al. Randomized phase 2a efficacy and safety trial of the topical Janus kinase inhibitor tofacitinib in the treatment of chronic plaque psoriasis. Br J Dermatol. 2013;169(1):137-45.
20. Papp KA, Bissonnette R, Gooderham M, et al. Treatment of plaque psoriasis with an ointment formulation of the Janus kinase inhibitor, tofacitinib: a phase 2b randomized clinical trial. BMC Dermatol. 2016;16(1):15.
21. Levy LL, Urban J, King BA. Treatment of recalcitrant atopic dermatitis with the oral Janus kinase inhibitor tofacitinib citrate. J Am Acad Dermatol. 2015;73(3):395-9.
22. Bissonnette R, Papp KA, Poulin Y, et al. Topical tofacitinib for atopic dermatitis: a phase IIa randomized trial. Br J Dermatol. 2016;175(5):902-11.
23. Liu LY, Craiglow BG, Dai F, et al. Tofacitinib for the treatment of severe alopecia areata and variants: a study of 90 patients. J Am Acad Dermatol. 2017;76:22-8.
24. Craiglow BG, Liu LY, King BA. Tofacitinib for the treatment of alopecia areata in adolescents. J Am Acad Dermatol. 2017;76(1):29-32.
25. Kennedy CM, Ko JM, Craiglow BG, et al. Safety and efficacy of the JAK inhibitor tofacitinib citrate in patients with alopecia areata. JCI Insight. 2016;1(15):e89776.
26. Dhayalan A, King BA. Tofacitinib citrate for the treatment of nail dystrophy associated with alopecia universalis. JAMA Dermatol. 2016;152(4):492-3.
27. Craiglow BG, King BA. Tofacitinib citrate for the treatment of vitiligo: a pathogenesis-directed therapy. JAMA Dermatol. 2015;151(10):1110-2.
28. Food and Drug Administration. (2016). Highlights of prescribing information. [online] Available from https://www.accessdata.fda.gov/drugsatfda_docs/label/2016/208246s000lbl.pdf. [Accessed December, 2017].
29. Souto A, Maneiro JR, Salgado E, et al. Risk of tuberculosis in patients with chronic immune-mediated inflammatory diseases treated with biologics and tofacitinib: a systematic review and meta-analysis of randomized controlled trials and long-term extension studies. Rheumatology (Oxford). 2014;53:1872-85.

Kingshuk Chatterjee

INTRODUCTION

Apremilast is an oral phosphodiesterase-4 (PDE4) enzyme inhibitor. It reduces the proinflammatory cytokine production by increasing the anti-inflammatory cytokines and the intracellular levels of cyclic adenosine monophosphate (cAMP). It was synthesized by Celgene Corporation (Summit, NJ, USA). Apremilast was approved by Food and Drug Administration in 2014 for the treatment of active psoriatic arthritis and moderate-to-severe plaque psoriasis.

PHARMACOLOGY

Apremilast is chemically identified as N-[2-[(1S)-1-(3-ethoxy-4-methoxyphenyl)-2-(methylsulfonyl) ethyl]-2, 3-dihydro-1, 3-dioxo-1H-isoindol-4-yl] acetamide. The empirical formula is $C_{22}H_{24}N_2O_7S$, with a molecular weight of approximately 460.5 g/mole (Fig. 27.1).

Absolute bioavailability of apremilast is ~73%. The peak plasma concentration (C_{max}) is achieved in a median time (t_{max}) of ~2.5 hours. Absorption is not altered by coadministration with food. Human plasma protein binding of apremilast is approximately 68%. Following oral administration, apremilast is metabolized by cytochrome (CYP) oxidative metabolism with subsequent glucuronidation as well as non-CYP-mediated hydrolysis. In vitro, the CYP metabolism is primarily mediated by CYP3A4, with minor contributions from CYP1A2 and CYP2A6. It is eliminated through urine and feces.

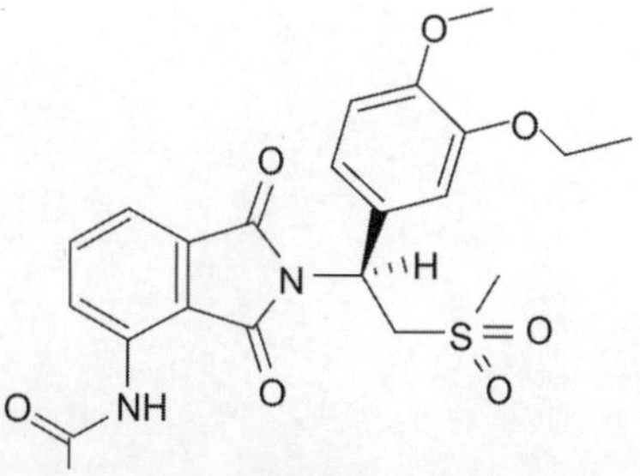

Fig. 27.1: Chemical structure of apremilast.[1]

MECHANISM OF ACTION

Apremilast regulates immune response that causes inflammation and skin disease associated with psoriasis and psoriatic arthritis, by selective inhibition of PDE4. By inhibition of PDE4, a key regulator of inflammatory processes, apremilast prevents degradation of cAMP. Elevated cAMP level, in turn, stimulates anti-inflammatory mediators and antagonizes the production of proinflammatory cytokines, e.g. tumor necrosis factor (TNF)-α, interleukin (IL)-23, IL-17, interferon (IFN)-γ and various chemokines from peripheral blood mononuclear cells (PBMC) and polymorphonuclear leukocytes, including neutrophils, monocytes, natural killer cells and plasmacytoid dendritic cells. Chemokines and cytokines produced by toll-like receptor (TLR-2 and TLR-4) stimulated PBMC are also susceptible to PDE4 inhibition. TNF-α produced by rheumatoid synovial membrane as well as keratinocyte in-vitro is also inhibited by apremilast due to expression of PDE4 in cell types resident in the joints and skin. An increase in anti-inflammatory cytokines, e.g. IL-10 is also caused by apremilast. Thus, apremilast leads to intracellular interruption of inflammatory cascade at an early point, in contrast to biologic agents that act as target specific (e.g. TNF-α) inhibitors.[2-4]

Currently, research is being conducted on PDE4 inhibitors and their immune-modulating effects in a variety of inflammatory conditions, such as chronic obstructive pulmonary disease (COPD), atopic dermatitis, asthma, psoriasis and psoriatic arthritis (PsA).[2,5]

USES

Food and Drug Administration-approved Indications

- Active psoriatic arthritis in adults
- Patients with moderate-to-severe plaque psoriasis who are suitable for phototherapy or systemic therapy.

Other Uses

- Atopic dermatitis[6]
- Lichen planus[7]
- Discoid lupus erythematosus[8]
- Sarcoidosis[9]
- Behcet's disease.[10]

Most of these indications are phase II study or open label pilot studies. Newer indications of apremilast are being explored.

ADMINISTRATION

Availability

- Trade name: Otezla® or Aprezo
- Marketed by:
  - Celgene Corporation (Summit, NJ, USA)
  - Glenmark Pharma in India.

Preparation

Oral diamond shaped, film-coated tablet available as 10 mg, 20 mg and 30 mg.

Storage and Handling

Below 30°C (86°F).

Dosage (Table 27.1)

The tablet should not be chewed or crushed and should be swallowed without regard to meals.

CURRENT EVIDENCE

Plaque Psoriasis

The efficacy of apremilast in management of chronic plaque psoriasis is discussed in Table 27.2. Another study conducted by Paul et al. (ESTEEM 2) in which safety and efficacy of apremilast was evaluated over 52 weeks. Subgroup analysis of this study revealed that Psoriasis Area and Severity

Table 27.1: Apremilast dosage.

Day 1	Day 2		Day 3		Day 4		Day 5		Day 6 and thereafter	
AM	AM	PM	AM	PM	AM	PM	AM	PM	AM	PM
10 mg	10 mg	10 mg	10 mg	20 mg	20 mg	20 mg	20 mg	30 mg	30 mg	30 mg

Table 27.2: Efficacy of apremilast in plaque psoriasis.

Dose	PASI-50	PASI-75	Reference
30 mg twice daily	58.7%	32.6% (16 weeks)	Papp et al. (2015)[11]
20 mg twice daily	33%	20% (after 16 weeks)	Edwards et al.
30 mg twice daily	41%	21%	(2016)[12]
	67%	33% (after 52 weeks)	

Index (PASI)-75 score with apremilast 30 mg BD was achieved in 33.3% patients when patient did not have any exposure to conventional therapy, 31.9% when patient did not have any previous biologic exposure and 22.8% in patients with previous biologic exposure.[13]

Psoriatic Arthritis

Psoriatic arthritis long-term assessment of clinical efficacy (PALACE) studies were conducted to assess efficacy of apremilast in treatment of psoriatic arthritis. In PALACE 1 study, an American College of Rheumatology 20% (ACR20) response rate was found to be 31.8% and 39.8% for 20 mg BD group and 30 mg BD group, respectively. This efficacy was maintained till 52 weeks across these studies.[14]

▌ADVERSE REACTIONS

Apremilast was generally well-tolerated up to 52 weeks in plaque psoriasis patients and possesses an acceptable safety profile. Majority of the adverse reactions encountered were mild-to-moderate in severity and no significant changes in laboratory values were observed in any of the trials.

- *Gastrointestinal*: Diarrhea (most common adverse reaction, requiring dose titration as mentioned before), upper abdominal pain, nausea, vomiting, frequent bowel movement, dyspepsia and gastroesophageal reflux disease. Nausea and diarrhea occur in first week of treatment and generally resolves by one month of treatment. Loperamide can be used in patient who developed diarrhea due to apremilast.
- *Respiratory*: Upper respiratory tract infection, nasopharyngitis, cough and bronchitis.
- *Nervous system*: Headache, depression or depressed mood has been reported in almost 1% of patients taking apremilast.
- *Immunological*: Hypersensitivity, skin rash.
- *Others*: Loss of weight, decreased appetite, fatigue, back pain, tooth abscess, insomnia.[15]

▌CONTRAINDICATIONS

- Known hypersensitivity to apremilast or the formulation excipients
- Renal impairment
- Hepatic impairment
- History of depression or suicidal ideation.

▌DOSE ADJUSTMENT[1]

Renal Impairment

Mild or moderate renal impairment: No dose adjustment required.

Severe renal impairment [creatinine clearance (CrCl) <30 mL/min]: Reduce dose to 30 mg OD.

Hepatic Impairment

No dose adjustment required.

▌DRUG INTERACTIONS[1]

Coadministration of cytochrome P450 enzyme inducers (e.g. phenobarbital, carbamazepine, phenytoin, rifampicin) with apremilast resulted in reduced levels of the drug with loss of its efficacy.

▌INVESTIGATIONS

- Weight of the patient
- Liver function test
- Renal function test
- *Chest X-ray:* However, no reactivation of tuberculosis has been reported in patients on apremilast.

▌SPECIAL SITUATIONS

Pregnancy Category C

The safety and efficacy of apremilast in patients less than 18 years of age has not yet been established.

▌CONCLUSION

Apremilast is an oral PDE-4 inhibitor and belongs to a new class of drug. Its novel mechanism of action, oral formulation and safety makes it an interesting drug for management of psoriasis and many other indications.

▌REFERENCES

1. Celgene Corporation. (2014). Otezla® (apremilast)—Highlights of full prescribing information. [online] Available from http://www.otezla.com/otezla-prescribing-information.pdf. [Accessed August, 2015].
2. Schafer P. Apremilast mechanism of action and application to psoriasis and psoriatic arthritis. Biochem Pharmacol. 2012;83(12):1583-90.

3. Kavanaugh A, Adebajo AO, Gladman DD, et al. Long-Term (156-Week) Efficacy and Safety Profile of Apremilast, an Oral Phosphodiesterase 4 Inhibitor, in Patients with Psoriatic Arthritis: Results from a Phase III, Randomized, Controlled Trial and Open-Label Extension (PALACE 1). Arthritis Rheumatol. 2015;67 (suppl 10).

4. Schafer PH, Parton A, Gandhi AK, et al. Apremilast, a cAMP phosphodiesterase-4 inhibitor, demonstrates anti-inflammatory activity in vitro and in a model of psoriasis. Brit J Pharm. 2010;159:842-55.

5. Baumer W, Hoppmann J, Rundfeldt C, et al. Highly selective phosphodiesterase 4 inhibitors for the treatment of allergic skin diseases and psoriasis. Inflamm Allergy Drug Targets. 2007;6(1):17-26.

6. Samrao A, Berry TM, Goreshi R, et al. A pilot study of an oral phosphodiesterase inhibitor (apremilast) for atopic dermatitis in adults. Arch Dermatol. 2012;148:890-7

7. Paul J, Foss CE, Hirano SA, et al. An open-label pilot study of apremilast for the treatment of moderate to severe lichen planus: A case series. J Am Acad Dermatol. 2013;68:255-61.

8. De Souza A, Strober BE, Merola JF, et al. Apremilast for discoid lupus erythematosus: Results of a phase 2, open-label, single-arm, pilot study. J Drugs Dermatol. 2012;11:1224-6.

9. Baughman RP, Judson MA, Ingledue R, et al. Efficacy and safety of apremilast in chronic cutaneous sarcoidosis. Arch Dermatol. 2012;148:262-4.

10. Hatemi G, Melikoglu M, Tunc R, et al. Apremilast for the treatment of Behcet's syndrome: A phase II randomized, placebo-controlled, double blind study. Arthritis Rheum. 2013;65(10 Suppl):S322.

11. Papp K, Reich K, Leonardi CL, et al. Apremilast, an oral phosphodiesterase 4 (PDE4) inhibitor, in patients with moderate to severe plaque psoriasis: Results of a phase III, randomized, controlled trial (Efficacy and Safety Trial Evaluating the Effects of Apremilast in Psoriasis [ESTEEM] 1). J Am Acad Dermatol. 2015;73:37-49.

12. Edwards CJ, Blanco FJ, Crowley J, et al. Apremilast, an oral phosphodiesterase 4 inhibitor, in patients with psoriatic arthritis and current skin involvement: a phase III, randomised, controlled trial (PALACE 3). Ann Rheum Dis. 2016;75:1065-73.

13. Paul C, Cather J, Gooderham M, et al. Efficacy and safety of apremilast, an oral phosphodiesterase 4 inhibitor, in patients with moderate-to-severe plaque psoriasis over 52 weeks: a phase III, randomized controlled trial (ESTEEM 2). Br J Dermatol. 2015;173(6):1387-99.

14. Cutolo M, Myerson GE, Fleischmann RM, et al. A Phase III, Randomized, Controlled Trial of Apremilast in Patients with Psoriatic Arthritis: Results of the PALACE 2 Trial. J Rheumatol. 2016;43:1724-34.

15. Crowley J, Thac D, Joly P, et al. Long-term safety and tolerability of apremilast in patients with psoriasis: Pooled safety analysis for ≥156 weeks from 2 phase 3, randomized, controlled trials (ESTEEM 1 and 2). J Am Acad Dermatol. 2017;77:310-7.

Riti Bhatia, Vishal Gupta

INTRODUCTION

Sirolimus is a pleiotropic molecule having immunosuppressive, anti-proliferative, and antifungal properties. It was named rapamycin after the native name of Easter Island, Rapa Nui, where *Streptomyces hygroscopicus* (a soil fungus) was discovered to produce this antibiotic. Its antifungal properties were also discovered here.[1] After receiving United States Food and Drug Administration (USFDA) approval for renal transplant in 1999, it has been used for preventing graft rejection in heart and liver transplant recipients as well.[1] It is also used in drug-eluting stents after cardiac procedures to prevent restenosis. Structurally, sirolimus is a crystalline lipophilic macrolide lactone. Its molecular weight is 290 kDa (914.2 g/mol) and the chemical formula is $C_{51}H_{79}NO_{13}$.[1]

MECHANISM OF ACTION

Sirolimus shares structural similarity with tacrolimus and cyclosporine. Like these molecules, it also acts by binding to immunophilins, which are intracellular binding proteins (FK506 binding protein or FKBPs), specifically FKBP-12. However, further mode of its action is different. While cyclosporine-immunophilin complex acts via calcineurin, rapamycin-immunophilin complex acts via another protein called the mammalian target of rapamycin (mTOR). mTOR is a 289 kDa multifunctional serine/threonine kinase involved in transduction of cytokines like interleukin (IL)-2 and cell growth. Thus, inhibition of mTOR leads to inhibition of cytokine-mediated immune response. Inhibition of mTOR also blocks its downstream pathways, resulting in arrest of cell cycle progression between G1 and S phase.[2] Newer mTOR inhibitors, like temsirolimus and everolimus have been developed with broader applications in oncology and transplant medicine. Flowchart 28.1 illustrates the various mechanisms of action of sirolimus.

PHARMACOKINETICS

Sirolimus is rapidly absorbed orally, reaching its peak serum concentration in 1 hour in healthy individuals and 2–3 hours in renal transplant recipients.[3]

Flowchart 28.1: Various mechanism of action of sirolimus.

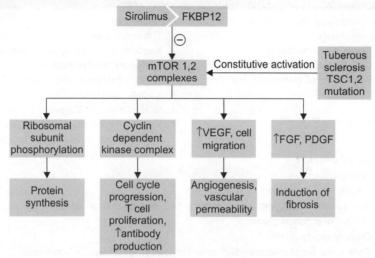

(FGF: Fibroblast growth factor; mTOR: Mammalian target of rapamycin; PDGF: Platelet-derived growth factor; VEGF: Vascular endothelial growth factor).

After oral absorption, 95% of the drug is bound to serum proteins, primarily albumin (97%). It is metabolized by the hepatic cytochrome P450 3A4 enzyme and p-glycoprotein intestinal pump.[4] Oral bioavailability is poor (approximately 14%), owing to extensive intestinal and hepatic first pass metabolism. It is primarily excreted by the fecal route (90%), and has a half-life of 57–62 hours.[5,6] Sirolimus is commercially available as oral tablets (1 mg, 2 mg, and 5 mg) and solution (1 mg/mL).

CLINICAL USES

There is no FDA approved dermatological indication of sirolimus at present. Some of its better known uses in dermatology include treating facial angiofibromas and vascular anomalies. Apart from these, it has shown encouraging results in various other skin disorders which is a subject of further investigation. The list of various indications for sirolimus in dermatology is summarized in Table 28.1.

TUBEROUS SCLEROSIS

In a serendipitous discovery, immunosuppressive treatment with sirolimus in a renal transplant recipient with tuberous sclerosis led to improvement in facial angiofibromas.[7] Defects in the gene products of TSC1 or TSC2 (mutations in these genes are implicated in tuberous sclerosis) lead to an unregulated activation of the downstream mTOR signaling pathway. Thus,

Table 28.1: Sirolimus—Indications in dermatology.

Food and Drug Administration (FDA) approved uses	Off-label uses
• None in dermatology • *Only FDA approved indication:* Prevention of transplant rejection	• Tuberous sclerosis • Kaposiform hemangioendothelioma • Lymphatic malformations • Kasabach-Merritt phenomenon • Kaposi's sarcoma • Graft-versus-host disease • Chemoprevention of cutaneous malignancies in transplant recipients

Investigational role
• Antiaging
• Keloids and hypertrophic scars
• Blue rubber bleb syndrome, capillary, and venous malformations
• Erosive oral lichen planus
• Chronic urticaria
• *Connective tissue disorders:* Systemic lupus erythematosus, scleroderma
• Pemphigus vulgaris
• Cutaneous T-cell lymphoma
• Melanoma
• *Other genodermatoses:* Pachyonychia congenita, neurofibromatosis, Birt-Hogg-Dubé syndrome, PTEN hamartoma syndrome, basal cell nevus syndrome, and Muir-Torre syndrome

sirolimus by virtue of its inhibitory effect on mTOR pathway can have a beneficial effect on different manifestations of tuberous sclerosis. Multiple studies have demonstrated the efficacy of topical sirolimus ointment in treating angiofibromas (level of evidence I).[8] As it is not available commercially, the topical formulation of sirolimus has to be compounded by mixing the crushed tablet in petrolatum. A split-face trial comparing the efficacy of topical sirolimus (gel, ointment) with emollient for 12 weeks on 11 patients with tuberous sclerosis showed significantly better improvement in the sirolimus-treated side. The gel form was found to be more effective and less irritating than the ointment. Higher percutaneous absorption of sirolimus in gel form than ointment was also demonstrated on a human skin model.[9] A wide variety of topical formulations, viz. ointment, gel, solution, and cream, in varying concentration (0.003–1%) have been tried. In a review, Balestri et al. concluded that ointment and gel formulations should be preferred, but optimum concentration is not clear.[8] A prospective single-blinded crossover split-face study on 12 patients comparing sirolimus ointment 0.1% with petrolatum for 12 weeks also found significantly better results with sirolimus. There was statistically significant reduction in the redness and size of the lesions. Notably, the facial angiofibromas started to increase in size after stopping the treatment for 6 months suggesting only a temporary effect of sirolimus. Retreatment with topical sirolimus again led to improvement.[10] The response may be better in early lesions, and may be apparent as early as few (4–8) weeks.[11,12] Side effects are minimal and include redness and irritation at the site of application, which can be managed with mild topical corticosteroid and Vaseline. Serum sirolimus levels with topical use are largely undetectable and no systemic side effects are observed. Good improvement with topical application of commercially available oral solution (1 mg/mL) once daily has also been reported in two patients.[13] Using commercially available oral solution may be more cost-effective than the compounded ointments, however, it causes more irritation. Apart from topical formulation, oral sirolimus has also been found to be effective in treating angiofibromas, renal angiomyolipomas, pulmonary lymphangiomyomatosis, and brain astrocytomas, and may even have a disease-modifying effect in patients with tuberous sclerosis.[14-16]

▌VASCULAR ANOMALIES

Based on the role of mTOR pathway in proliferation and growth of endothelial cells, sirolimus can have antiangiogenic effects. Successful use of sirolimus in the treatment of refractory kaposiform hemangioendothelioma and Kasabach-Merritt phenomenon was first reported by Blatt et al. in 2010.[17] Since then, reports of good results with sirolimus in the treatment of different vascular anomalies, mainly kaposiform hemangioendothelioma and lymphatic malformations have emerged in the literature (level of evidence II).[18,19] In a retrospective review of six children with different vascular anomalies (kaposiform hemangioendothelioma n = 2, lymphatic-venous malformation n = 2, pulmonary lymphangiectasias n = 1, and orbital lymphatic malformation n = 1), oral sirolimus (0.05 mg/kg twice daily, and subsequently dose adjusted to achieve serum levels between 5 ng/mL and 15 ng/mL) produced complete and partial remission in three patients each (median duration 10 months, range 3–53 months). The coagulation profile and platelet counts in three patients with Kasabach-Merritt phenomenon normalized within 1 month. Mild reversible leukopenia was seen in all the patients. In a phase II trial involving patients with complicated vascular anomalies (like lymphatic malformations, lymphangiomatosis, kaposiform hemangioendotheliomas), oral sirolimus (0.8 mg/m^2 twice daily) administered for 12 courses; each course lasting 28 days was found to be effective. Of the 61 patients enrolled, 57 could be evaluated. Partial improvement was seen in 47 (of 57, 83%) patients after six courses and 45 (of 53, 85%) patients after 12 courses. Stability was achieved in three (5%) patients at 6 months, while lesions remained progressive in seven (12%) and eight (15%) patients at 6 and 12 months, respectively. None of the patients had a complete clinical response. Bone marrow toxicity was seen in 27% of patients, gastrointestinal toxicity in 3%, and metabolic/laboratory toxicity in 3%. Dose reduction was needed in two patients due to toxicity and two patients were taken off the study for the same reason. No toxicity-related deaths occurred.[20] As many patients achieve only partial improvement at the end of study period, the optimum duration for complete remission needs further investigation. The initial results suggest that the improvement may be sustained after cessation of treatment.[21] Oral sirolimus has been reported to be effective in treating Kasabach-Merritt phenomenon refractory to previous treatment (including steroids and vincristine) as well, in the dose of 0.8 mg/m² twice daily with subsequent dose adjustments to maintain trough levels of 10–15 ng/mL.[19,22] In a series of six patients with refractory kaposiform hemangioendothelioma with life-threatening Kasabach-Merritt phenomenon, the average time to respond was only 5.3 days (range 4–7 days) and platelet counts stabilized on an average of 15 days (range 5–28 days),[19] though it may take as long as 3–4 months.[22] A phase II clinical trial comparing sirolimus and vincristine for the treatment of kaposiform hemangioendothelioma complicated with Kasabach-Merritt phenomenon is currently recruiting patients.[23]

Topical sirolimus has also been used in the treatment of microcystic lymphatic malformations. Topical sirolimus 0.8% ointment in petrolatum used on microcystic lymphatic malformation on scrotum once daily led to complete resolution in 3 months. No recurrence was noted in the next 2 months of follow-up.[24]

CHEMOPREVENTION IN TRANSPLANT RECIPIENTS

Organ transplant recipients are at a higher risk of developing cutaneous malignancies; the risk being highest for squamous cell carcinoma. Immunosuppression with sirolimus, as opposed to cyclosporine, to prevent graft rejection reduces the risk of nonmelanoma skin cancers (level of evidence I). In a recent meta-analysis involving 20 randomized controlled trials (RCTs) and two observational studies, including 39,039 kidney recipients overall, sirolimus was associated with 51% lower incidence of nonmelanoma skin cancer [incidence rate ratio (IRR) = 0.49, 95%; confidence interval (CI) = 0.32–0.76]. This protective effect of sirolimus on nonmelanoma skin cancer risk was most notable in studies comparing sirolimus against cyclosporine (IRR = 0.19, 95%; CI = 0.04–0.84).[25,26]

KAPOSI'S SARCOMA

Because of its antiangiogenic properties, sirolimus has been used in the treatment of Kaposi's sarcoma (KS) (level of evidence III). In addition, sirolimus has been demonstrated to suppress human herpesvirus-8 (HHV-8) lytic master switch protein, thereby impairing virion production.[27] In a series of 15 renal transplant recipients with KS treated with sirolimus (0.15 mg/kg, followed by a dose of 0.04–0.06 mg/kg to maintain drug trough levels of 6–10 ng/mL), complete clinical and histological remission was seen in all the patients after 3 months and 6 months, respectively.[28] It has also been used in human immunodeficiency virus (HIV) patients with KS: three patients out of seven had partial improvement. All these three patients were on protease inhibitor-based regimens, which led to higher serum sirolimus levels, due to drug interactions. No change was observed in HIV load, but CD4 count decreased transiently in five (out of six) patients.[29] In a patient of pemphigus vulgaris with iatrogenic KS, clinical and histological remission was maintained at 24 months with low-dose prednisone, dapsone, and sirolimus.[30]

▌ PSORIASIS

A RCT compared oral sirolimus (0.5, 1.5, and 3 mg/m^2), cyclosporine (5 mg/kg), and a combination of the two agents (sirolimus 3 mg/m^2 and subtherapeutic dose of cyclosporine 1.25 mg/kg) for 8 weeks in the treatment of severe plaque psoriasis [Psoriasis Area Severity Index (PASI) ≥ 12] of duration of at least 6 months in 150 patients. While the combination treatment was comparable to cyclosporine monotherapy (63.7% and 70.5% reduction in PASI, respectively), sirolimus monotherapy led to less than 30% reduction in PASI for any dose. These results suggest that sirolimus monotherapy is ineffective, but adding sirolimus to cyclosporine may reduce its dose (level of evidence I).[31] Another randomized double-blind, left-right comparative clinical trial tested the efficacy of topical sirolimus versus its vehicle in the treatment of stable chronic plaque psoriasis. In vitro studies showed topical sirolimus to penetrate the skin and decrease the number of CD4$^+$ T cells in the epidermis. Twenty-four patients were treated first with a lower concentration of 2.2% for 6 weeks, followed by a higher concentration of 8% for additional 6 weeks. The area treated with sirolimus showed significant reduction in a composite clinical score based on erythema, induration, and scaling, but there was no significant change in plaque thickness (measured by ultrasound) and redness (reflectance erythema meter).[32]

▌ GRAFT-VERSUS-HOST DISEASE

Sirolimus has been found to be a safe and effective alternative to glucocorticoids in graft-versus-host disease (GVHD). Similar response rate as with glucocorticoids (of 50%) was found in a series of 32 cases with acute GVHD. These patients were also on tacrolimus and methotrexate/mycophenolate mofetil in addition, for prophylaxis of acute GVHD.[33] It was also found to be effective in steroid refractory acute GVHD with a response rate of 44% for a minimum of 1 month, without additional immunosuppressants.[34] In a retrospective review of 22 cases with steroid refractory acute GVHD, sirolimus treatment produced sustained remission rate of 72%.[35]

OTHER DERMATOLOGICAL INDICATIONS

Apart from the above-mentioned indications, utility of sirolimus is being studied in a variety of other conditions as well. As it downregulates K6A gene, it has been tried in three patients of pachyonychia congenita with improvement clinically as well as in the quality of life.[36] With the evidence for involvement of mTOR pathway in aging, there is a growing interest in sirolimus and its analogs as antiaging agents. Sirolimus has been found to enhance the lifespan of genetically engineered mice.[37] Post-transplant immunosuppression with cyclosporine or tacrolimus but not with sirolimus, in patients with Muir-Torre syndrome was seen to exacerbate sebaceous adenomas.[38] Sirolimus appears to have the advantage of reducing the risk of malignancies over cyclosporine in transplant recipients. It is being investigated for its role in keloids and hypertrophic scars, blue rubber bleb nevus syndrome, capillary and venous malformations, erosive oral lichen planus, chronic urticaria, systemic lupus erythematosus, scleroderma, pemphigus vulgaris, cutaneous T-cell lymphoma, melanoma and genodermatoses like basal cell nevus syndrome, neurofibromatosis, PTEN hamartoma syndrome, and Birt-Hogg-Dubé syndrome.[39]

ADVERSE EFFECTS AND MONITORING

Common side effects seen in more than 30% cases, include anemia, thrombocytopenia, fever, arthralgia, hypertension, hypertriglyceridemia, hypercholesterolemia, headache, gastrointestinal effects, such as anorexia, abdominal pain and diarrhea, impaired wound healing, lymphedema and infections like urinary tract infections, and reactivation of latent viral infections.[39] Serious adverse events include upper respiratory infections and noninfective pneumonitis. Common cutaneous side effects include acneiform eruption, oral ulcers, and nail changes. In a study involving 80 renal transplant patients receiving sirolimus, 79 (99%) patients experienced cutaneous side effects, including pilosebaceous apparatus disorders like acneiform lesions (46%), scalp folliculitis (26%), and hidradenitis suppurativa (12%); edematous complaints including chronic edema (55%) and angioedemas (15%); mucosal involvement like aphthous ulcers (60%), epistaxis (60%), chronic gingivitis (20%), and chronic fissuring of lips (11%); nail involvement like chronic dystrophic nails (74%) and periungual infections (16%). Serious events were seen in 20 (25%) patients, while six

Box 28.1: Monitoring guidelines for oral sirolimus.
Investigations prior to starting sirolimus treatment: • Complete blood count, liver and renal function tests, and fasting lipid profile • Blood pressure measurement • *Consider screening for infections in high-risk patients:* Tuberculosis, hepatitis B, hepatitis C, and human immunodeficiency virus (HIV). *Investigations while on sirolimus treatment:* • Complete blood count, liver and renal function tests, and fasting lipid profile • Blood pressure measurement • Serum or whole blood sirolimus trough levels; dose adjustment to maintain trough levels 5–15 ng/mL (every week in the 1st month, every 2 weeks in the 2nd month; thereafter, can be done only in patients who undergo dose changes or may have drug interactions).

(7%) patients stopped sirolimus primarily due to cutaneous adverse effects.[40] The recommended monitoring guidelines for sirolimus are summarized in Box 28.1. Most of this information comes from the experience of using sirolimus in renal transplant patients.

CONCLUSION

Sirolimus, the mTOR inhibitor, appears to be a promising new agent for the treatment of many often difficult-to-treat skin diseases, including inflammatory skin disorders, vascular tumors and malformations, and genodermatoses. Good-quality evidence supporting its use in tuberous sclerosis and vascular anomalies is gradually emerging. Topical application, which can bypass the side effects of oral treatment, may be preferred for superficial cutaneous lesions. The optimum formulation and concentration of topical sirolimus is not clear and warrants further investigation. Prospective clinical trials evaluating the efficacy and safety of oral as well as topical sirolimus in various dermatological conditions are currently being conducted. Randomized placebo-controlled studies are required to validate its status in dermatology pharmacotherapeutics.

REFERENCES

1. Vénzina C, Kudelski A, Sehgal SN. Rapamycin (AY-22,989), a new antifungal antibiotic. I. Taxonomy of the producing streptomycete and isolation of the active principle. J Antibiot (Tokyo). 1975;28(10):721-6.
2. Sehgal SN. Sirolimus: its discovery, biological properties, and mechanism of action. Transplant Proc. 2003;35(3):S7-14.
3. Wyeth TM. (2014). Rapamune® (Sirolimus oral solution and tablets). [online] Available from www.pfizer.ca/sites/g/files/g10017036/f/201410/Rapamune_0.pdf. [Accessed December, 2017].

4. Zimmerman JJ, Kahan BD. Pharmacokinetics of sirolimus in stable renal transplant patients after multiple oral dose administration. J Clin Pharmacol. 1997;37(5):405-15.

5. Paghdal KV, Schwartz RA. Sirolimus (rapamycin): from the soil of Easter Island to a bright future. J Am Acad Dermatol. 2007;57(6):1046-50.

6. MacDonald A, Scarola J, Burke JT, et al. Clinical pharmacokinetics and therapeutic drug monitoring of sirolimus. Clin Ther. 2000;22(Suppl B):B101-21.

7. Hofbauer GF, Marcollo-Pini A, Corsenca A, et al. The mTOR inhibitor rapamycin significantly improves facial angiofibroma lesions in a patient with tuberous sclerosis. Br J Dermatol. 2008;159(2):473-5.

8. Balestri R, Neri I, Patrizi A, et al. Analysis of current data on the use of topical rapamycin in the treatment of facial angiofibromas in tuberous sclerosis complex. J Eur Acad Dermatol Venereol. 2015;29(1):14-20.

9. Tanaka M, Wataya-Kaneda M, Nakamura A, et al. First left-right comparative study of topical rapamycin vs. vehicle for facial angiofibromas in patients with tuberous sclerosis complex. Br J Dermatol. 2013;169(6):1314-8.

10. Cinar SL, Kartal D, Bayram AK, et al. Topical sirolimus for the treatment of angiofibromas in tuberous sclerosis. Indian J Dermatol Venereol Leprol. 2017;83(1):27-32.

11. Samanta D. Topical mTOR (mechanistic target of rapamycin) inhibitor therapy in facial angiofibroma. Indian J Dermatol Venereol Leprol. 2015;81(5):540-1.

12. Salido R, Garnacho-Saucedo G, Cuevas-Asencio I, et al. Sustained clinical effectiveness and favorable safety profile of topical sirolimus for tuberous sclerosis—associated facial angiofibroma. J Eur Acad Dermatol Venereol. 2012;26(10): 1315-8.

13. Mutizwa MM, Berk DR, Anadkat MJ. Treatment of facial angiofibromas with topical application of oral rapamycin solution (1mgmL(-1)) in two patients with tuberous sclerosis. Br J Dermatol. 2011;165(4):922-3.

14. Micozkadioglu H, Koc Z, Ozelsancak R, et al. Rapamycin therapy for renal, brain, and skin lesions in a tuberous sclerosis patient. Ren Fail. 2010;32(10):1233-6.

15. Bissler JJ, McCormack FX, Young LR, et al. Sirolimus for angiomyolipoma in tuberous sclerosis complex or lymphangioleiomyomatosis. N Engl J Med. 2008;358(2):140-51.

16. Sadowski K, Kotulska K, Schwartz RA, et al. Systemic effects of treatment with mTOR inhibitors in tuberous sclerosis complex: A comprehensive review. J Eur Acad Dermatol Venereol. 2016;30(4):586-94.

17. Blatt J, Stavas J, Moats-Staats B, et al. Treatment of childhood kaposiform hemangioendothelioma with sirolimus. Pediatr Blood Cancer. 2010;55(7):1396-8.

18. Lackner H, Karastaneva A, Schwinger W, et al. Sirolimus for the treatment of children with various complicated vascular anomalies. Eur J Pediatr. 2015;174(12):1579-84.

19. Kai L, Wang Z, Yao W, et al. Sirolimus, a promising treatment for refractory kaposiform hemangioendothelioma. J Cancer Res Clin Oncol. 2014;140(3):471-6.

20. Adams DM, Trenor CC, Hammill AM, et al. Efficacy and safety of sirolimus in the treatment of complicated vascular anomalies. Pediatrics. 2016;137(2):e20153257.

21. Yesil S, Bozkurt C, Tanyildiz HG, et al. Successful treatment of macroglossia due to lymphatic malformation with sirolimus. Ann Otol Rhinol Laryngol. 2015;124(10):820-3.

22. Wang Z, Li K, Dong K, et al. Refractory Kasabach-Merritt phenomenon successfully treated with sirolimus and a mini-review of the published work. J Dermatol. 2015;42(4):401-4.

23. National Institutes of Health (NIH). (2014). A Study to Compare Vincristine to Sirolimus for Treatment of High Risk Vascular Tumors. [online] Available from www.clinicaltrials.gov/ct2/show/NCT02110069. [Accessed December, 2017].

24. Ivars M, Redondo P. Efficacy of topical sirolimus (rapamycin) for the treatment of microcystic lymphatic malformations. JAMA Dermatol. 2017;153(1):103-5.

25. Mathew T, Kreis H, Friend P. Two-year incidence of malignancy in sirolimus-treated renal transplant recipients: results from five multicenter studies. Clin Transplant. 2004;18(4):446-9.

26. Yanik EL, Siddiqui K, Engels EA. Sirolimus effects on cancer incidence after kidney transplantation: A meta-analysis. Cancer Med. 2015;4(9):1448-59.

27. Nichols LA, Adang LA, Kedes DH. Rapamycin blocks production of KSHV/HHV8: insights into the anti-tumor activity of an immunosuppressant drug. PLoS One. 2011;6(1):e14535.

28. Stallone G, Schena A, Infante B, et al. Sirolimus for Kaposi's sarcoma in renal-transplant recipients. N Engl J Med. 2005;352(13):1317-23.

29. Krown SE, Roy D, Lee JY, et al. Rapamycin with antiretroviral therapy in AIDS-associated Kaposi sarcoma: An AIDS Malignancy Consortium study. J Acquir Immune Defic Syndr. 2012;59(5):447-54.

30. Saggar S, Zeichner JA, Brown TT, et al. Kaposi's sarcoma resolves after sirolimus therapy in a patient with pemphigus vulgaris. Arch Dermatol. 2008;144(5):654-57.

31. Reitamo S, Spuls P, Sassolas B, et al. Efficacy of sirolimus (rapamycin) administered concomitantly with a subtherapeutic dose of cyclosporin in the treatment of severe psoriasis: a randomized controlled trial. Br J Dermatol. 2001;145(3):438-45.

32. Ormerod AD, Shah SA, Copeland P, et al. Treatment of psoriasis with topical sirolimus: preclinical development and a randomized, double-blind trial. Br J Dermatol. 2005;152(4):758-64.

33. Pidala J, Tomblyn M, Nishihori T, et al. Sirolimus demonstrates activity in the primary therapy of acute graft-versus-host disease without systemic glucocorticoids. Haematologica. 2011;96(9):1351-6.

34. Benito AI, Furlong T, Martin PJ, et al. Sirolimus (rapamycin) for the treatment of steroid-refractory acute graft-versus-host disease. Transplantation. 2001;72(12):1924-9.

35. Ghez D, Rubio MT, Maillard N, et al. Rapamycin for refractory acute graft-versus-host disease. Transplantation. 2009;88(9):1081-7.

36. Hickerson RP, Leake D, Pho LN, et al. Rapamycin selectively inhibits expression of an inducible keratin (K6a) in human keratinocytes and improves symptoms in pachyonychia congenita patients. J Dermatol Sci. 2009;56(2):82-8.

37. Harrison DE, Strong R, Sharp ZD, et al. Rapamycin fed late in life extends lifespan in genetically heterogeneous mice. Nature. 2009;460(7253):392-5.

38. Levi Z, Hazazi R, Kedar-Barnes I, et al. Switching from tacrolimus to sirolimus halts the appearance of new sebaceous neoplasms in Muir-Torre syndrome. Am J Transplant. 2007;7(2):476-9.

39. Fogel AL, Hill S, Teng JM. Advances in the therapeutic use of mammalian target of rapamycin (mTOR) inhibitors in dermatology. J Am Acad Dermatol. 2015;72(5):879-89.

40. Mahé E, Morelon E, Lechaton S, et al. Cutaneous adverse events in renal transplant recipients receiving sirolimus-based therapy. Transplantation. 2005;79(4):476-82.

Index